Proceedings in Life Sciences

First International Congress on Medicinal Plant Research, held at the University of Munich, Germany, September 6—10, 1976.
Section B: Plant Tissue Culture and Its Bio-technological Application. Eds.: W. Barz/E. Reinhard/M. H. Zenk.
Published by Springer-Verlag Berlin Heidelberg New York 1977.

New Natural Products and Plant Drugs with Pharmacological, Biological or Therapeutical Activity

Proceedings of the First International Congress on Medicinal Plant Research, Section A, held at the University of Munich, Germany September 6—10, 1976

Edited by
H. Wagner and P. Wolff

With 152 Figures

Springer-Verlag Berlin Heidelberg New York 1977

Prof. Dr. H. WAGNER
Dr. P. WOLFF
Institut für Pharmazeutische Arzneimittellehre
Universität München
Karlstraße 29, 8000 München 2/FRG

Cover motive: Left: a shoot of *Maytenus buchananii*, a bush or tree growing in Central West Africa, belonging to the Celastraceae. Right: structure of maytansin, isolated from the plant.

ISBN 3-540-08292-1 Springer-Verlag Berlin Heidelberg New York
ISBN 0-387-08292-1 Springer-Verlag New York Heidelberg Berlin

Library of Congress Cataloging in Publication Data. International Congress on Medicinal Plant Research, 1st, University of Munich, 1976. New natural products and plant drugs with pharmacological, biological or therapeutical activity. (Proceedings in life sciences) Includes bibliographies and index. 1. Materia medica, Vegetable—Congresses. I. Wagner, Hildebert, 1929—. II. Wolff, Peter Maria, 1932—. III. Title. [DNLM: 1. Drugs—Congresses. 2. Plants, Medicinal—Congresses. W3 IN632M 1976/QV766 161 1976n]. RS164.I56.1976. 615'.32. 77-8846.

Offsetprinting and bookbinding: Brühlsche Universitätsdruckerei Lahn-Gießen.
2131/3130-543210

Preface

The fact that, of the approximately 600,000 plant species existing on the earth, only some 5 % have been specifically investigated chemically or pharmacologically, is a challenge to chemists spezializing in natural substances and to pharmacologists. In view of the limited number of research capacities and the ever-diminishing financial means, this challenge can only be met if, together with an improvement and refinement of methods of analysis, medicinal plant research is carried out on a broader interdisciplinary basis, with comparable, scientifically recognized screening methods, and if it is better coordinated, with greater use of modern documentation means. It is thus necessary in the future to concentrate specifically on projects leading to the development of new medicinal preparations.

The plenary lectures hold in the present symposium of the 1st International Congress for Research on Medicinal Plants reflect these efforts and tendencies. At the same time they provide a survey of some of the fields of medicinal plant research which are at present most actual and most intensively researched. They range from plant screening, isolation and structure elucidation of new principles, to the therapeutical optimization of a natural product.

The lectures given at this congress show clearly the necessity, in addition to national phytochemical societies, for a central international organisation, in which all active medicinal plant researchers in the world are included. Their aim should be to provide the impulse for more optimal, rational research, aimed at the solution of specific projects.

The symposium was generously supported by the Deutsche Forschungsgemeinschaft (Bonn) and various chemical and pharmaceutical industries.

June, 1977

H. WAGNER
P. WOLFF

Contents

List of Contributors

ACHENBACH, H., Prof. Dr., Chemisches Institut der Universität, Albertstraße 21, 7800 Freiburg / FRG

BINGEL, A.S., Dr., College of Pharmacy, University of Illinois, P.O. Box 6998, Chicago, Illinois 60680 / USA

CORDELL, G.A., Prof. Dr., College of Pharmacy, University of Illinois, P.O. Box 6998, Chicago, Illinois 60680 / USA

FARNSWORTH, N.R., Prof. Dr., College of Pharmacy, University of Illinois, P.O. Box 6998, Chicago, Illinois 60680 / USA

GOTTLIEB, O.R., Prof. Dr., Instituto de Quimica, Universidade de Sao Paulo, Caixa Postal 20780, 01000 Sao Paulo / Brasilia

GOVINDACHARI, T.R., Prof. Dr., 8, Crescent Park St., T. Nagar, Madras 60017 / India

MALONE, M.H., Prof. Dr., School of Pharmacy, University of the Pacific, Stockton, California 95211 / USA

SCHWARTING, A.E., Prof. Dr., University of Connecticut, School of Pharmacy, Storrs, Connecticut 06268 / USA

SHIBATA, S., Prof. Dr., Faculty of Pharmaceutical Sciences, University of Tokyo, Hongo, Bunkyo-ku, Tokyo 113 / Japan

STICHER, O., Prof. Dr., Pharmazeutisches Institut der Eidgenössischen Technischen Hochschule, Clausiusstraße 25, 8006 Zürich / Schweiz

TAMM, CH., Prof. Dr., Institut für Organische Chemie der Universität Basel, St. Johannes-Ring 19, 4056 Basel / Schweiz

THIES, P.W., Dr., Hans-Böckler-Allee, 3000 Hannover / FRG

VOGEL, G., Prof. Dr., Firma Dr. Madaus und Co., Ostmerheimer Straße 198, 5000 Köln 91 / FRG

Problems and Prospects of Discovering New Drugs from Higher Plants by Pharmacological Screening

N. R. FARNSWORTH and A. S. BINGEL

A. Introduction

There are probably very few in attendance at this Congress who have not experienced the frustrations of initiating research on plants alleged to have interesting biological activity, only to find that the activity could not be confirmed or demonstrated in animal models. Perhaps even more frustrating to most of you, has been the often nonreproducible nature of biological effects initially shown by a plant extract. Difficulties involved in preparing plant extracts into suitable dosage forms that would allow accurate amounts of the extract to be administered to an animal are further complications that bring frustration to this type of research. A difficult-to-explain phenomenon, associated with the administration of active plant extracts to animals, is the failure to produce consistent dose-response curves such as those usually obtained when pure chemical compounds are evaluated. Behind all of these problems, we find the most important deterrent to the search for new potential drugs in plants, i.e. apathy on the part of industrial firms, foundations, academic institutions, and government agencies to provide adequate funds for long enough periods of time so that a program of this type would be expected to yield clinically useful agents.

It is our suspicion that the organizers of this Congres invited us to prepare this manuscript for one of two reasons. First, there may have been a desire to confirm the rumor that the presentation would be illustrated with visual aids designed to prevent the frequently sedative atmosphere characteristic of many scientific meetings. Second, these same organizers may have felt that we would be able to provide answers to the universal problems associated with the search for new drugs from higher plants alluded to previously. While we may be able to provide the hoped-for visual aids, it may not be possible to provide the hoped-for answers.

Perhaps the most important aspect of this presentation will be to provide evidence that the current misconceptions attributed to the lack of importance of plant products as drugs have little basis, and that the problems alluded to above may not really be insurmountable.

B. Value of Drugs Obtained from Higher Plants

I. Commercial Value of Plant-Derived Drugs

To the best of our knowledge, data are not available outside the U.S.A. that allow one to calculate the actual number of prescriptions dispensed to patients that contain plant-derived drugs, nor the monetary value of such prescriptions. However, we can now document rather well that in the United States in the year 1973, the American public paid about $3 billion for prescription drugs that are still extracted from higher plants.

Recent data (1) claim that domestic sales of ethical drugs (*at the manufacturer's level*) in the U.S.A. totaled \$6.3 billion in 1974 for human dosage forms, and that worldwide sales of combined veterinary and human dosage forms totaled \$11.3 billion in the same year. One can probably double these industry figures to estimate the cost of human and/or veterinary drugs to the consumer.

We have analyzed the National Prescription Audit (NPA) data in the U.S.A., which includes total new and refilled prescription sales for community pharmacies in the United States. Of the 1.532 billion prescriptions (3) dispensed during 1973, 25.2 % contained one or more active constituents obtained from higher plants (seed plants). If one considers that in 1973 the average prescription price to the consumer was \$4.13 (2), then total prescription sales in community pharmacies for drugs from higher plants for that year amounted to about \$1.59 billion. Further, microbial products (antibiotics, ergot alkaloids, immunizing biologicals, etc.) accounted for about 13.3 % of all prescriptions. Animal-derived prescriptions accounted for about 2.7 % of the total.

In order to determine whether or not 1973 was an atypical year, a computerized analysis was carried out on the American prescription market from NPA data each year for the period 1959 through 1973. Although the total number of prescriptions increased dramatically over this 15-year period, the percentage of natural-product prescriptions remained rather constant (Table 1), indicating perhaps two major points: (1) that natural products represent an extremely stable market in the United States, and (2) that, because of this stability, it can be safely assumed that the drugs represented in the survey are heavily relied on (prescribed) by physicians.

Table 1. Comparison of natural-product containing prescriptions dispensed in community pharmacies (1959 and 1973)

Year	Higher plants	Microbes	Animals	Total
1959	25.5 %	21.4 %	2.3 %	49.2 %
1973	25.2 %	13.3 %	2.7 %	41.2 %

While it is true that the total percentage of prescriptions containing natural products decreased from 49.2 % in 1959 to 41.2 % in 1973, it is clear from Table 1 that the drop was attributed solely to a decreased use of microbial products, chiefly antibiotics. Thus, it can be stated that over the period 1959 to 1973, drugs from *higher plants* did not increase or decrease in frequency of use in the American prescription market. This is of interest because no new drugs from higher plants were introduced during the same span of time. It is our opinion that industry research and development investment for higher drug plant research during this same period of time *decreased* substantially. During the period 1959 to 1973, it is known that in the U.S.A. research programs in the pharmaceutical industry relating to the search for new drugs from higher plants were either phased out or reduced at Ciba, Smith Kline and French, Riker, G.D. Searle, and Eli Lilly and Co., and perhaps at other pharmaceutical companies as well.

National Prescription Audit figures for 1973 (3) indicate that 1.532 billion new and refilled prescriptions were dispensed from community pharmacies in the United States. At an average cost to the consumer of \$4.13 per prescription (3), one can calculate a dollar value of \$6.327

billion for the market in 1973. Thus, if a predicted 25.2 % of these prescriptions contained active principles of higher plant origin, the dollar cost to the consumer in 1973 would be estimated at $1.594 billion.

Now, how does one obtain the figure of $3 billion as the current value of higher plant medicinals in the U.S.A.? It can be estimated that somewhat less than the dollar volume representing the community pharmacy prescription market may be *added* to the $1.594 billion prescription market to account for the value of drugs dispensed in hospitals, government agencies, and the like. Thus, it seems logical and convenient to consider $3 billion as the annual value of drugs at the consumer level that are obtained from higher plants.

There is no way to estimate the importance and/or commercial value of drugs obtained from plants that are available to individuals without prescription, either in the U.S.A. or elsewhere, but this figure would probably be staggering.

Although our data are restricted to the U.S.A., it is safe to assume that plant-derived drugs are at least of equal importance in other countries of the world. Thus, it is safe to claim that there is little justification for the pharmaceutical industry to neglect plants as sources of new drugs on the base of infrequency of use, lack of importance of therapeutic effects, or inacceptability by the medical profession. That neglect could be based on a low dollar value, or poor profit potential, likewise, seems unjustified.

II. Role of Plant-Derived Drugs as Therapeutic Agents

To illustrate the importance of many higher plant drugs, the 12 most commonly encountered pure compounds, derived from higher plants and tabulated from the 1973 NPA prescription data, are presented in Table 2.

Table 2. Most commonly-encountered pure compounds from higher plants used as drugs in 1973 in the U.S.A.

Active plant principle	Total number of Rxs[a]	Percent of total Rxs
Steroids (95 % from diosgenin)	225,050,000	14.69
Codeine	31,099,000	2.03
Atropine	22,980,000	1.50
Reserpine	22,214,000	1.45
Pseudoephedrine[b]	13,788,000	0.90
Ephedrine[b]	11,796,000	0.77
Hyoscyamine	11,490,000	0.75
Digoxin	11,184,000	0.73
Scopolamine	10,111,000	0.66
Digitoxin	5,056,000	0.33
Pilocarpine	3,983,000	0.26
Quinidine	2,758,000	0.18

[a]Total number of Rxs in 1973 was 1.532 billion. [b]Produced commercially by synthesis, all others by extraction from plants

Another interesting note is that in 1973, a total of 76 different chemical compounds of known structure, derived from higher plants, were represented in the prescriptions analyzed. Further, the assumption by many people is that most, if not all, of the higher plant-derived drugs of known structure are now produced commercially by synthesis. Nothing could be further from the truth. Of the 76 individual drugs just indicated, only seven are commercially produced by synthesis, emetine, caffeine, theobromine, theophylline, pseudoephedrine, ephedrine, and papaverine. This is not to imply that most of the naturally occurring drugs have not been synthesized; indeed they have. However, practical industrial syntheses for such important drugs as morphine, codeine, atropine, digoxin, etc. are not available. The alkaloid, reserpine, for example, can be commercially extracted from natural sources for about $0.75/g, whereas a multistep and difficult synthesis is available that yields reserpine at about $1.25/g. It should be obvious which of the two sources is used to produce this pharmaceutical.

Even more interesting information can be derived from the 1973 survey data. For example, 99 different crude plant drugs, or types of extracts from crude plant drugs, were found to be present in the prescriptions analyzed, involving about 38,300,000 prescriptions in 1973 (2.5 % of the total). Those found in the greater number of prescriptions are listed in Table 3.

Table 3. Most commonly encountered higher plant extracts used in prescriptions in 1973[a]

Crude botanical or extract	Total number of Rxs	Per cent of total Rxs[b]
Belladonna *(Atropa belladonna)*	10,418,000	0.68 %
Ipecac *(Cephaelis ipecacuanha)*	7,047,000	0.46 %
Opium *(Papaver somniferum)*	6,894,000	0.45 %
Rauwolfia *(Rauvolfia serpentina)*	5,822,000	0.38 %
Cascara *(Rhamnus purshiana)*	2,451,000	0.16 %
Digitalis *(Digitalis purpurea)*	2,451,000	0.16 %
Citrus Biflavonoids *(Citrus* spp.*)*	1,379,000	0.09 %
Veratrum *(Veratrum viride)*	1,072,000	0.07 %

[a]Compounded prescriptions represented less than 2.0 % of total prescriptions (3) and were excluded from the survey data that were compiled and analyzed. The drugs indicated above were in standard dosage forms and not in multicomponent, extemporaneously prepared prescriptions. [b]Total Rx volume in 1973 was 1.532 billion prescriptions

One only needs to open the pages of any standard textbook of pharmacology to be impressed by the fact that virtually every pharmacological class of drug includes a natural product prototype that exhibits the classical effects of the pharmacological category in question; most of them are plant-derived (see Table 4).

Table 4. Typical plant principles used to illustrate pharmacological principles in standard textbooks

Type of pharmacological action	Type of compound	Name of compound
Centrally acting skeletal muscle relaxant	Alkaloid	Bulbocapnine
Analgesic	Alkaloid	Morphine, codeine
Smooth muscle relaxant	Alkaloid	Papaverine
Antigout	Alkaloid	Colchicine
CNS stimulant	Monoterpene	Camphor
	Sesquiterpene	Picrotoxin
	Alkaloid	Strychnine, caffeine, theobromine, theophylline
Local anesthetic	Alkaloid	Cocaine
Parasympatholytic	Alkaloid	Atropine, scopolamine
Parasympathomimetic	Alkaloid	Pilocarpine, physostigmine
Peripherally acting skeletal muscle relaxant	Alkaloid	*d*-Tubocurarine
Sympathomimetic	Alkaloid	Ephedrine
Ganglionic blocker	Alkaloid	Nicotine, lobeline
Cardiotonic	Cardiac glycoside	Digitoxin, digoxin
Antiarrhythmic	Alkaloid	Quinidine
Uterine stimulant	Alkaloid	Sparteine, ergot alkaloids
Antihypertensive	Alkaloid	Reserpine, *Veratrum* alkaloids
Psychotropic	Alkaloid	Reserpine
Cathartic	Anthraquinone	Anthraquinone glycosides
	Mucilages	Psyllium, agar
	Fixed oil	Castor Oil
Antimalarial	Alkaloid	Quinine
Antiamebic	Alkaloid	Emetine

III. Uses Other than as Drugs for Plant-Derived Chemicals

Natural drug products, many of which have been derived from higher plants, play an important role as useful investigative tools in pharmacological studies. Some such compounds are included in Table 4. Others are mescaline and LSD-derivatives in the study of psychiatric disorders; various toxins, e.g. tetrodotoxin, in the study of nerve transmission; cyclopamine in the study of teratogenesis; phalloidin for induction of hepatoxicity; and phorbol myristate acetate as a standard cocarcinogen in the investigation of potential carcinogens and cocarcinogens.

Other useful applications of plant derived chemicals can be cited; e.g. bixin as a coloring agent for foods; nordihydroguaiaretic acid as an antioxidant in lard; essential oils and their derived terpenes as perfumes and flavoring agents, etc. The economic value of these materials is difficult to estimate, but surely must be in the billion dollar category on a worldwide basis.

A number of laboratories feel that the major purpose for finding in plants new structures with biological activity is to provide templates for the synthesis of analogs and/or derivatives which will have equivalent or better activity than the parent molecule. This may indeed be an admirable purpose, and from a practical point of view, it may be advantageous with regard to patent protection. However, history shows that it is an exceptionally rare instance when a naturally occurring chemical compound that has found utility as a drug in man, will yield a derivative on structure modification that exceeds the value of the parent compound in drug efficacy.

This also does not discount the value of such model compounds as cocaine, yielding information that led chemists to produce related local anesthetics such as procaine and its congeners, nor the value of the large number of synthetic anticholinergic drugs that were designed from the tropane nucleus and which have their own specific advantages.

Finally, the value of plant-derived chemical compounds as building blocks for semisynthetic derivatives cannot be underestimated. The classical example is the use of diosgenin as the primary starting material for the synthesis of the majority of steroidal hormones currently used in medicine.

C. Apathy in Plant-Derived Drug Development

Although estimates vary, the most commonly-quoted figure as to the number of species of higher plants that can be found growing on planet Earth is 250,000 to 500,000. One also often hears educated "guestimates" that "less than 5 % (or 10 % or 15 %) of these plants have been investigated for pharmacologically active principles." However, no one has adequately determined what parameters must be considered before one can state that a particular plant has indeed been "investigated for pharmacologically active principles." With respect to attempting to estimate how many plants have been investigated *as potential sources of new drugs*, our more than *six* years experience at computer coding the world literature concerning chemical constituents and pharmacological activities of living organisms leads us to believe that no reasonable estimate can be made.

For example, for the past dozen or so years, what might be considered to be the most extensive pharmacological investigation of plants ever, has been carried out by the National Cancer Institute (Drug Research and Development Branch). About 20,525 different species of plants were screened for animal antitumor activity (4). However, the fact that 90 % of these were shown to be devoid of antitumor effects against the one or two tumor systems (of several hundred known) selected for the "screen" surely does not preclude the sample plants from having chemical entities of potential use as medicaments in a variety of other diseases or conditions. Therefore, although one might be able to say that 4 - 8 % of higher plants have been investigated for *antitumor* activity, these plants must still be considered "uninvestigated" with respect to the many other important drug actions that they might possess.

What is the financial gamble in developing a new drug, synthetic or natural? This figure is difficult to determine, mainly because of the complications involved in assessing and calculating drug development costs. Do we consider the cost of discovering the compound? of pre-clinical testing? of clinical evaluation? of preparing FDA approval forms? One cannot use the figure of $722.7 million, published by the U.S. drug industry as indicative of its total 1974 budget for company-financed research and development of human pharmaceuticals in the United States (1). This figure is not specific for new drug entities, but includes costs for developing "me too" products, new dosage forms, etc. If we nevertheless did use that figure and considered also that in 1973, only 19 single *new* drugs were introduced on the market in the United States (5), then the research and development costs per drug would amount to $38 million. Since other sources (6), however, state that, taking into consideration the factors mentioned above, the total cost of research and development of each new drug before it reaches the market may be only from $2.5 to $4.5 million, then it becomes obvious that the total research and development costs of pharmaceuticals, published by the drug industry, are far from being atributable primarily to NEW drugs.

If one accepts the more conservative figure, ca. $3 million, as the cost to develop a new drug to a marketable form (estimated cost from inception to marketable dosage form, including clinical trials, etc.), and if the industry currently invests a maximum of $0.15 million per year for research on drugs from higher plants, then one could expect, on an average, that only *one* new drug from higher plants would be marketed every 20 years. From our experience it seems doubtful that more than three or four pharmaceutical firms in the U.S.A. are currently engaged in any type of meaningful research on higher plants as sources of new drugs. We further suggest that $0.15 million annually is a generous estimate of the current cost of such research to the American pharmaceutical industry. What might happen if the financial commitment to research in this area were at the same level as for the development of synthetic drugs?

Let us now consider the fact that in the U.S.A. during the period 1954 to 1973, eight new drugs from higher plants were introduced as prescription items; reserpine, deserpidine, rescinnamine, sparteine, Rauwolfia whole root, alseroxylon fraction products, vincaleukoblastine (vinblastine), and leurocristine (vincristine). One might argue that, during the past 20 years, even at a low level of research funding for developing new drugs from higher plants, one new drug has been marketed every 2.5 years, on the average. Because the expectation by the parameters previously discussed is one plant-derived drug every 20 years, while the actual situation is one every 2.5 years, research and development costs in this area appear to be a "bargain."

Why have the pharmaceutical industry and government agencies turned their heads against further exploitation of a market now estimated in the U.S.A. at $3 billion at the consumer level? The answer can be expressed simply that there are major examples, from the not-too-distant past, in which modest investments of time, money, and effort, have not paid off. Let me cite just a few to illustrate the point.

A few years ago, one of our leading pharmaceutical houses in the U.S.A. made the decision to initiate a modest effort in the search for new drugs in plants. At that time, the company had no staff trained in the problems and approaches to developing such a program. Thus, it surveyed the employment records of its Ph.D staff of chemists, and determined that one individual had indicated on his employment form that he was also interested in natural products chemistry. He was an excellent organic chemist and had decided that the best approach would be to collaborate with a trained botanist in a country rich in medicinal folklore. This botanist was directed to ship several plants each month to the pharmaceutical firm where extracts were made and subjected to a broad array of pharmacological screens. It should be noted that, in many instances, the pharmacological screens did not include animal models to detect the type of activity for which the plant was allegedly used by the natives, i.e. the tests were restricted to those currently available for all compounds being "screened." As time passed, the pharmacology staff became irritated at "thick, black, sticky extracts that clogged up their syringes, and which, for the most part, did not give dramatic activity."

After about two years the program was dropped, and the results of the pharmacological evaluation of one hundred or more of the plants were published. An examination of the fine print in the article revealed that indeed many of these plants elicited remarkable pharmacological effects, and it was difficult to envision a pharmaceutical firm making such information known to the scientific community without following through on the isolation of the active principles. An inquiry brought to light the fact that since cooperation of the pharmacologists could not be enlisted, and because the results of the crude extract testing were not dramatic enough, the program was dropped and the chemist was allowed to publish the data.

It was subsequently determined, through talking with colleagues of the botanist, that many of the plants eventually published as having interesting activity, had been only tentatively identified. Indeed, several plants were eventually found to have been incorrectly identified. The botanist had not been consulted prior to publication of the results to determine the exactness of the identifications; thus, even though many interesting pharmacological leads appear to be apparent in this publication, a follow-up by other interested investigators would probably result in utter frustration.

A second example can be cited in which another pharmaceutical firm in the U.S.A. initiated a program for which leads were obtained by searching books on medical botany concerning the flora of primitive countries. Interesting uses of plants were noted, and orders were placed for the collection of 1 kg quantities of each plant for initial pharmacological screening. Commercial plant suppliers usually operate by notifying their botanist collaborators to collect specific plants (giving them the Latin name and any other pertinent information). In most cases, the botanist recognizes the Latin name of the plant as one which is known popularly by the natives under some common (vernacular) name. A native in the area who is knowledgeable in herbal medicine is dispatched to collect 2 kg of "the bark of capinuri" (as a hypothetical example).

The native collects what to him is "capinuri," but a native in an adjoining village or province might have collected an entirely different plant that he knew as "capinuri." This is not too difficult to understand; even in Europe, if a person were asked to collect 2 kg of "periwinkle," that person could conceivably return with any one of four or five different species of plants, each quite distinctly unrelated. Thus, the shipment of "capinuri" is shipped to the pharmaceutical firm (invariably the collector does not supply for future reference, a *voucher herbarium specimen* of the plant being collected). The extract from the "capinuri" shows very interesting pharmacological effects, and the commercial supplier is requested to obtain 500 kg of the bark of the specified Latin name plant. Our supplier again notifies his contact (usually several months or years later), and perhaps a different native is dispatched to collect the 500 kg of "capinuri." Again, no voucher specimen is made and the 500 kg of bark, after extraction and testing for confirmation of the original activity, is found to be devoid of that activity!

Several years ago, more than 20 plants with extremely interesting pharmacological effects were obtained by the aforementioned pharmaceutical firm, but the pharmacological effects shown by most of the plants could not be duplicated when recollected samples were tested subsequently. The obvious answer to the mystery (by those in charge of the operation) was that this simply represented the trials and tribulations of botanical-chemical-pharmacological research and/or biological variation from one batch of plant material to the next. Could not all of this have been avoided if all parties concerned had been more aware of the need for proper precautions in documenting botanical specimens so that identical collections could have been made at a later date?

A third vivid and unfortunate example, and perhaps the most costly one known to us, is that concerning a physician who approached a major pharmaceutical firm in the U.S.A. stating that for a modest sum (ca. $500,000), he would spend some time in a primitive jungle area and observe medicine men using plants as drugs. He, as a physician, would be able to ascertain the condition of the patient, confirm the diagnosis of the disease, and assess the effects of the herbal remedies prescribed by the medicine man. In cases where the herbal remedy was judged effective, the physician would then collect large quantities of the plants and ship them to the drug firm.

Because this was a novel approach, the physician was funded, and he went off to the jungle. He did everything that he agreed to do. He collected several large samples of plant material, carefully numbered each sample, and prepared pressed voucher specimens of each sample so that botanists could later identify each sample. He identified each of the voucher specimens by writing the correct identifying number on a leaf of each specimen with a ball point pen! The voucher specimens were carefully dried (concurrently the leaves became brittle), and the bulk samples of plant material and the voucher specimens (not carefully packaged) were shipped to the drug firm. The voucher specimens were turned over to a botanist who found either that many of the leaves had crumbled, or that the identifying numbers were illegible; virtually none of the voucher specimens was found to be identifiable. The company had no further interest in testing the bulk samples collected because if any were to have shown interesting activity, it would probably have been impossible to recollect larger samples for additional studies without repeating the whole study.

A fourth example of more recent vintage concerns a major pharmaceutical firm in the U.S.A. that was approached by a scientist from another country who indicated that a plant used in his country in folkloric medicine had been shown under his direction to have what appeared to be a very promising drug action. The pharmaceutical firm obtained some of the plant but could not show these effects in its laboratories. At some expense, they requested a university pharmacology laboratory to attempt to duplicate the effects described by this scientist. This laboratory also failed to ascertain any type of biological effects.

Since that time, a small pharmaceutical firm in the U.S.A. has isolated the active principle from this plant, after assigning 50 % of its research staff (about 40 people) to the problem. They have also synthesized the compound and prepared a number of active derivatives.

Why did one group succeed and the others fail? Perhaps we will never know, but the writers would like to venture a guess that it might have been due to a difference in attitude in their approaches to the problem. In the former instance, the investigators might have looked at the problem with a great deal of skepticism, whereas the latter group perhaps may have had a more positive outlook.

These are only a few of the many examples that could be cited if space were available, and surely such examples must be widely known. Is it any wonder that administrators allocating funds for research programs are reluctant to initiate projects to explore the possibility of finding new drugs from plants? On the other hand, is it not more reasonable to look at the tremendous untapped potential of new drug development from higher plants from a positive viewpoint, and to make a *commitment* to a *major* program that would include sufficient time, adequate funds, and the acquisition of a variety of properly trained specialists who could recognize the problems inherent in this area, so that the obvious oversights in the examples cited, could be avoided?

D. Current Level of Worldwide Research on Plant-Derived Drugs

No one to date has compiled accurate figures for a given year, concerning the number of novel compounds vs. the number of compounds of known structure reported from plants, fungi, and animals. Since in our laboratory we now are computerizing the world literature on all aspects of natural products, we are able to present some interesting data that we consider to be quite accurate. Before presenting the data, however, an explanation will be given regarding the extent of the literature covered. Our sources are *Chemical Abstracts*, *Biological Abstracts*, and current issues of 70 journals which we have found by experience to contain the majority of new information concerning natural products. From these sources, we computerize all reports concerning new biological activities for novel or known compounds from natural sources, and all reports concerning biological activities reported for extracts prepared from organisms. We computerize, rather completely, reports in which a secondary metabolite has been isolated from, or detected in, any living organism. Unfortunately, due to lack of funds, we have not been able to include many articles concerned with only primary metabolites e.g. simple sugars, amino acids, proteins, and the like; we do hope to be able to do so in the future, however.

The data to be cited are from about 10,000 articles, the contents of which we computerized in the year 1975. No 1976 literature will be discussed; however, a large segment of 1974, and even some earlier, data are represented, in addition to data published in 1975, because of the fact that many references in abstracting services tend to be less than current.

The figures to be cited now represent numbers of compounds of already known and of novel structure, reported isolated from various groups of organisms in the 1975 literature as defined above. Compounds identified by chromatographic procedures, without being actually isolated, are not included.

As indicated in Table 5, 1650 compounds of novel structure were reported, as well as 3077 of known structure, from higher plants, i.e. monocots, dicots, and gymnosperms. From the remaining groups (Table 6), 749 additional compounds of novel structure were isolated, as well as 888 of known structure. Thus, from all classes of organisms, a total of 2399 compounds were reported isolated and their structures determined, for the first time. An additional 3965 compounds of known structure were also reported isolated. The latter category probably represents in fact only about 3000 - 3500, since there is some duplication among the compounds isolated from organisms in Tables 5 and 6.

Table 5. Numbers of compounds of known structure isolated from higher plants as determined from the 1975 literature

Plant group	New	Known
Monocots	97	277
Dicots	1504	2579
Gymnosperms	49	221
Totals	1650	3077

Table 6. Numbers of compounds of known structure isolated from lower plants and marine organisms as determined from the 1975 literature

Plant group	New	Known
Pteridophytes	29	90
Bryophytes	17	32
Lichens	14	44
Fungi and bacteria	479	523
Marine organisms	210	199
Totals	749	888

To say that these compounds have little commercial importance would not be true; in 1975 more than 400 patents were issued for substances isolated from higher plants alone.

It may be of some interest to learn also that syntheses were published for about 1000 natural products, and that the structures of 275 natural products were determined by X-ray analysis during 1975.

A total of 325 compounds of known structure, isolated from higher plants only, was reported in the 1975 literature as having one or more types of biological activity in some system(s) having relevance to their potential use as a drug. Of the 325, 93 were compounds of novel structure reported for the first time, and 232 were previously known structures (Table 7). As would be expected, the majority of these biologically active plant principles were alkaloids (73/325), followed by sesquiterpenes (47/325), diterpenes (26/325), triterpene saponins (22/325), triterpene aglycones (18/325), flavonoids (18/325), coumarins and quinones (15/325 each), sterols (17/325) and monoterpenes (13/325).

The various categories of biological activity for these 325 compounds are summarized in Table 8. As can be seen, various categories of chemotherapeutic agents (antibacterial, antiprotozoan, antifungal, antiviral) were most frequently cited, followed by tumor inhibitors and cytotoxic agents, antiinflammatory agents, tumor promoters and/or cocarcinogens, hypocholesterolemics, hypoglycemics, antiulcer agents, and toxic plant principles.

It was not possible to determine how many of these activities were published from laboratories of pharmaceutical firms, but it would be safe to estimate that perhaps less than 10 % would be categorized as such.

Table 7. Summary of classes of plant products showing biological activity from the 1975 literature[a]

Class of compounds	Total No.	New[b]	Old[c]	Class of compound	Total No.	New	Old	Class of compounds	Total No.	New	Old
Alkaloids	73	24	49	Monoterpenes	13	1	12	Thiophenes	2	0	2
Sesquiterpenes	47	19	28	Simaroubolides	9	8	1	Sulfides	2	0	2
Diterpenes	26	12	14	Phenolic acids	8	2	6	Nitro derivatives	2	0	2
Triterpene saponins	22	2	20	Amino acids	8	0	8	Phenylpropanoids	2	0	2
Triterpenes	18	5	13	Lignans	6	2	4	Steroid saponins	2	0	2
Flavonoids	18	2	16	Carbocyclic comps.	5	0	5	Cardenolides	2	0	2
Coumarins	15	1	14	Benzenoid deriv.	4	2	2	Cyano derivatives	1	1	0
Quinones	15	4	11	Fatty acid and esters	4	1	3	Naphthalenes	1	0	1
Sterols	17	7	10	Isothiocyanates	2	0	2	Xanthones	1	0	1

[a]Total number is 325; [b]total number is 93; [c]total number is 232

Table 8. Numbers of biologically interesting plant products from the 1975 literature by category of activity

Type of biol. activity	Number	Type of biol. activity	Number	Type of biol. activity	Number
Analgesics	8	Cardiovascular (Misc.)	5	Hypocholesterolemics	22
Anorexics	2	Cathartics	1	Hypoglycemics	13
Antiarrhythmics	2	Chemother.-anthelmintics	5	Hypotensives	8
Antiazotemics	1	Chemother.-antibacterial	30	Immunosuppressants	1
Anticonvulsants	3	Chemother.-antifungal	28	Insecticides	2
Antiemetics	1	Chemother.-antimycoplasmics	2	Insect feeding deterrants	1
Antifertility agents	4	Chemother.-antiprotozoan	30	Psoriasis ameloriating agents	1
Antihepatotoxic agents	3	Chemother.-antiviral	8	Spasmolytics	7
Antihistaminics	4	Choleretics	5	Spermicides	3
Antiinflammatory agents	32	Cholinomimetics	1	Teratogens	6
Anti-sickling agents	4	CNS active agents	14	Toxic plant principles	12
Antitussives	3	Coronary vasodilators	1	Tumor inhibitors	63
Antiulcer agents	12	Diuretics	4	Cytotoxic agents	49
Capillary antihemorrhagic	2	Fish poisons	1	Tumor promoters	25
Cardiotonics	1	Gonadotropics	1	Uterine stimulants	1
				Vasodilators	1
				Miscellaneous	3

These data do not include a large number of reports concerning interesting biological activities of extracts from organisms which remain to be studied for their active principle(s). Although it is perhaps of little interest to most people since they personally would have no need for such a drug, it may be of some interest to others that a recent preliminary report concerns an unusual biological activity for a crude extract prepared from *Dryopteris filix-mas* (7). The title of the article "Preliminary Report on an Unexpected Effect of an Extract from *Dryopteris filix-mas*" would not attract much attention from the casual reader. The article, however, states that: "In male mice and rats, one drop of an extract from *Dryopteris filix-mas*, administered orally pure or suspended in sunflowerseed oil, caused a spectacular enlargement of the penis. This unexpected effect cannot be explained so far and will have to be elucidated by further experiments."

There are many other similar published reports that could provide stimuli for research projects by interested phytochemists, but for some reason many remain uninvestigated.

In concluding this section of the presentation, it may be significant to point out that less than 5 % of the new structures isolated from higher plants as determined from the 1975 literature were reported to have been evaluated for any type of biological activity.

E. Pharmacological Screening Programs for Plant Extracts

In any program in which the end-product is to be a drug, some type of pharmacological screening, or pharmacological evaluation, must obviously be used. This will be discussed later. Preliminary to the actual pharmacological testing, however, one must decide which plants to collect. As was indicated previously, there are probably from 250,000 to 500,000 species of higher plants from which to make the selection; thus, some decision must be made as to which procedure will yield the highest number of extracts showing the sought-after activity in an animal or in an in vitro system.

It is very difficult to obtain exact data as to the effectiveness of any of the procedures that have been used in recent years. There are few programs of sufficient magnitude to be used as examples. Those of which we have some personal knowledge will be discussed.

I. Random Selection Approach

The program of the National Cancer Institute (NCI) in the U.S.A. selects plants on a random basis and evaluates the extracts against one or more in vitro tumor systems, and also evaluates them for in vitro cytotoxicity. Since its inception, the program has screened about 20,525 species, and extracts from 1127 species have shown activity in one or more of the screens, based on the criteria selected for that program (4). It is difficult to evaluate the overall productivity of the total program; perhaps some idea can be gained as to the productivity and cost-benefit ratio that can be expected from such an approach by using the published data of one of the laboratories involved in the NCI program.

Kupchan and co-workers have reported on the isolation of 92 active compounds from 42 species of plants. If in the total program, 10.4 % of all species randomly selected were to show activity (4), then it would be expected that Kupchan's 42 active species had resulted from screening about 405 plants. This may be entirely accurate, since the active compounds may have been isolated from plants available that had shown the most promising activity, whereas low-activity plants may have been set aside. However, of the 92 active compounds isolated from 42 species, about six were judged of sufficient activity to undergo preclinical pharmacological investigation. Two of the six are currently in the clinic. Thus, if only one of the six selected for preclinical pharmacological investigation shows promise as an antitumor agent in humans, we can say that this single compound resulted from a random selection and biological evaluation of only 405 species (or more, depending on the factors indicated above).

Obviously, as a program such as this gains in experience, the selection of candidate plants for antitumor testing can become more selective, resulting in a better possibility of selecting from taxa, plants which would be expected to show higher activity.

It is generally thought by most that this type of approach is too expensive for profit-making pharmaceutical firms. However, as demonstrated above, this does not appear to be the case. If one would compare the number of synthetic compounds that are prepared and tested in order to obtain six candidates for clinical testing, the natural-products random selection-pharmacological screening approach would seem to compare very favorably.

In our own laboratories, we randomly selected 163 species of higher plants and evaluated them for antiinflammatory activity in the carrageein-induced rat pedal edema assay (8). Extracts from 73 of the species displayed inhibition of inflammation of 25 % or greater at doses of 5 - 100 mg/kg of *crude plant extract*. Seventeen species exhibited between 30 and 39 % inhibition, 21 species between 40 and 49 % inhibition, 15 species between 50 and 59 % inhibition, four species between 60 and 69 % inhibition, and two species between 70 and 79 % inhibition. Although we recognize that this particular animal model can often yield false-positive results, it is not unreasonable to believe that many of the active extracts could yield interesting antiinflammatory compounds.

II. Selection of Plants Containing Specific Types of Chemical Compounds

The Smith Kline and French Laboratories in the U.S.A. carried out a rather extensive program for about a ten-year period. The general procedure was for a chemist to go into the field and test various parts of plants for the presence of alkaloids. Any plant showing good positive tests for this group of substances was collected and shipped to the main laboratory. The total alkaloid fraction was extracted and subjected to a variety of pharmacological screens. Very little has been published on the exact details of this program, even to the extent that little is known of the types of pharmacological screens employed. It is generally known (though not published) that the program yielded several compounds which were very close to being marketed, yet in spite of this, the program was terminated. The reasons for this are not clear, even to this day.

Presumably the program concentrated only on alkaloidal substances because of the high proportion of members of this group that show biological effects. Also, of course, a large percentage of useful drugs already obtained from plants are members of this class. Also, the ease of manipulation of alkaloids, hence less problems in the extraction, purification, and separation of active compounds, undoubtedly must have been a major factor in the decision. In addition, the problems involved in preparing water-soluble dosage forms of many "neutral" plant constituents could have been a feature that was important in restricting the program to alkaloids. One can only speculate on the number of potentially useful drugs missed by the program because of a lack of attention to alkaloid-free plants.

It is indeed unfortunate that programs such as this one have not been fully documented in the literature so that others contemplating similar programs could benefit from the vast experience that a 10-year effort of this type must surely have produced.

III. Selection of Plants Based on a Combination of Criteria

At Eli Lilly and Company in Indianapolis, a program was set up in 1956, in which three scientists selected the plants to be collected. Extracts were submitted to the general pharmacological screen available at Lilly at that time. The screen was made up of the following, and some details have been published (9).

1. Antitumor screen (3 - 5 animal tumors)
2. CNS screen ("mouse behavior")
3. Antimicrobial screen (in vitro, including human and plant pathogens, bacteria, fungi, protozoa, algae, yeasts, etc.)
4. Antiviral screen (tissue culture, 3 viruses)
5. Insecticide screen

Further details regarding the program are not available. However, one of the scientists involved, Dr. Gordon H. Svoboda, selected his plants primarily on the basis of interesting folkloric medicinal uses recorded for the plants, and secondarily on his knowledge that the plant contained alkaloids.

The following serves to point out the risk-benefit ratio of this approach. Svoboda claims that to date he has submitted about 400 species of plants to the screen (1956 - 1976). The most well-known plant screened in this program, *Catharanthus roseus (Vinca rosea)*, was submitted for biological evaluation on December 23, 1957. The antitumor activity of extracts from this plant was reported in January, 1958, and vincaleukoblastine (vinblastine, Velban^R, VLB), currently used for Hodgkin's disease, choriocarcinoma, and other human neoplasms, was marketed in the U.S.A. in March, 1961. Leurocristine (vincristine, Oncovin^R, VCR), was marketed in the U.S.A. in July, 1963, and is currently one of the most useful clinical antitumor agents available. Of Svoboda's 400 selections for this program, *C. roseus* was the 40th.

The 175th submission to the program was *Ochrosia maculata*, extracts of which showed marked antileukemic activity in animals; subsequently, Svoboda isolated 9-methoxyellipticine as the active antitumor agent. Although Lilly did not pursue this alkaloid further into the clinic, it is receiving widespread attention, especially in France.

The 250th submission to the screen was *Acronychia baueri (Bauerella australiana)*, which eventually yielded acronycine, an alkaloid originally discovered by the Australians, and which is now being evaluated clinically both by the Lilly group, and by the National Cancer Institute.

Thus, we can summarize this selection approach based on combination criteria as yielding two clinically useful drugs of commercial interest, as well as a third drug now being clinically evaluated, and a fourth drug having high interest as a potential drug.

F. Problems in the Pharmacological Screening of Extracts from Higher Plants

One problem with pharmacological screening programs is that very often one expects too much. The ideal pharmacological screen would identify only those extracts or pure compounds that are highly active and non-toxic. Such a screen does not exist. Thus, the screen must be one that will accommodate the largest number of samples in the shortest period of time and for the least possible cost, the hope being that the variability of the data will be minimal and that the screen will be sensitive enough to detect active principles that may be present in crude extracts at low concentrations. Any screen with these parameters may also identify false-positive activities. To exclude false-negatives seems too much to expect.

In addition, in order to isolate the active compound(s), it is necessary to use the screen, or a modification of it, to monitor the initial biological activity throughout the fractionation procedure. This necessitates that the screen will utilize only small amounts of extracts and fractions. If the screen requires gram quantities of material for evaluation, it most often becomes impractical. Using reasonable quantities of starting material, one can expect that after chromatographic separation of such fractions, gram quantities of column cuts are unrealistic to expect. This problem will be commented upon subsequently.

The problems in failing to duplicate results from one lot of plant material to another, or from different samples prepared from the same lot of plant material can perhaps be summarized briefly as follows:

I. Variation from Sample to Sample

Failure to duplicate pharmacological results obtained with extracts from one lot of plant material with an extract from subsequent lots of plant material is a real problem. However, there is very little evidence, based on controlled experimental data, to support the contention that the problem must be based primarily on variation in the concentration of active principle(s) from one lot to another. Perhaps the least expected factor may be the most responsible, i.e. failure to collect the same specimen on separate occasions as discussed above in Section C. The extreme importance of documenting collections with voucher specimens, in order to avoid such a problem, should be obvious.

However, a look at the 1975 literature concerning the isolation of new chemical entities from higher plants alone revealed the following. Only 160 of the 2399 novel chemical compounds reported were isolated from plants for which the author(s) indicated that a voucher specimen was available for reference to the plant material investigated. Until such time that editors of journals recognize the importance for documenting investigational material from natural sources with voucher specimens, in scientific articles, this problem will undoubtedly continue. There is even a 1975 paper, published in a reputable chemical journal, in which a new compound was reported isolated from a plant that was identified only as "probably belonging to the Menispermaceae!"

II. Unexpected Dose-Response Relationships

In Table 9, one can see the normal type of dose - response relationship that is expected. In this instance, the data were derived from the evaluation of a plant extract against the P-388 lymphocytic leukemia system in mice. On the other hand, Table 10 illustrates the type of dose - response relationship often seen in the same type of evaluation. The data shown in Table 10 were obtained with a different plant extract from that shown in Table 9.

What might be the explanation(s) for the type of dose - response results seen in Table 10? It is possible that a compound might exhibit one type of activity at a lower dose and an opposite type of activity at a higher dose; i.e. compounds can be antiestrogenic at low doses, for example, and estrogenic at high doses (11). Furthermore, almost all clinically useful antitumor agents have been shown to be carcinogenic (12). Other possible explanations exist. However, it is the opinion of the authors that improper preparation of samples of water-insoluble crude extracts injected into animal models may be the primary reason for failure to elicit normal dose - response relationships. Invariably plant extracts are only partially soluble, or insoluble, in the usual nontoxic diluents available to the pharmacologist. Thus, the pharmacologist is forced to utilize aqueous suspensions; a suspending or solubilizing agent may or may not have to be added. Shaking of the vial prior to withdrawing a dose of the suspension into a hypodermic syringe should result in an injection being made into the test animal of the calculated mg/kg dose. However, the suspension may settle out rather rapidly, and if the pharmacologist neglects to mix the contents of the vial thoroughly prior to withdrawing *each* dose, subpotent, and eventually suprapotent injections, as the vial empties, could be made.

Table 9. Normal dose-response curve of plant extract vs. P-388 leukemia in mice

Dose (mg/kg, i.p.)	Activity (% T/C)
50	133
33	125
22	110

Table 10. Abnormal dose-response curve of plant extract vs. P-388 leukemia in mice

Dose (mg/kg, i.p.)	Activity (% T/C)
400	110
200	88
100	144

Thus, as simple a matter as inadequately mixing a sample prior to filling a syringe could result in a very frustrating and expensive problem in this type of research.

III. Variation Within Samples from the Same Lot of Plant Material

Perhaps even more frustrating is the type of data shown in Table 11. Two samples, fractionated separately from the same lot of plant material, were evaluated in the same in vivo antitumor test system. Only the petroleum ether fraction showed activity the first time the plant was fractionated, and the order of activity was barely marginal. When another sample from the same lot was fractionated subsequently, two other fractions showed moderate degrees of activity, and the water-soluble fraction proved toxic.

How might these results be explained? One might first wonder whether the fractionation schemes were identical. If so, were the conditions, e.g. temperature, length of time for extraction, volumes of solvent, length of time the plant material was stored before the second sample was fractionated and tested, etc. identical? In this specific example, the fractionations were carried out within two months of each other, and to the best of our knowledge, all extraction conditions were identical, within the normal limits of control for this type of work. Subsequent fractionations resulted in results quite similar to those obtained with the second sample shown in Table 11, i.e. where activity was seen in the methanol and chloroform fractions. Thus, when test result differences cannot be explained by differences among fraction schemes and/or extraction conditions, one must again look at the animal testing procedure as indicated above in Section F.II.

Table 11. Test data from two samples fractionated from the same lot of plant material

Type of fraction	First fractionation	Second fractionation
	mg/kg % T/C	mg/kg % T/C[a]
Petroleum ether	200/126	200/153
	100/116	100/103
	50/90	50/103
Methanol	200/119	200/140
	100/124	100/113
	50/124	50/113
Chloroform	200/116	200/163
	100/104	100/150
	50/100	50/130
Water	200/104	200/Toxic
	100/100	100/97
	50/98	50/96

[a]Treated/Control against P-388 leukemia in mice. T/C $\geq$ 125 indicates an active extract

IV. Failure to Obtain Positive Results with an Extract Containing Active Principles

That false-negative results may be obtained in pharmacological screens was already pointed out at the beginning of Section F. There are, indeed, a few cases reported in the literature of active compounds being isolated from plant extracts, even though the extracts themselves were shown to be devoid of activity (10). A logical explanation would seem to be that the active compound(s) was(were) present in insufficient quantity in the crude extract to manifest activity at the dose levels employed. If they were present at sufficient concentration, then one must search for an alternative explanation, such as the presence of other compound(s) in the extracts that were able to antagonize, somehow, the effects of the active compound(s). Perhaps that might explain the lack of antitumor activity of fractions of *Catharanthus lanceus*, from which we nevertheless were able to isolate significant quantities of the highly active antitumor alkaloid, leurosine (10).

Because of the possibility of having antagonistic substances present in an extract prepared with a single solvent, i.e. ethanol, it is our feeling that such extracts should not be pharmacologically evaluated until fractionated in some manner. Fractionation according to the procedure of (1) first extracting with petroleum ether, followed by (2) extraction of the marc of the drug with methanol, or ethanol, followed by (3) partition of the methanol extract between chloroform and water, and extraction of the water extract with 1-butanol, would seem to be a reasonable alternative. In this way one would crudely separate the low from the higher polarity components, and the higher polarity compounds (methanol-soluble) into medium (chloroform-soluble) and high polarity (water-soluble) components. Further separation of the high polarity materials, with 1-butanol, could be achieved. Although this procedure would give no assurance that antagonistic substances would be separated completely, it seems to offer a reasonable alternative to a single-solvent extract. The obvious disadvantage is that one would have to evaluate several fractions, and in a broad screening program, this would be expensive.

V. Miscellaneous Considerations in Screening Plant Extracts

There are a number of additional problems associated either directly or indirectly with interpretation of data from the pharmacological evaluation of crude extracts from higher plants. Professor Malone will treat many of these in greater detail. However, it would seem appropriate to touch briefly on certain of these that we have encountered in our laboratory.

It has been our experience that pharmacological screening in general, including the screening of synthetic compounds, is not always treated seriously. Since screening, by definition, implies that one may expect to miss some interesting activities, this philosophy may not be entirely unjustified. On the other hand, one should not deliberately approach the problem with this attitude. Very often, pharmacological screening is assigned to technical assistants who are trained to observe for a predetermined set of responses in a given biological system. If the screen is an in vitro one, this practice is perhaps without fallacy. On the other hand, when observing for gross effects in an intact animal, it is often the subtle and unpredictable responses elicited by plant extracts that become the most significant. Technical assistants not having a good background and understanding of pharmacology cannot usually function effectively in such cases. Thus, we propose that when organizing an in vivo pharmacological screening program, the interpretation of data be assigned to persons having a complete pharmacological understanding of all types of drug effects.

Even well-trained pharmacologists who are not experienced in working with crude extracts must reorient their way of thinking to the fact that what they are injecting into an animal or other biological system is not a 100 % pure substance. Thus, if a crude extract contains only 0.1 to 0.01 % or less of an active principle, the interpretation of observed responses must take this into account. In other words, if one normally expects to see a CNS depressant response with a synthetic compound at doses of 1 - 2 mg/kg, perhaps 200 or more mg/kg of a plant extract would need to be administered to an animal in order to elicit a response comparable with that shown by pure compounds.

We are reminded of a paper published several years ago which reported on rather remarkable CNS depressant and tranquilizing activity for crude extracts of *Bixa orellana* (13). The procedures used included activity cage studies, rotorod studies, and the like. Since the active principle had not been identified, we obtained some of the plant material, prepared comparable extracts as reported in the paper just cited, and indeed observed quite similar effects. On further study, however, it was apparent that the extract being evaluated also contained irritant substances. Following i.p. administration, irritant substances frequently cause small animals to become immobile, which by some observers could be mistaken for CNS depressant effects. This specific problem reinforces our previous suggestion that single solvent plant extracts should be pharmacologically evaluated with caution.

One of the major problems, alluded to previously, is that of solubilizing plant extracts prior to parenteral administration to animals. This is especially important if the extract is to be administered intravenously. To date, no one has solved this problem satisfactorily; few specific studies concerning it have been published, suggesting that not many investigators are even concerned with this problem. One can often find one, or a combination of several, nontoxic solvents that will solubilize a pure chemical compound without affecting the pharmacological effect of the substance being evaluated. However, when extracts are being solubilized, one is never certain how much solvent is needed; large concentrations of insoluble, inert materials may remain in the supposedly solubilized extract. This is surely a field of investigation that deserves high priority attention on the part of those engaged in the pharmacological evaluation of plant extracts.

The length of the work day can also affect test results. In many instances a substance is injected into an animal, and if some type of gross effect is not observed within a 6 - 7 h period of time (the normal work day), the material is said to be "inactive." How many compounds having delayed effects do we miss by adhering to a rigid work schedule? How many do we miss because they have a cumulative effect that can be seen only if *repeat* injections are given?

In fact, how many are missed because of an effect at the *biochemical level* that is not detected in an intact animal by observation of gross effects?

Finally, a major problem inherent in pharmacological screening is the cost involved. We propose that whenever possible an in vitro prescreen be utilized to establish the presence of an effect, and that the most promising of the prescreen actives be reevaluated in more sophisticated intact animal models. Should the activity be reproducible, the prescreen could then be used as a rapid and inexpensive means for monitoring the isolation procedures. This approach has been used extensively in studies with biologically active microbial extracts, but has been rarely used with extracts from higher plants.

G. Prospects for the Future

In this presentation we have attempted to convey the following points:

1. Higher plants are an untapped and neglected source of potential drugs for use by man.
2. Higher plants are indeed an important source of drugs currently used by man, and have been for at least the past 15 years; they represent at least a $3 billion annual market in the U.S.A. alone.
3. The amount of private and governmental financial support of programs designed to uncover new drugs from higher plants, based on their current and historical importance, is negligible.
4. The few major programs that have been organized to study higher plants as sources of new drugs have probably been considered as failures due to lack of support in providing these programs with: (a) experienced leadership; (b) well-trained and experienced personnel; (c) adequate funding for periods of time sufficient to expect the program to yield new drugs.

5. Those few programs that have been successful in yielding marketable drugs derived from higher plants are generally thought to be cost-prohibitive. A careful look at the productivity of some of these programs shows that they are perhaps at least as productive as are comparable synthetic programs.
6. For programs designed to yield new drugs from higher plants to be successful, industrial firms must be interested in such programs and be willing to support and participate in them.

In summary, it is our opinion that we are approaching a new era in drug development from higher plants and indeed, from natural sources in general. Higher plants are an untapped reservoir, only waiting to be investigated. For many classes of drugs widely employed in humans, syntheses of novel structures have not yielded entities with novel mechanisms of action; nor have they yielded entities with fewer side effects and/or activities improved over those of drugs currently available. In essence, it appears that the chemist has run into a dead-end street. Because of this, it is our feeling that those concerned with new drug development must initiate major programs to explore higher plants for biologically active structures that up to now have eluded the imagination of the synthetic chemist.

If those involved with decision-making processes in organizations, the primary concern of which is drug development, would read and appreciate the papers presented at this Congress, there is no doubt that a resurgence of interest in this area would result. Or are we overestimating the logic, imagination, and wisdom of these astute individuals?

References

1. Anon.: Annual survey report, 1973 - 1974, Pharmaceutical Manufacturers Association, Washington, D.C. 1975
2. Anon.: National Prescription Audit Ten Year Summary, 1959 - 1968, and subsequent supplements. Dedham: R.A. Gosselin Co., and Ambler: Lea Inc., 1969
3. Anon.: National Prescription Audit General Information Report, 12th ed., Ambler: Lea Inc., 1972
4. Spjut, R.W., Perdue, Jr., R.E.: Plant folklore: A tool for predicting sources of antitumor activity? Cancer Treatment Rep. 60, 979-985 (1976)
5. DeHaen, P.: Non-proprietary Name Index. New York: Paul DeHaen, Inc., 1974
6. Clymer, H.A.: The changing costs of risks of innovation in drug development. IN: Research Management. New York: John Wiley and Sons, Inc., 1970, pp. 375-388
7. Kantemir, I., Akder, G., Tulunay, O.: Vorläufige Mitteilung über die Wirkung von Extractum *Dryopteris filix-mas*. Arzneim.-Forsch. 26, 261-262 (1976)
8. Benoit, P.S., Fong, H.H.S., Svoboda, G.H., Farnsworth, N.R.: Biological and phytochemical evaluation of plants. XIV. Antiinflammatory evaluation of 163 species of plants. Lloydia 39, 260-271 (1976)
9. Farnsworth, N.R., Henry, L.K., Svoboda, G.H., Blomster, R.N., Yates, M.J., Euler, K.L.: Biological and phytochemical evaluation of plants. I. Biological test procedures and results from two hundred accessions. Lloydia 29, 101-122 (1966)
10. Farnsworth, N.R.: Anomalous isolation of an active antitumor alkaloid from a fraction of *Catharanthus lanceus* devoid of antitumor activity. J. Pharm. Sci. 61, 1840-1841 (1972)
11. Emmens, C.W.: Antifertility agents. Ann. Rev. Pharmacol. 10, 237-251 (1970)
12. Casarett, L.J., Doull, J.: Toxicology, the Basic Science of Poisons. New York: Macmillan, 1975
13. Dunham, N.W., Allard, K.R.: A preliminary pharmacologic investigation of the roots of *Bixa orellana*. J. Am. Pharm. Assoc. Sci. Ed. 49, 218-219 (1960)

Pharmacological Approaches to Natural Product Screening and Evaluation

M. H. MALONE

When dealing with synthetic compounds, the usual sequence of pharmaceutical development continues to be (1) primary pharmacological screening, (2) secondary and tertiary acute pharmacological/toxicological evaluations, (3) chronic pharmacological/toxicological evaluations, (4) product formulation, (5) the various stages of clinical trials, and (6) release in commerce for therapeutic utilization. When dealing with natural drug products with centuries of ethnotherapeutic use, one can consider that the clinical trials for all practical purposes have been conducted successfully before screening even begins. The major problem for natural-product researchers then becomes how to define and isolate the useful chemical activity -- activity which frequently may be unlike that of existing drugs on the market.

This paper will concentrate upon the pharmacological screening of crude plant drugs and their extractives. Screening implies the evaluation of multiple samples in a ritualized fashion using a standardized single technique or a battery of standardized techniques. The pharmacological screening of a single plant or drug sample can sometimes proceed using rather extemporaneous techniques, but this decision is accompanied by (1) some loss of efficiency coupled with an increase in relative expense, (2) the inability to make interexperiment comparisons using previously obtained data for both known and test drugs, and (3) some real risk of missing unexpected, unique activities because of experimental bias.

Since a battery of tests is proportionally more expensive and time-consuming, emphasis in recent years has been placed upon the use of a single, standardized, multipurpose, very discriminating procedure as the primary or beginning screen. Several of such procedures with high predictive value presently exist.

A. Ideal Requirements for a Primary Screen

If crude drugs are to be evaluated, the ideal requirements which a primary screen should possess are the following (listed roughly in the order of importance): (1) results must be able to be extrapolated to man either directly or by analogy with clinically effective drugs which have also been screened by the procedure; (2) potentially useful pharmacological activity must not go undetected even though the activity may be either unexpected or unique; (3) the probable nature of the activity should be indicated so that subsequent research can be organized intelligently; (4) the procedure must be unbiased and allow for the coding of all samples, including both "known" reference materials and "unknown" test materials; (5) results obtained should be reproducible if second or third "runs" are conducted; (6) the screen should detect both rapid-onset and delayed-onset activity; (7) the procedure should be a multilevel dose-response experiment; (8) the procedures for setting up the experiment and collecting data should be standardized so as to allow cross-comparisons with known pure and crude drugs; (9) the screen should allow the use of both crude material and extractives so that the procedure can be used to direct extraction, isolation and purification procedures for the phytochemist; (10) completion of a single screen should not require more than 1.0 - 2.0 g of crude dry plant material; (11) with sufficient replication and the concurrent testing of a standard drug, statistically sound bioassays should result, i.e. data from the primary screen can be incorporated into larger scale, more definitive (publishable) research; (12) potential toxic activity should be indicated by the procedure so that subsequent research does not ignore this aspect; (13) a single dosing vehicle should be used which does not affect screening results either qualitatively or quantitatively; (14) the procedure should not require expensive equipment or sophisticated laboratory environments so that primary-level experiments might be conducted more near the sites of collection -- especially in the case of natural products containing very labile active constituents; (15) the procedures should be capable of being taught easily to technicians so that highly trained and educated scientists are not required for the day-to-day operation of the program; (16) the screen should utilize an intact, unanesthetized test animal -- intact so that all body systems are exposed to the injected test materials as in the clinical situation; (17) the test animal should be easily obtainable, easily handled, easily bred (if necessary), and resistant to infection; (18) the procedure should not be time-consuming; and (19) lastly, the screen should be relatively inexpensive to conduct over a sustained period of time -- the whole purpose of screening is lost if one selects a slightly cheaper, somewhat less efficient screen and then proceeds to miss "useful" activity.

B. Past Approaches to Primary Pharmacological Screening

An excellent survey of the phytochemical and pharmacological screening of plants has been published by Farnsworth et al. (1966). The majority of the literature cited in that manuscript (59 %) represented only phytochemical research -- the seeking of specific chemical types (e.g., alkaloids, glycosides, unsaturated sterols, steroidal sapogenins, flavonoids, etc.) without resorting to biological screening. Furthermore, that survey indicated that the biological screening which has been done has in the main (34 % of the citations) been directed towards chemotherapeutic goals (e.g. the detection of antimicrobial, antiviral, antifungal, antimalarial, antineoplasic principles). Chemotherapeutic research lies somewhat outside the mainstream of pharmacological research, which traditionally has been concerned with principles affecting the organ systems of the body itself (CNS and autonomic agents, cardiotonics and depressants, diuretics, autacoids and antiautacoids, endocrines and antiendocrines, etc.). Of the literature cited by Farnsworth et al. (1966), only 7 % could be considered pharmacologically oriented in the classical sense. A search of the literature to date, reveals that phytochemical and chemotherapeutic screening remain the dominant trends for screening programs seeking medicinals from crude drugs. This lack of interest in phytopharmacology remains inexplicable, since 14 years ago Gosselin (1962) pointed out that almost half of the prescriptions dispensed in the U.S.A. were derived from natural products.

The scant pharmacological screening that has been reported to date can be divided into four styles of approach: (1) the use of a single technique to search for only one particular type of activity; (2) the use of a battery of specific techniques with each procedure searching for a different type of useful activity; (3) the use of a single technique designed to detect multiple activities; and (4) the use of a variety of procedures -- some to detect specific activities and some to detect multiple activities. The use of a battery of techniques each designed to detect multiple activities has not been done in phytopharmacology for routine primary screening.

I. Single Technique - Single Goal Screening

The limited-observation, single-technique approach to primary screening can be illustrated by the work of Sharaf et al. (1963) where alloxan-diabetic rats were used to screen plants for their antidiabetic potential. After the problems of collection and authentication of plant material, it appears inefficient to screen for only one pharmacological end-point -- the lowering of blood glucose. Another study in this fashion was that reported by Krider et al. (1957) where cardiotonic activity on the frog heart was sought to the exclusion of all other activities. Orgell (1963) studied aqueous extracts of 256 species of plants for their capacity to inhibit human plasma cholinesterase, and recently Benoit et al. (1976) screened 177 plant extracts for anti-inflammatory potential using only the carrageenin-induced pedal-edema assay in the rat.

II. Screening Using a Battery of Specific Procedures

The use of multiple specific tests to define the pharmacological activity of a crude drug can be illustrated by the work reported by Feng et al. (1962). These workers utilized seven different isolated-organ preparations to screen aqueous extracts of 55 West Indian plants. These preparations were: guinea-pig ileum, rat uterus, rat hind limb, rat phrenic nerve-diaphragm, rat stomach fundus, rabbit duodenum, and rabbit heart (in the manner of Langendorff). In addition, a simple intraperitoneal lethality estimate was obtained in mice (no gross observations were made of drug-induced symptomatology) and intravenous doses were screened for effects on blood pressure in the intact anesthetized dog. In a subsequent paper screening 61 more West Indian plants, Feng et al. (1964) revised their battery of tests, reducing the number of isolated-organ preparations to only four: guinea-pig ileum, rat uterus, rat hind limb, and toad *rectus abdominis* muscle.

The philosophy of a battery approach to the screening of pure compounds has been elegantly defined and defended by Janssen (1964) and Janssen et al. (1965a, b). Decisions usually are held back pending completion of all the tests constituting the primary evaluation which can be very time consuming. As defined by Janssen (1964), this approach would be absolutely unwieldly if used to direct extraction, isolation, and purification procedures for the phytochemist. Frequently such pharmacological procedures can be combined into fewer tests to reduce time- and animal-expense without the loss of desired data or procedural sensitivity -- as this happens, then the resultant technique becomes more like the primary screens to be discussed in Sections B.III. and B.IV.

III. Single Technique - Multiple Goals Screening

An illustration of the multiple observation - single technique used to search for virtually any and all pharmacological activities in a single crude drug can be illustrated by Malone et al. (1967) who reported on the multidimensional screening of 66 species of higher fungi using the intact unanesthetized rat. This investigation involved intraperitoneal injections of powdered whole carpophores or 70 % ethanol extracts (solvent removed) suspended/dissolved in a dosing vehicle of 0.25 % agar. Recording of drug-induced symptomatology was facilitated by the use of the standardized data-sheet of Malone and Robichaud

(1962). Activity for these species were sorted into 10 different pharmacological categories based upon dose-response patterns: (1) generally inactive; (2) CNS depressant; (3) tranquilizing activity; (4) psychotropic; (5) skeletal muscle relaxant; (6) sympathetic stimulant; (7) parasympathetic stimulant; (8) peripheral vasodilator; (9) diuretic; and (10) metabolic poison. Other categories were possible but were not documented in the species studied. This approach and its variations will be discussed subsequently in Section C in some detail.

IV. Combinations of Specific and Multipurpose Procedures

In Australia, the screening of native crude drugs for medicinal potential was divided by Thorp (1951) into three main areas of effort: (1) general screening for activity; (2) testing for chemotherapeutic potential; and (3) determining the effects of chronic feeding. The general screening was further subdivided into two distinct phases. Phase I consisted of toxicity testing in mice with observations made for CNS stimulation and depression, cardiac effects, and cause of death. Phase II involved blood pressure and respiration recording in an anesthetized mammalian preparation. Secondary and tertiary testing of the test materials involved a logical succession of specific tests -- the selection and sequence based on all previous results.

Hooper and Leonard (1965) investigated the aqueous extracts of 47 West Indian plants using four isolated-organ preparations: rabbit duodenum, rat phrenic nerve-diaphragm, Langendorff rabbit heart, and guinea-pig ileum (pharmacodynamic design). Intraperitoneal toxicity was determined grossly in mice and (most importantly) records were kept on symptomatology observed after injection -- specifically: general behavior, respiration, reflexes (pinna, corneal, righting), grip strength, capacity to stay on a 45°-inclined plane and on a rotating rod. Those extracts showing CNS effects were further screened for their capacity to alter barbiturate sleeping-time in mice, and those extracts displaying effects in the Langendorff preparation were further screened for their effects on blood pressure when given intravenously to an anesthetized cat.

Perhaps the most comprehensive and well coordinated study to date is that of Jiu (1966) who surveyed 94 species of plants indigenous to Mexico using a spectrum of 25 techniques adapted for phytopharmacologic screening: CNS activity (general observational screens in mice, cats and dogs, plus exploratory behavior and spontaneous activity screens in rats); appetite inhibition; hypotensive capacity; antiatherogenic activity (cockerels and rats); diuretic ability; antimicrobial *(Escherichia coli, Bacillus subtilis, Trichophyton mentagrophytes, Candida albicans)* and antileukemic capacity; antiinflammatory activity (yeast-induced foot edema and cotton-pellet granuloma in rats); and endocrine-antiendocrine capability (anabolic, androgenic, progestational, fertility).

Farnsworth et al. (1966, 1968) and Fong et al. (1972) have also employed a broad spectrum approach to the biological evaluation of 600 plants for potentially useful principles. The approach in this laboratory involved: (1) an observational screen in mice for all gross drug-induced symptomatology, plus (2) antineoplastic, (3) antimicrobial (20 bacteria, 2 yeasts, 16 fungi, 4 protozoa, 2 algae, 3 viruses), and (4) insecticide (*Aedes aegypti* larvae) screening. Subsequent work from this laboratory has emphasized phytochemical screening.

Zealous young researchers usually adopt a primary screening design utilizing a number of both specific and multipurpose procedures in order to insure that useful and unique pharmacologic activity will not escape detection. However, the expense and the time involved can all too often outstrip the possible benefits of this increased comprehensiveness -- especially if a large number of crude drugs are to be evaluated. When a primary screening program has been completed and there is neither money nor energy left to conduct the chemical isolations and the necessary in-depth pharmacological evaluations of the medically interesting plants, this completed program becomes a Pyrrhic "victory." The budding phytopharmacologist eschews all future plant research, avoids all those who continue to investigate medicinal plants, drops the "phyto" from his title, and simply becomes a rather traditional pharmacologist working only with pure synthetics.

Primary screening should unequivocally detect activity and roughly categorize it, but primary screening should *never* attempt to replace more sophisticated and more specific secondary and tertiary pharmacological evaluations.

C. Multidimensional Primary Screening

Multipurpose or multidimensional primary screens involving the observation of drug-induced effects in intact unanesthetized animals (see Sect. B.III) were developed independently in several USA drug companies in the beginning years of the 1950 - 1960 decade. The original impetus was to document the changes in spontaneous behavior produced by the newly introduced psychopharmaceuticals of this period. The early versions were modeled upon the traditional "open field" observational techniques used in experimental psychology and introduced by Hall (1934). Two techniques are widely employed presently for primary screening -- one using the rat as the experimental subject, and the other using the mouse. The former appears best suited for natural-product research.

I. The Rat "Hippocratic" Screen

The rat multidimensional screen was proposed in 1954 by Dr. Bradford N. Craver of the Squibb Institute for Medical Research when the present author was employed there in the Pharmacodynamics Section as one of the natural products team under the direction of Dr. Bernard Rubin. Within a year, the rat screen had been accepted as a primary screen, and mouse, dog, and monkey (*Macaca mulatta* mulatta) versions had been developed as effective secondary screens. Bioassays of *Rauvolfia serpentina* Benth and reserpine were published by Rubin et al. (1956) using some of the data so generated. The present author proposed that the rat version be included in abridged form in a student pharmacology laboratory manual (Holck et al., 1959) since he had found the procedure was unexcelled in developing a student's capacity to observe and to make logical deductions based upon drug-induced symptomatology. In 1962, the present author coined the term "hippocratic" to designate the pharmacological principles involved in all multidimensional observational screens. This name derives from the classical observation-and-deduction method (hippocratic) used by physicians to diagnose a patient. The standardized procedures for the rat hippocratic screen have been published in detail (Malone and Robichaud, 1962). This version, as published, has been used by the present author with very few changes since that time (Malone, 1973). The present two-page version of the standardized work-sheet is illustrated in Figure 1 (front) and Figure 2 (back). The blanks have been filled in with data obtained during a recently completed projet involving *Brunfelsia hopeana* Benth.

Date: 5/29/76 Notebook No. 43, pp. 20

Hippocratic Qualitative/Semiquantitative Screen and Toxicity Report of: # 760529CY Lot/Identification No. CI-ME/2

Dosage: 100.0 mg/kg; Dosage Vehicle: 0.25% AGAR; Conc.: 20 mg/ml

Parameters	Con-trol	+5 min	+10 min	+15 min	+30 min	+60 min	+2 h	+4 h	+ h	+24 h	+48 h	+4 days	+7 days	*
Decr. Motor Activity	0	0	+	3+	3+	3+	2+	2+		0	0	0	0	
Decr. Resp. Rate/30''	33	0	±	+	+	+	+	±		0	0	0	0	
Decr. Resp. Depth	0	0	0	0	0	0	0	0		0	0	0	0	
Dyspnea	0	0	0	0	0	0	0	0		0	0	0	0	
Cheyne-Stokes Resp.	0	+	+	+	+	+	+	+		0	0	0	0	
Analgesia	0	+	+	2+	2+	2+	2+	2+		0	0	0	0	
Anesthesia	0	0	0	±	±	±	±	±		0	0	0	0	
Loss Corneal Reflex	0	0	0	0	0	0	0	0		0	0	0	0	
Loss Pinna Reflex	0	0	0	0	0	0	0	0		0	0	0	0	
Back Plasticity	0	0	0	0	0	0	0	0		0	0	0	0	
Ataxia	0	0	0	0	0	0	0	0		0	0	0	0	
Hind Leg Grip Loss	0	+	+	+	+	+	+	+		0	0	0	0	
Foreleg Grip Loss	0	0	+	+	+	+	+	+		0	0	0	0	
Hind Leg Paralysis	0	0	0	0	±	±	±	0		0	0	0	0	C
Foreleg Paralysis	0	0	0	0	0	0	0	0		0	0	0	0	
Neck Paralysis	0	0	0	0	0	0	0	0		0	0	0	0	
Incr. Motor Activity	0	0	0	0	0	0	0	0		0	0	0	0	
Inc. Resp. Rate/30''	33	0	0	0	0	0	0	0		0	0	0	0	
Inc. Resp. Depth	0	0	0	0	0	0	0	0		0	0	0	0	
Fine Body Tremors	0	0	0	0	0	0	0	0		0	0	0	0	
Coarse Body Tremors	0	+	+	+	+	+	+	+		0	0	0	0	A
Back Tonus	0	0	0	0	0	0	0	0		0	0	0	0	
Tonic Convulsions	0	0	0	0	0	0	0	0		0	0	0	0	
Clonic Convulsions	0	0	0	0	0	0	0	0		0	0	0	0	

Project Code: IYER: 2. Reader Signature: CHRIS, IYER

Test Animal: RAT; Fasted/Nonfasted: N.F.; Sex: M; Weight: 230 g

Mark: B; Dye Color: YELLOW; Cage No. 2; Special Treatment: X

Injection Volume: 1.15 ml; Injection Route: IP; Clock Time: 11:15

Parameters	Con-trol	+5 min	+10 min	+15 min	+30 min	+60 min	+2 h	+4 h	+ h	+24 h	+48 h	+4 days	+7 days	*
Tail Erection	0	0	0	0	0	0	0	0		0	0	0	0	
Tail Grasping	0	0	0	0	0	0	0	0		0	0	0	0	
Tail Lashing	0	0	0	0	0	0	0	0		0	0	0	0	
Enophthalmos	0	+	+	2+	2+	+	0	0		0	0	0	0	
Exophthalmos	0	0	0	0	0	0	0	0		0	0	0	0	
Palpebral Ptosis	0	0	0	0	0	0	0	0		0	0	0	0	B
Pupil Size, mm	1/2	1/2	5/8	3/4	3/4	3/4+	3/4	5/8		1/2	1/2	3/8	3/8	
Pupil Size (Light)	1/8	1/8	1/8	1/4	1/4	1/4	1/8	1/8		1/8	1/8	1/8	1/8	
Nystagmus	0	0	0	0	0	0	0	0		0	0	0	0	
Chromodacryorrhea	0	0	0	0	0	0	0	0		0	0	0	0	
Ear Blanching	0	0	0	0	0	0	0	0		0	0	0	0	
Ear Hyperemia	0	0	0	0	0	0	0	0		0	0	0	0	
Ear Cyanosis	0	0	0	0	0	0	0	0		0	0	0	0	
3-4 Ear Metachrosis	0	0	0	0	0	0	0	0		0	0	0	0	
Fasciculation	0	0	0	0	0	0	0	0		0	0	0	0	
Thick Salivation	0	0	0	0	0	0	0	0		0	0	0	0	
Watery Salivation	0	0	0	0	0	0	0	0		0	0	0	0	
Pilomotor Erection	0	0	0	0	0	0	0	0		0	0	0	0	
Robichaud Positive	0	0	0	0	±	+	+	+		0	0	0	0	
Writhing Movements	0	0	0	0	0	0	0	0		0	0	0	0	
Râles	0	0	0	0	0	0	0	0		0	0	0	0	
Micturition	0	0	+	+	+	2+	+	+		±	0	0	0	D
Colored Micturition	0	0	0	0	0	0	0	0		0	0	0	0	
Diarrhea	0	0	0	0	0	0	0	0		0	0	0	0	

Fig. 1. Front side of the present version of the standardized work-sheet used for hippocratic screening in the rat (Malone and Robichaud, 1962). The illustrative data entered upon the sheet correspond to one dose of test material 760529CY -- an extract from *Brunfelsia hopeana* Benth

Parameters	Response Rating (0 - +4) or Measurement Con-trol	+5 min	+10 min	+15 min	+30 min	+60 min	+2 hrs	+4 hrs	+ hrs	+24 hrs	+48 hrs	+4 days	+7 days	*
Sterotypy	O	O	O	O	+	+	+	+	↑	O	O	O	O	↑
Circling Motions	O	O	O	O	O	O	O	O		O	O	O	O	
Disorientation	O	O	+	+	+	+	+	+		O	O	O	O	
Statue Positions	O	O	O	O	O	O	O	O		O	O	O	O	
Startle Sensivity	O	O	O	O	O	O	O	O		O	O	O	O	
Head Tap: Aggressive	O	O	O	O	O	O	O	O		O	O	O	O	
Head Tap: Fearful	O	O	O	O	O	O	O	O		O	O	O	O	
Head Tap: Passive	+	+	+	+	+	+	+	+		+	+	+	+	
Body Grasp: Aggressive	O	O	O	O	O	O	O	O		O	O	O	O	
Body Grasp: Fearful	+	+	O	O	O	O	O	O		+	+	+	+	
Body Grasp: Passive	O	O	±	+	+	+	+	±		O	O	O	O	
Persistent Grooming	O	O	O	O	O	O	O	O		O	O	O	O	
Priapism/Colpectasia	O	O	O	O	O	O	O	O		O	O	O	O	
——														
Rectal Temp., °C	38.0	x	x	x	38.0	37.5	37.5	38.0		38.5	38.0	38.5	38.0	
Body Weight, g	230	x	x	x	230	228	225	224		232	235	240	242	
——														
——									↓					↓

Death and Necropsy Notes:

Heart: beating: rhythm ✓, nonrhythm ___; stopped: systole ___, diastole ___

Intestines: motile ✓, nonmotile ___, blanched ___, hyperemic ___, empty X

Blood: aleady clotted ___, prompt clotting ✓, will not clot ___

Color: liver NORMAL; spleen NORMAL
lungs NORMAL; kidneys NORMAL

Gall Bladder: extended ___, normal ✓, empty ___; Liver: friable ___ OK

Urinary Bladder: extended ___, normal ✓, empty ___; color OK

Other: ⟶

Other Observations: Note Time After Injection For Each

A: COARSE TREMORS VERY APPARENT: +5/+10/+15 MIN. +30/+60 (VERY NOTABLE IN TAIL)/+2 HRS/+4 HRS. —

B: NO TRUE BLEPHAROSPASM, BUT PREFERS TO KEEP EYES CLOSED: +10/+15/+30 MIN./ +60 MIN. —

C: DEFINITE LOSS OF SCREEN GRIP STRENGTH/ CO-ORDINATION PRESENT/ PARALYSIS OF HIND LEGS EQUIVOCAL: +30 MIN./+60/ +120 MIN —

D: UNEQUIVOCAL CONTINUING DIURESIS: +60/+120 MIN/+4 HRS. —

6/4/76
CHRIS IYER

Fig. 2. Reverse side of the standardized work-sheet shown in Figure 1, and again containing illustrative data corresponding to one dose of an extract of *Brunfelsia hopeana* Benth

1. Variations of Hippocratic Screening

Hippocratic testing in rats satisfies all of the ideal requirements specified earlier (Sect. A) for a primary screen. Hippocratic evaluation represents a standardized dose-response experiment in rats conducted using code-identified materials. Unbiased evaluation can be facilitated by the periodic submission of known materials as coded "unknowns" and the use of computer evaluation (see Sect. C.I.2 and F). Hippocratic screening provides an estimate of the general pharmacological/toxicological nature of the active principles in a crude drug and a rough estimate of the safety ratio. The actual screen is an observational one (no expensive equipment) and can be executed by trained technicians. It requires the equivalent of one working day for one technician to test one sample. Crude drug materials, extractives, and pure chemicals can be tested equally well, and there is no need to solublize test materials for injection (0.25 % agar is the specified vehicle for dosing). No more than 1.0 g of crude material is generally necessary to complete the screening procedure. Experience has shown its usefulness in guiding extraction, isolation, and purification procedures, and the method has been used to advantage in makeshift laboratories in relatively primitive areas (e.g. its use by the Amazon Natural Products Drug Company in Iquitos, Peru). Repeated testing of the same material to increase the population at each dose level coupled with the concurrent testing of a reference standard allows several statistically sound, graded-response bioassays to be conducted simultaneously on one batch of rats (Rubin et al., 1956; Malone et al., 1961). The data from a single study can be handled as a series of traditional analysis-of-variance assays or as a single multivariate analysis. While such quantitative studies are clearly publishable, the goal of the hippocratic screen really is not quantitation but qualitative orientation -- to guide the pharmacologist and toxicologist in launching more specific studies (secondary and tertiary evaluations) and to guide the pharmacognosist in extraction/isolation procedures. Orientation data are rarely published, but this has been done in certain instances where the limited availability or the pharmacological/toxicological nature of the test material has indicated that more extensive research would not be feasible (Tyler and Malone, 1960; Tyler et al., 1963; Robichaud et al., 1964; Mileski et al., 1965; Khanna et al., 1965; Carrano and Malone, 1966, 1967; Kaplan and Malone, 1966; Miyata et al., 1966; Marozzi and Malone, 1968; Dewey et al., 1968; Sklar et al., 1971; Nucifora and Malone, 1971; Chilton et al., 1973; Buckley et al., 1973; Brady et al., 1975; Tutupalli et al., 1975).

While salicylates and other antiinflammatory agents present recognizable profiles of activity upon hippocratic screening, our laboratory often applies a modified hippocratic/antiinflammatory screen to any crude drug with some suggestion of analgesic and/or antiinflammatory activity in its ethnomedical history. Control observations are obtained in the usual way, and the test drug is administered orally to male rats using the usual 0.25 % aqueous agar vehicle. All observations are collected using the standardized worksheet at +15, +30, and +60 min, after which the left hind foot receives a subplantar injection of 0.10 ml of 1 % carrageenin in sterile 0.9 % saline similar to the method described by Winter et al. (1962). Injected-foot volume is measured immediately and +1, +3, and +5 h later using the volume displacement method of van Arman et al. (1965). Normally drug injections are made intraperitoneally for hippocratic screening; but in this special version, dosage is done orally so as to avoid the subtle "counter-irritant" effects that in certain instances can affect the reliability of the pedal edema screen (Benitz and Hall, 1963).

Almost every classic pharmacological technique requiring a one- or two-hour premedication of rats (or other species) can be similarly modified to yield useful hippocratic data, which would not otherwise be collected.

2. Computerized Hippocratic Evaluation

Hippocrates, the father of medicine, introduced diagnosis by observation as a method, and it is still the most powerful tool of todays physicians. The clinically well-trained physician views the entire patient and notes such things as mental attitude, gross physical appearance, muscle tone and coordination, autonomic-related items such as pupil size, skin temperature, skin color, etc. and then correlates these observations with measurements of blood pressure, heart rate, urinalysis, and blood analysis. The physician mentally integrates his subjective impressions with his measurements and compares this multidimensional data with his past experience to achieve the diagnosis. There is really no important difference between this method and that of the rat screen except that in the rat screen the pharmacologist can integrate the "diagnoses" of several "patients" with different degrees of the same drug-induced "disease" and at several different time intervals.

Since five equally spaced log-dose levels are required for a complete hippocratic screen and since the parameters to be observed are fixed in number (58 ratings specified for the original work-sheet and 63 ratings in Figs. 1 and 2), and since the observation times are fixed, a standard multiparameter matrix of dose/effect/time is achieved which design lends itself to computer analysis and computer matching with known "library" drugs. Each crude or pure drug has a characteristic multiple symptomatology/dose/effect/time matrix which is distinctive in much the same way that a infrared absorption spectrum for a pure chemical is distinctive and recognizable. While a single specific symptom can be found to be common to a variety of different drugs and drug classes, the matrix profile allows a very sensitive differentiation between pharmacological classes and generally also between drugs of a single chemical class. In consultation with the present author, Carrano and Truax (1968) of Atlas Chemical Industries Inc. (now ICI America Inc.) devised the first computer evaluation method for the superabundance of data produced by the rat screen when conducted on a regular basis. The final version was published in full detail by Malone and Carrano (1970). The original worksheet of Malone and Robichaud (1962) was modified to conform to the restricted working hours of the company, and further altered so as to be compatible with punch-card data storage and retrieval methods. Failure to perform on a rotarod and effects on blood glucose levels were added as new parameters for measurements. The resultant two-page form is illustrated in Figure 3 (front) and Figure 4 (back). The blanks have been filled in with data for a "library" drug, pilocarpine hydrochloride, a somewhat nontypical parasympathomimetic in the rat (e.g. note the effects on pupil diameter).

The goals for the computerized hippocratic screen were to provide a rapid data retrieval system and a rapid and unbiased in-depth comparison of each test substance against a "library" of similarly tested prototype drugs with known clinical utility. The computer evaluation program was not to replace human evaluation of data, since the various computer outputs were structured to facilitate independent human evaluation by a professional pharmacologist. The Addendum (Sect. F) reproduces for the first time in the literature one complete computer output -- the illustrative compound tested (code: Z11162021; subcode: 680508) is actually pilocarpine hydrochloride submitted as an "unknown." As indicated earlier, this compound represents a rather nontypical parasympathomimetic. The program illustrated was developed on an IBM 360/30 computer using a combination of Fortran IV and BAL (basic assembly language).

Initially there is a reorientation of the experimental data whereby the actual scores are corrected for control values and conflicting data (e.g. even though a test rat loses righting reflex, ataxia would be noted on the work-sheet with a 0 value; however, since the animal is really maximally "ataxic," a corrected value of 3 would be issued by the computer).

Output A (i.e. in the Addendum designated as RAT SCREEN OUTPUT A) consists of a simple printout of the necropsy data and the technician's general comments arranged per dose level.

Output B (designated as RAT SCREEN OUTPUT B) presents a summary of calculations made to indicate the general gross category of the drug's activity (ANS: autonomic drug; CNS STIM: central nervous system stimulant; CNS DEP: CNS depressant; MISC: other activity). This output results from a weighting of certain parameters to accentuate those found from experience to be the most discriminating. The weighted totals are expressed as a percent of the maximum possible weighted score for each category. Final figures are only meaningful within a specific category -- one cannot directly compare a CNS DEP value to an ANS value. Moreover, a 5 % score does not necessarily mean that there is only slight activity within that category. Dose-related increases within a category are considered essential for the presence of true pharmacologic activity. This output does very clearly predict the potential for side effects and toxic effects if the material were to be used as a drug. While textbooks in pharmacology tend to classify pilocarpine simply as a parasympathomimetic, any toxicologist can testify that the drug taken internally has a variety of activities which are less easily classified.

Output C represents a summary of the corrected data for each symptom noted and is intended to assist human evaluation of the dose-response and time-response relationships. The weighting factors used in Output B are noted for each parameter.

Output D lists those symptoms which should be considered to be dose-related and indicates the dose at which these symptoms first appeared. The therapeutic potential of the test material is suggested by the symptoms appearing at the lowest doses tested. Output D also recognizes that reverse dose-response relationships are important pharmacologically and that ascending and descending relationships can exist for scores of a single parameter.

Output E indicates the results of matching dose-related and important symptoms for the test substance with the computer's "library" of reference drugs. The unknown tested under the code designation of Z11162021 (actually pilocarpine hydrochloride) most closely matches the library drug pilocarpine hydrochloride, with reserpine acetate being the next closest match. Both matching and nonmatching symptoms are listed in Output E to facilitate human evaluation. The output is designed to draw attention to any test agent with apparent advantages over the reference or "library" drugs. At the end of Output E, the computer "diagnoses" the probable pharmacological class of the compound --

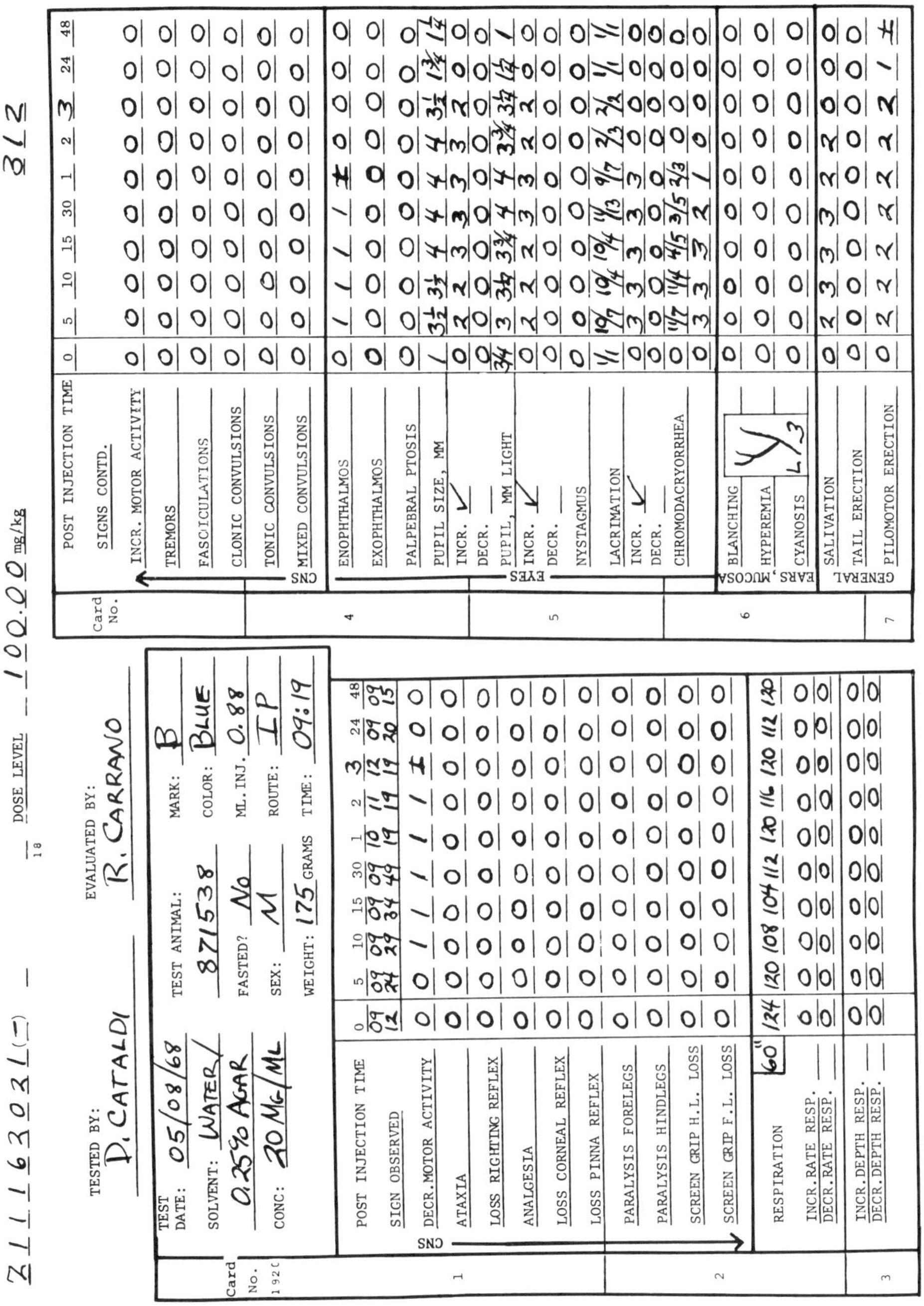

Fig. 3. Front side of the standardized work-sheet used for the computerized version of the rat hippocratic screen (Carrano and Truax, 1968; Malone and Carrano, 1970). The illustrative data entered upon the sheet correspond to one dose of test material Z11162021 (actually pilocarpine hydrochloride run as an unknown)

date 05/08/68 dose level 100.00 mg/kg Z111162021(-) — 312

Card No.	POST INJECTION TIME / SIGNS CONTD.	0	5	10	15	30	1	2	3	24	48
7	URINATION	0	0	0	0	0	0	0	0	0	0
	DIARRHEA	0	1	1	2	2	2	2	1	0	0
	ROBICHAUD TEST	0	±	0	1	±	0	0	0	0	0
	CIRCLING MOTIONS	0	0	0	0	0	0	0	0	0	0
	TAIL LASHING	0	0	0	0	0	0	0	0	0	0
GENERAL	WRITHING	0	0	0	0	0	0	0	0	0	0
	RECTAL TEMP °C	37.9	x	x	38.1	38.9	38.0	38.1	37.9	38.2	38.0
	INCR. 0	0	x	x	0	0	0	0	0	0	0
8	DECR. 0 (DEGREE)	0	x	x	0	0	0	0	0	0	0
	BODY WEIGHT	175	x	x	x	168	167	164	163	172	174
	INCR.	0	x	x	x	0	0	0	0	0	0
	DECR. ✓	0	x	x	x	1	1	2	3	0	0
	ROTAROD	0	1	2	2	2	1	0	0	0	0
	BODY TONE	0	↑	↑	↑	↑	↓	↓	0	0	0
	INCR. ✓	0	1	2	2	1	0	0	0	0	0
	DECR. ✓	0	0	0	0	0	1	1	0	0	0
SUBJECTIVE	HEAD TAP, AGGRESSIVE	0	0	0	0	0	0	0	0	0	0
9	HEAD TAP, PASSIVE	0	2	2	2	2	2	1	1	0	0
	HEAD TAP, FEARFUL	1	0	0	0	0	0	0	0	1	1
	BODY TOUCH, AGGRESSIVE	0	0	0	0	0	0	0	0	0	0
	BODY TOUCH, PASSIVE	0	2	2	2	2	2	1	1	0	0
	BODY TOUCH, FEARFUL	1	0	0	0	0	0	0	0	1	1
10	CATALEPSY	0	0	0	0	0	0	0	0	0	0
	EXCESS CURIOSITY	0	0	0	0	0	0	0	0	0	0
OTHER	BLOOD GLUCOSE ↑	0	X	X	X	X	X	2	2	1	X
	BLOOD GLUCOSE ↓	0	X	X	X	X	X	0	0	0	X

[✓] survived to completion of experiment

[2] DEATH AND NECROPSY — time (3 4 5 6) — units (8 9 10) POST INJECTION

[✓] SACRIFICED — time 48 — units HRS POST INJECTION

[4] found dead — time (3 4 5 6) — units (8 9 10), no necropsy

HEART: [✓] beating; [ ] not beating; [ ] size increased; [ ] size decreased
COMMENT

LIVER: [ ] normal; [ ] petechial hemorrhage; [✓] engorged; [ ] enlarged
COMMENT

SPLEEN: [✓] normal; [ ] engorged; [ ] enlarged; [ ] atrophied
COMMENT

INTESTINES: [✓] motile; [ ] immotile; [ ] empty
COMMENT:

LUNGS: [ ] normal; [✓] petechial hemorrhage; [ ] rhexis hemorrhage
COMMENT

PERITONEAL WALL
COMMENT

KIDNEY: [✓] normal; [ ] petechial hemorrhage; [ ] rhexis hemorrhage
COMMENT

CONSTANT HEAD SCRATCHING: +5/+10/+15/+30 MIN.
HEAD ROTATION: +5/+10/+15/+30 MIN.
05/09/76 D. CATALDI

Fig. 4. Reverse side of the standardized work-sheet shown in Figure 3 and again containing illustrative data corresponding to one dose of pilocarpine hydrochloride run as an "unknown"

in this case, Z11162021 has been classified tentatively as a potential parasympathomimetic. The human evaluator will compare the results of Output E with Output G very carefully before coming to his final evaluation.

Output F rank-orders all drug-induced symptoms in a dose-response manner while Output G compares the dose/effect/time matrix of the test material with the corresponding matricies of all library drugs and converts the data to a new scheme which reflects a weighting for every corresponding match of the test drug with a library drug. The totals are then ranked by the computer and a "gap-jump" comparison (Carrano and Malone, 1970) made to indicate which of the library drugs statistically match with the test drug. In this instance, Z11162021 significantly matches only with pilocarpine hydrochloride. Reserpine acetate, which was ranked by Output E as the most similar drug to Z11162021 in the library on a pharmacological basis, now becomes the twenty-ninth in similarity. The unbiased ranking produced by Output G continually provokes the pharmacologist into new insights relative to both the test and the library drugs. Commercially available drugs run as "unknown" are cumulatively added to the library of the computer (e.g. see the designation Reserpine Acetate-Combined-II), which progressively increases the sensitivity of Output G. The printout in Section F dates back to the early postdevelopment year of 1968; consequently the illustrative Output G presented here is relatively crude.

In spite of computerization, it is the trained pharmacologist who makes the final evaluation of the assembled data. Virtually inactive and almostly completely toxic materials are easily identified and shelved. Hippocratic testing identifies potentially useful activity while also pointing out the potential side effects and toxic effects. Once hippocratic screening and evaluation has been completed, the pharmacologist has some working theories and can purposely get on with secondary and tertiary evaluations -- if the drug seems worthy of this effort.

II. The Mouse Multidimensional Screen

In 1959, Irwin at Schering Corporation independently developed an observational screen using the intact cat, dog, and monkey (Irwin et al., 1959). Although not cited in the publication, the inspiration for this paper may have been the widely discussed report of Norton and DeBeer (1956) regarding the effects of certain psychopharmaceuticals upon the spontaneous behavior of the cat. In August, 1959, Irwin described at the Gordon Research Conferences a "multidimensional screening-evaluative" procedure using both the mouse and the cat (Irwin, 1959). The philosophy of generalized observational procedures as primary screens has been discussed very effectively by Irwin (1962), but the various procedures recommended have never been published in detail (Irwin, 1964). Nevertheless, these reports have stimulated many to create their own versions, thus leading to the popularity of the mouse multidimensional screen. Notable variations on the mouse primary screen have been published by Bastian (1961) and Campbell and Richter (1967). None of these publications have addressed the problems of using the mouse screen for crude drug evaluation.

III. Relative Merits of the Mouse and Rat Primary Screens

Observational screens involving cats, dogs, and monkeys require relatively expensive animals and significant amounts of test materials, so workers have concentrated on adopting either the mouse or the rat as subjects for primary screening.

Both the mouse (Irwin, 1964) and rat (Malone and Robichaud, 1962) screens are observational and require a standardized worksheet. Both require technicians trained-on-the-job to be consistent in rating the drug-induced symptomatology. Neither demands expensive equipment to perform. Only the rat screen requires that all blanks on the work-sheet must be filled in to be sure that some parameter has not been inadvertently overlooked. This requirement (although merely one of procedure) is important in that the absence of symptomatology is virtually as important as the presence of symptomatology in evaluating the data.

While both techniques use log-doses, the mouse technique specifies fixed doses (0.01, 0.03, 0.10, 0.30, etc., 300, and 1000 mg/kg) while the rat version insists on the operator determining the actual dose-response curve based upon where ineffective and lethal doses occur. This later requirement respects the fact that there are both flat and steep dose-response curves and that the slope of the dose-response curve for a drug is an important and nonvarying pharmacologic characteristic.

The mouse version specifies 44 parameters to be observed, but only peak drug effects are recorded at the required nonlog-times. The scores for parameters which can either show an increase or a decrease range from 4 - 0 for depression and 4 - 8 for stimulation. Scores for symptoms normally absent (e.g. ataxia) range from 0 to 8. The rat version (Figs. 1 and 2) specifies 63 parameters, with all to be rated at all log-time intervals to form a matrix (kinetic dimensions). All scoring is on the scale of 0 to 4 (no effect to maximum effect), which facilitates both human interpretation and computerization. Equivocal responses are given a value of $\pm$ with the operator knowing that with higher doses, this value must change to a + or ++ if it is to be considered in making the final evaluation. Hippocratic screening requires that a noninjected rat be in the observation rink with the injected test rat at all times. This allows the technician to make cross-comparisons with a control animal while rating, and also allows some assessment of drug effects on the socialization process.

Although the mouse screen may appear at first to use less drug material, three mice are required for each of the specified doses while only five rats can complete the minimum hippocratic screen. In addition, the rat is more resistant to infection than the mouse, and (because of its size) the rat is easier to observe, safer to handle, and its changes in behavior and personality are more easily apparent. Also because of its size, injection volumes are larger, allowing more precise measurement of injection volume and placement upon injection.

The mouse screen was designed to facilitate the evaluation of new synthetic drugs, consequently a wide variety of dosing vehicles have been used in the past with most workers attempting to solublize the test drugs before injection. Worthley and Schott (1966) have reviewed the literature in regard to the intrinsic toxicity of dosing vehicles. They also determined the intraperitoneal toxicities of a number of common vehicles for injection using mice as the test subjects. Listed in descending order of toxicity, they are: ethanol, polyethylene glycol-200, propylene glycol, dimethylsulfoxide, sterol diluent (benzyl alcohol, Tween-80, sodium carboxymethylcellulose, and sodium chloride in water), distilled water, 0.5 % methylcellulose, isotonic saline, and 3.0 % polyvinylpyrrolidone in isotonic saline. Even if administered in their insoluble form, the present author has found that potentially useful drugs (i.e. those with reasonable Meyer-Overton ratios) are rapidly mobilized from the peritoneal cavity into the circulation if suspended in the form of very fine particles. Consequently, hippocratic screening demands only one dosage vehicle: sterile 0.25 % aqueous agar. If prepared correctly, this vehicle lacks viscosity, yet has excellent suspending capacity for solvent-free extractives and for finely divided (> 200 mesh) plant materials. This vehicle is virtually nontoxic intraperitoneally for rats. A constant dosage volume of 5 ml/kg is specified for all dose levels so there are no volume effects in regard to the onset of drug-induced symptomatology. In the rat, the presence of up to 10 % of tannins in crude drug material has been shown not to affect the response patterns -- even in the case of tannin-precipitated alkaloids (Malone and Robichaud, 1962). Having worked with both the mouse and the rat screens, the present author believes that the rat hippocratic screen is more reliable than the mouse version for natural-product research and that the final costs are quite comparable.

D. Multidimensional Secondary Screening of Extracts and Pure Compounds

Primary screening is always conducted using only minimum amounts of carefully authenticated crude drug. The screening of an unauthenticated sample is a waste of time and money. If promising activity has been found during primary screening, then a sizeable quantity of authenticated plant material is acquired and secondary evaluations are organized. The present author believes it neither wise nor economically sound to conduct primary, secondary, and tertiary research using only one batch of crude drug. Taxonomists can make mistakes. Occasionally chemically distinct varieties can exist within a single species. Multiple acquisitions of a natural product -- each containing the activity -- can establish that a predictable commercial source is possible.

Secondary testing should confirm in another species of laboratory animal the activity noted in the primary screen and should consist (at least in part) of drug/drug-interaction (pharmacodynamic) experiments. Secondary evaluations should also be multidimensional if at all possible and certainly standardized so as to allow comparisons with known, clinically useful, "library" drugs.

Secondary testing is conducted to support a major decision which *must* be rendered at the completion of this phase. All secondary testing should be conducted using either solvent-free extractives (prechecked for activity by hippocratic testing) or semipure/pure chemicals (also prechecked in a similar manner). Since phytochemical investigations must be conducted to provide these materials needed for secondary testing, the phytochemist can during this process make rough estimates as to the potential yield of active material(s) from the crude drug and can formulate some ideas as to the physicochemical characteristics of the active principle(s). If an active principle corresponds physicochemically with a known drug, all further research is terminated.
If secondary pharmacological testing confirms the activity and indicates some unique potential, and if the active principle also appears to be chemically new (i.e. patentable), then an all-or-none decision will have to be made whether or not to launch the very expensive, very time-consuming tertiary investigations. Tertiary investigation consists of (1) chemical structure determination and (2) what the present author regards as classical pharmacological and toxicological research. Many expert (and expensive) scientists will have to work together in a

team-effort; consequently tertiary biological investigation must be done using only chemically pure material. Large amounts of authentic crude material will be needed on a regular basis until a synthetic or semisynthetic procedure can be developed and patented. Tertiary biological investigation of a drug compound never really ceases -- even after the drug is released for sale.

I. The Dog Pharmacodynamic Screen

The one technique which the present author believes is essential for secondary evaluation is the dog pharmacodynamic screen. This standardized multidimensional technique utilizes only one urethan-anesthetized, intact dog; consequently the procedure is quite economical to execute and very desirable if only limited amounts of test material are available. The methodology has been published in detail by Morton and Malone (1967).

The design of the screen involves the continuous repetition of a test cycle consisting of four pharmacologically significant (but transient) physiological challenges. These challenges consist of the intravenous injection of individually standardized doses of l-epinephrine, acetylcholine, and histamine, plus a 45-s-duration, bilateral carotid artery occlusion. All responses to the challenges are documented by continuous polygraphic recording of systolic/diastolic blood pressure, heart rate, electrocardiogram, respiratory rate and depth (including minute volume), as well as core temperature. If the test animal does not respond in a predictable manner to these physiological challenges, it is considered abnormal and sacrificed without injection of any of the test material. If the responses to the challenges are within normal limits, a surely ineffective dose of the test material is injected at a fixed rate intravenously. This first dose is usually estimated as 1/10th of the lowest mg/kg intraperitoneal dose used for hippocratic testing in the rat. The test cycle of epinephrine/acetylcholine/histamine/carotid-occlusion is then repeated -- to be followed sequentially by the injection of the same dose of the test drug (representing a two-fold cumulative dose). Another cycle is performed, another cumulative injection of the test compound, etc. until death occurs. Continuous polygraphic recording is done.

It appears that the first reported use of physiological challenges for drug screening can be attributed to Nieschulz et al. (1956, 1957), and the first use of such challenges (in a format like the one described above) for mass drug screening can be attributed to Domer and Schueler (1958). The advantages and disadvantages have been debated by Morton and Malone (1967) and by Domer (1971).

Conclusions as to the test material's qualitative activity are based upon (1) its immediate effects upon injection (all recorded parameters plus gross observations of the entire animal), (2) its residual or so-called "resting" effects measured just before the next cumulative injection, and (3) its dose-related effects on the physiological responses of the dog to the four challenges. This data assembles into a multidimensional matrix which can be evaluated using computer technology, although such a method has not appeared in the literature to date. In addition, all visible changes from the control state of the dog are considered (e.g. thick/thin salivation, fasciculation, miosis/mydriasis, changes in muscle tone, vomiting, defecation, urination, reversal of anesthesia, convulsions, etc.). Insight into the pharmacological mechanisms of the test material is achieved by evaluation of its effects on the standardized challenges. Some resolution is made as to which physiologic sites are affected or not affected by the test material. It is this active interplay of drug-induced changes at specific physiological sites by the challenges that led to the technique being designated a "pharmacodynamic" screen (Morton and Malone, 1967).

In the absence of a computerized method, data are usually presented for interpretation using graphical means. This technique is swift if the respective graphs (test material and library prototype reference drug) are overlaid and viewed simultaneously. Figure 5 illustrates (in part) the pharmacodynamic profile of cryogenine, while Figure 6 illustrates one comparison of the pharmacodynamic profiles of cryogenine and nesodine (Kaplan and Malone, 1966). These compounds are structurally-related alkaloids isolated from *Heimia salicifolia* Link and Otto.

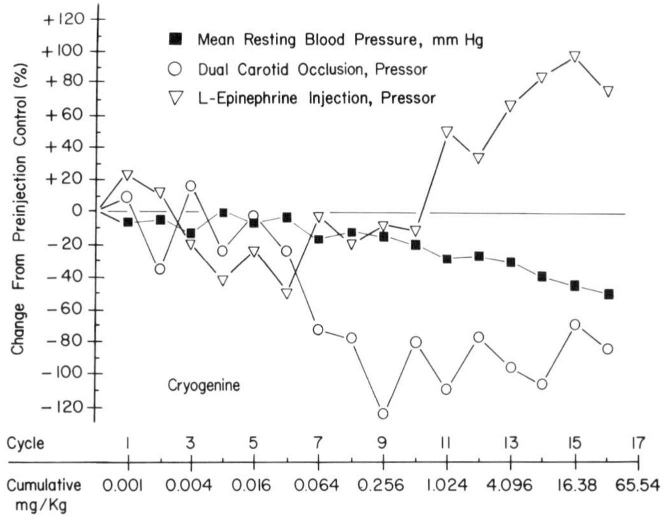

Fig. 5. Simulated overlay of three graphs obtained with cryogenine (Kaplan and Malone, 1966) when screened using the cumulative-injection and physiological-challenges format of the dog pharmacodynamic screen (Morton and Malone, 1967). Such overlays are used during the data evaluation process to suggest possible mechanism(s) of action for the test drug

II. Other Approaches to Secondary Evaluation

An experienced pharmacologist can devise an almost endless variety of pharmacodynamic screens by varying the challenges used for the test cycle, but each challenge to be valid must (1) be with some physiological and pharmacological significance, (2) be of a very transient nature so as to not increase the duration of time for a single cycle, and (3) be sufficiently innocuous so that the physiological integrity of the animal is not changed in some cumulative fashion. Too many challenges per cycle can draw the complete experiment out to an unphysiological length of time. Other vital recordings can be made de-

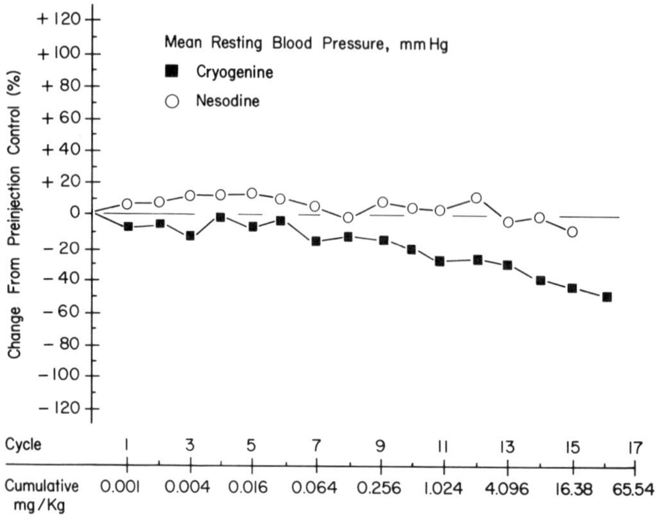

Fig. 6. Simulated overlay of the resting-blood-pressure graphs for cryogenine and nesodine -- obtained in each case using the dog pharmacodynamic screen. Such overlays are used during the evaluation process to compare a new test drug (nesodine) with a known reference drug (cryogenine) in an attempt to elucidate their pharmacological differences and similarities. Both alkaloids were isolated from Mexican *Heimia salicifolia* Link and Otto. Cryogenine alkaloid (MW = 435.53) should not be confused with the trade name product Cryogénine (phenylsemicarbazide; MW = 151.2) distributed by Laboratoires Sarbach of Châtillon, France

pending upon the surgical skill of the investigator and the sophistication of the recording apparatus (Domer and Schueler, 1958). However, it is important for the animal to be functionally intact from a physiological point of view.

The use of hippocratic variants in intact, unanesthetized larger animals (dog, cat, monkey) continues to be popular during the secondary evaluation phase.

E. Tertiary Evaluation

As indicated in Section D, tertiary evaluation is expensive and time-consuming. The course taken for a single drug depends on the data accumulated during the primary and secondary phases of evaluation. Tertiary investigation never truly ends as there always remains some facet left unexplained and open for further research.

Many books have now been written which conveniently mass together and discuss the many techniques which can be used during tertiary evaluation to pharmacologically and toxicologically define the activity of a drug (Ther, 1948; Burn, 1952; Smith, 1961; Laurence and Bacharach, 1964; Nodine and Siegler, 1964; Turner, 1965; Siegler and Moyer, 1967; Perry et al., 1968; McLeod et al., 1970; Turner and Hebborn, 1971; Domer, 1971; Schwartz, 1971; Chignell, 1972; Danile and Paton, 1975). These extremely useful "idea" books allow for the experimental definition of all drug types -- except the unique new drug. For this unique specimen, the pharmacologist still must fall back upon observation and reasoning, working systematically from generalized screens to specific testing and on to more specific testing, etc. As pointed out by Gosselin (1962), unique new drugs continue to come from research on natural products more frequently than from synthetic-only research programs -- which will undoubtedly continue to be the case.

F. Addendum -- Sample Print-Out of Computerized Hippocratic Evaluation

```
RAT SCREEN OUTPUT A

Z11162021     UNKNOWN 680508

                NECROPSY DATA

DOSE LEVEL      3.00 MG/KG

   SURVIVED TO COMPLETION OF EXPERIMENT
   SACRIFICED    0048 HRS  POST INJECTION
   HEART               BEATING
   LIVER               NORMAL
   SPLEEN              NORMAL
   INTESTINES          MOTILE
   LUNGS               NORMAL
   PERITONEAL WALL     NORMAL
   KIDNEY              NORMAL
      GENERAL COMMENTS

DOSE LEVEL     10.00 MG/KG

   SURVIVED TO COMPLETION OF EXPERIMENT
   SACRIFICED    0048 HRS  POST INJECTION
   HEART               BEATING
   LIVER               NORMAL
   SPLEEN              NORMAL
   INTESTINES          MOTILE
   LUNGS               PETECHIAL HEMORRHAGE
   PERITONEAL WALL     NORMAL
   KIDNEY              NORMAL
      GENERAL COMMENTS

DOSE LEVEL     31.00 MG/KG

   SURVIVED TO COMPLETION OF EXPERIMENT
   SACRIFICED    0048 HRS  POST INJECTION
   HEART               BEATING
   LIVER               ENGORGED
   SPLEEN              NORMAL
   INTESTINES          MOTILE
   LUNGS               NORMAL
   PERITONEAL WALL     NORMAL
   KIDNEY              NORMAL
      GENERAL COMMENTS   CONSTANT SCRATCHING OF HEAD ROTATING FROM
         ONE SIDE TO OTHER (5-10 & 15 MIN)

DOSE LEVEL    100.00 MG/KG

   SURVIVED TO COMPLETION OF EXPERIMENT
   SACRIFICED    0048 HRS  POST INJECTION
   HEART               BEATING
   LIVER               ENGORGED
   SPLEEN              NORMAL
   INTESTINES          MOTILE
   LUNGS               PETECHIAL HEMORRHAGE
   PERITONEAL WALL     NORMAL
```

KIDNEY NORMAL
GENERAL COMMENTS CONSTANT SCRATCHING OF HEAD ROTATING FROM ONE SIDE TO OTHER (5-10-15 & 30 MIN)

DOSE LEVEL 316.00 MG/KG

SURVIVED TO COMPLETION OF EXPERIMENT
SACRIFICED 0048 HRS POST INJECTION

HEART	BEATING
LIVER	ENGORGED
SPLEEN	ENGORGED
INTESTINES	MOTILE
LUNGS	NORMAL
PERITONEAL WALL	NORMAL
KIDNEY	NORMAL

GENERAL COMMENTS CONSTANT SCRATCHING OF HEAD ROTATING FROM ONE SIDE TO OTHER (5-10-15-30 MIN & 1 HR)

//

RAT SCREEN OUTPUT B

Z11162021 UNKNOWN 680508

TESTED 8 MAY 68 RECORD NO. 016812260

SOLVENT WATER ROUTE IP

WEIGHTED SCORES EXPRESSED AS % MAXIMUM RESPONSE

TEST COMPOUND	ANS	CNS STIM	CNS DEP	MISC
3.00 MG/KG	1.69	0.0	0.23	2.67
10.00 MG/KG	4.76	0.0	3.32	2.67
31.00 MG/KG	11.96	0.82	4.86	3.91
100.00 MG/KG	18.94	2.47	6.40	7.41
316.00 MG/KG	16.83	2.88	11.50	9.05

MAXIMUM SUBLETHAL DOSE GREATER THAN 316.00 MG/KG

//

RAT SCREEN OUTPUT C

Z11162021 UNKNOWN 680508

RAW DATA (CORRECTED FOR CONTROL READINGS)

(1) DECR. MOTOR ACTIVITY WEIGHTING FACTOR = 1.0

DOSE	C	5	10	15	30	1	2	3	24	48
			TIME							
3.00 MG/KG	0	0	0	0	0	0	0	0	0	0
10.00 MG/KG	0	1	1	1	0	0	0	0	0	0
31.00 MG/KG	0	1	1	1	0	0	0	0	0	0
100.00 MG/KG	0	0	1	1	1	1	1	0	0	0
316.00 MG/KG	0	1	2	2	2	1	1	0	0	0

(9) SCREEN GRIP H.L.LOSS WEIGHTING FACTOR = 1.5

DOSE	C	5	10	15	30	1	2	3	24	48
			TIME							
3.00 MG/KG	0	0	0	0	0	0	0	0	0	0
10.00 MG/KG	0	0	0	0	0	0	0	0	0	0
31.00 MG/KG	0	0	0	0	0	0	0	0	0	0
100.00 MG/KG	0	0	0	0	0	0	0	0	0	0
316.00 MG/KG	0	1	2	2	1	0	0	0	0	0

(21) ENOPHTHALMOS WEIGHTING FACTOR = 1.5

DOSE	C	5	10	15	30	1	2	3	24	48
			TIME							
3.00 MG/KG	0	0	0	0	0	0	0	0	0	0
10.00 MG/KG	0	0	0	0	0	0	0	0	0	0
31.00 MG/KG	0	1	0	0	0	0	0	0	0	0
100.00 MG/KG	0	1	1	1	1	0	0	0	0	0
316.00 MG/KG	0	1	1	1	1	0	0	0	0	0

(24) INCR. PUPIL SIZE WEIGHTING FACTOR = 0.5

DOSE	C	5	10	15	30	1	2	3	24	48
			TIME							
3.00 MG/KG	0	1	1	1	2	1	1	1	0	0
10.00 MG/KG	0	1	1	2	2	2	2	1	0	0
31.00 MG/KG	0	1	2	2	2	2	2	2	0	0
100.00 MG/KG	0	2	2	3	3	3	3	2	0	0
316.00 MG/KG	0	2	2	2	2	2	2	1	0	0

(26) INCR. PUPIL SIZE-WL WEIGHTING FACTOR = 0.5

DOSE	C	5	10	15	30	1	2	3	24	48
			TIME							
3.00 MG/KG	0	1	1	1	2	1	1	1	0	0
10.00 MG/KG	0	1	1	2	2	2	2	1	0	0
31.00 MG/KG	0	2	2	3	3	2	2	2	0	0
100.00 MG/KG	0	2	2	2	3	3	2	2	0	0
316.00 MG/KG	0	2	2	3	3	2	2	1	0	0

(29) INCR. LACRIMATION WEIGHTING FACTOR = 0.5

DOSE	C	5	10	15	30	1	2	3	24	48
			TIME							
3.00 MG/KG	0	0	0	0	0	0	0	0	0	0
10.00 MG/KG	0	1	1	0	0	0	0	0	0	0
31.00 MG/KG	0	3	3	2	3	1	1	0	0	0
100.00 MG/KG	0	3	3	3	3	3	0	0	0	0
316.00 MG/KG	0	3	3	3	3	1	0	0	0	0

(31) CHROMODACRYORRHEA WEIGHTING FACTOR = 1.5

DOSE	C	5	10	15	30	1	2	3	24	48
			TIME							
3.00 MG/KG	0	0	0	0	0	0	0	0	0	0
10.00 MG/KG	0	2	1	0	0	0	0	0	0	0
31.00 MG/KG	0	3	1	1	1	0	0	0	0	0
100.00 MG/KG	0	3	3	3	2	1	0	0	0	0
316.00 MG/KG	0	3	3	1	1	0	0	0	0	0

(33) EAR/MUCOSA-HYPEREMIA WEIGHTING FACTOR = 1.0

DOSE	C	5	10	15	30	1	2	3	24	48
			TIME							
3.00 MG/KG	0	0	0	0	0	0	0	0	0	0
10.00 MG/KG	0	0	0	0	0	0	0	0	0	0
31.00 MG/KG	0	0	0	0	0	0	0	0	0	0
100.00 MG/KG	0	0	0	0	0	0	0	0	0	0
316.00 MG/KG	0	0	0	0	1	0	0	0	0	0

(35) SALIVATION WEIGHTING FACTOR = 2.0

DOSE	C	5	10	15	30	1	2	3	24	48
			TIME							
3.00 MG/KG	0	0	0	0	0	0	0	0	0	0
10.00 MG/KG	0	1	1	1	0	0	0	0	0	0
31.00 MG/KG	0	2	1	2	1	1	0	0	0	0
100.00 MG/KG	0	2	3	3	3	2	2	0	0	0
316.00 MG/KG	0	2	2	3	2	2	2	0	0	0

(37) PILOMOTOR ERECTION WEIGHTING FACTOR = 0.5

DOSE	C	5	10	15	30	1	2	3	24	48
			TIME							
3.00 MG/KG	0	1	2	2	2	2	2	2	0	0
10.00 MG/KG	0	2	2	2	2	2	2	1	0	0
31.00 MG/KG	0	2	2	2	2	2	2	1	0	0
100.00 MG/KG	0	2	2	2	2	2	2	2	1	0
316.00 MG/KG	0	3	3	3	3	2	2	1	0	0

(39) DIARRHEA WEIGHTING FACTOR = 1.0

DOSE	C	5	10	15	30	1	2	3	24	48
			TIME							
3.00 MG/KG	0	0	0	0	0	0	0	0	0	0
10.00 MG/KG	0	0	0	0	0	0	0	0	0	0
31.00 MG/KG	0	1	1	2	2	2	2	1	0	0
100.00 MG/KG	0	1	1	2	2	2	2	1	0	0
316.00 MG/KG	0	0	2	2	3	3	3	1	0	0

(40) ROBICHAUD TEST WEIGHTING FACTOR = 1.5

DOSE	C	5	10	15	30	1	2	3	24	48
			TIME							
3.00 MG/KG	0	0	0	0	0	0	0	0	0	0
10.00 MG/KG	0	0	0	0	0	0	0	0	0	0
31.00 MG/KG	0	0	0	0	0	0	0	0	0	0

100.00 MG/KG	0	0	0	1	0	0	0	0	0	0
316.00 MG/KG	0	1	1	1	1	0	0	0	0	0

(47) DECR. BODY WEIGHT WEIGHTING FACTOR = 1.5

			TIME							
DOSE	C	5	10	15	30	1	2	3	24	48
3.00 MG/KG	0	0	0	0	0	0	0	0	0	0
10.00 MG/KG	0	0	0	0	0	0	0	0	0	0
31.00 MG/KG	0	0	0	0	0	0	1	1	0	0
100.00 MG/KG	0	0	0	0	1	1	2	3	0	0
316.00 MG/KG	0	0	0	0	1	2	3	3	0	0

(48) ROTAROD FAILURE WEIGHTING FACTOR = 1.0

			TIME							
DOSE	C	5	10	15	30	1	2	3	24	48
3.00 MG/KG	0	0	0	0	0	0	0	0	0	0
10.00 MG/KG	0	0	0	0	0	0	0	0	0	0
31.00 MG/KG	0	0	1	1	0	0	0	0	0	0
100.00 MG/KG	0	1	2	2	2	1	0	0	0	0
316.00 MG/KG	0	2	2	2	2	1	0	0	0	0

(49) INCR. BODY TONE WEIGHTING FACTOR = 2.0

			TIME							
DOSE	C	5	10	15	30	1	2	3	24	48
3.00 MG/KG	0	0	0	0	0	0	0	0	0	0
10.00 MG/KG	0	0	0	0	0	0	0	0	0	0
31.00 MG/KG	0	1	1	0	0	0	0	0	0	0
100.00 MG/KG	0	1	2	2	1	0	0	0	0	0
316.00 MG/KG	0	2	2	2	1	0	0	0	0	0

(50) DECR. BODY TONE WEIGHTING FACTOR = 1.5

			TIME							
DOSE	C	5	10	15	30	1	2	3	24	48
3.00 MG/KG	0	0	1	0	0	0	0	0	0	0
10.00 MG/KG	0	1	1	1	0	0	0	0	0	0
31.00 MG/KG	0	0	0	0	2	1	0	0	0	0
100.00 MG/KG	0	0	0	0	0	1	1	0	0	0
316.00 MG/KG	0	0	0	0	0	2	2	1	0	0

(52) HEAD TAP-PASSIVE WEIGHTING FACTOR = 1.0

			TIME							
DOSE	C	5	10	15	30	1	2	3	24	48
3.00 MG/KG	0	0	0	0	0	0	0	0	0	0
10.00 MG/KG	0	1	1	1	1	1	1	1	0	0
31.00 MG/KG	0	1	2	2	2	2	1	1	0	0
100.00 MG/KG	0	2	2	2	2	2	1	1	0	0
316.00 MG/KG	0	3	3	3	3	2	2	1	0	0

(55) BODY TOUCH-PASSIVE WEIGHTING FACTOR = 1.0

			TIME							
DOSE	C	5	10	15	30	1	2	3	24	48
3.00 MG/KG	0	0	0	0	0	0	0	0	0	0
10.00 MG/KG	0	1	1	1	1	1	1	1	0	0
31.00 MG/KG	0	1	2	2	2	2	1	1	0	0
100.00 MG/KG	0	2	2	2	2	2	1	1	0	0
316.00 MG/KG	0	3	3	3	3	2	2	1	0	0

//

RAT SCREEN OUTPUT D

Z11162021 UNKNOWN 680508

LIST OF DOSE-RELATED AND IMPORTANT SYMPTOMS

1 DECR. MOTOR ACTIVITY
2 ENOPHTHALMOS
3 INCR. PUPIL SIZE
4 INCR. PUPIL SIZE-WL
5 INCR. LACRIMATION
6 CHROMODACRYORRHEA
7 SALIVATION
8 PILOMOTOR ERECTION
9 DIARRHEA
10 ROBICHAUD TEST
11 DECR. BODY WEIGHT
12 ROTAROD FAILURE

13 INCR. BODY TONE
14 DECR. BODY TONE

LIST OF SYMPTOMS FOR WHICH THERE WAS MARKED DECREASE IN ACTIVITY (E.G. 0,4,1,1)

NONE

SYMPTOMS THAT SHOW AT DOSAGE INDICATED

1	INCR. PUPIL SIZE	3.00 MG/KG
2	INCR. PUPIL SIZE-WL	3.00 MG/KG
3	PILOMOTOR ERECTION	3.00 MG/KG
4	DECR. BODY TONE	3.00 MG/KG
5	DECR. MOTOR ACTIVITY	10.00 MG/KG
6	INCR. LACRIMATION	10.00 MG/KG
7	CHROMODACRYORRHEA	10.00 MG/KG
8	SALIVATION	10.00 MG/KG
9	ENOPHTHALMOS	31.00 MG/KG
10	DIARRHEA	31.00 MG/KG
11	DECR. BODY WEIGHT	31.00 MG/KG
12	ROTAROD FAILURE	31.00 MG/KG
13	INCR. BODY TONE	31.00 MG/KG
14	ROBICHAUD TEST	100.00 MG/KG

///

RAT SCREEN OUTPUT E

Z11162021 UNKNOWN 680508

RANKED INDICATIONS OF PHARMACOLOGIC ACTIVITY
(SYMPTOMS SHOWING A MARKED DECREASE IN ACTIVITY ARE COUNTED AS A MATCH WHEN THAT SYMPTOM IS DOSE-RELATED IN THE COMPARED DRUG)

RANK	PERCENTAGE MATCH AVERAGE	TEST BASE	LIB. BASE	DRUG NAME
1	80.36	85.71	75.00	PILOCARPINE HCL-STANDARD DRUG

MATCHING SYMPTOMS
1 DECR. MOTOR ACTIVITY
2 ENOPHTHALMOS
3 INCR. PUPIL SIZE
4 INCR. PUPIL SIZE-WL
5 INCR. LACRIMATION
6 CHROMODACRYORRHEA
7 SALIVATION
8 PILOMOTOR ERECTION
9 DIARRHEA
10 DECR. BODY WEIGHT
11 ROTAROD FAILURE
12 INCR. BODY TONE

SYMPTOMS OF THE TEST DRUG THAT DID NOT MATCH WITH LIBRARY DRUG
1 ROBICHAUD TEST
2 DECR. BODY TONE

SYMPTOMS OF THE LIBRARY DRUG THAT DID NOT MATCH WITH THE TEST DRUG
1 ANALGESIA
2 LOSS CORNEAL REFLEX
3 TREMORS
4 CLONIC CONVULSIONS

RANK	AVERAGE	TEST BASE	LIB. BASE	DRUG NAME
2	69.05	71.43	66.67	RESERPINE ACETATE-COMBINED-II

MATCHING SYMPTOMS
1 DECR. MOTOR ACTIVITY
2 ENOPHTHALMOS
3 INC. LACRIMATION
4 PILOMOTOR ERECTION
5 DIARRHEA
6 ROBICHAUD TEST
7 DECR. BODY WEIGHT
8 ROTAROD FAILURE
9 INCR. BODY TONE
10 DECR. BODY TONE

SYMPTOMS OF THE TEST DRUG THAT DID NOT MATCH WITH LIBRARY DRUG
1 INCR. PUPIL SIZE
2 INCR. PUPIL SIZE-WL
3 CHROMODACRYORRHEA
4 SALIVATION

SYMPTOMS OF THE LIBRARY DRUG THAT DID NOT MATCH WITH THE TEST DRUG
1 DECR. RATE RESP.
2 PALPEBRAL PTOSIS
3 DECR. PUPIL SIZE
4 DECR. PUPIL SIZE-WL
5 DECR. RECTAL TEMP-C

3 68.75 50.00 87.50 INDOMETHACIN-STANDARD DRUG

MATCHING SYMPTOMS
1 DECR. MOTOR ACTIVITY
2 ENOPHTHALMOS
3 INCR. PUPIL SIZE
4 INCR. PUPIL SIZE-WL
5 ROBICHAUD TEST
6 DECR. BODY WEIGHT
7 DECR. BODY TONE

SYMPTOMS OF THE TEST DRUG THAT DID NOT MATCH WITH LIBRARY DRUG
1 INCR. LACRIMATION
2 CHROMODACRYORRHEA
3 SALIVATION
4 PILOMOTOR ERECTION
5 DIARRHEA
6 ROTAROD FAILURE
7 INCR. BODY TONE

SYMPTOMS OF THE LIBRARY DRUG THAT DID NOT MATCH WITH THE TEST DRUG
1 DECR. RECTAL TEMP-C

4 67.86 35.71 100.00 MEPROBAMATE-STANDARD DRUG

MATCHING SYMPTOMS
1 DECR. MOTOR ACTIVITY
2 ENOPHTHALMOS
3 PILOMOTOR ERECTION
4 ROBICHAUD TEST
5 DECR. BODY TONE

SYMPTOMS OF THE TEST DRUG THAT DID NOT MATCH WITH LIBRARY DRUG
1 INCR. PUPIL SIZE
2 INCR. PUPIL SIZE-WL
3 INCR. LACRIMATION
4 CHROMODACRYORRHEA
5 SALIVATION
6 DIARRHEA
7 DECR. BODY WEIGHT
8 ROTAROD FAILURE
9 INCR. BODY TONE

SYMPTOMS OF THE LIBRARY DRUG THAT DID NOT MATCH WITH THE TEST DRUG
NONE

5 66.76 64.29 69.23 RESERPINE-COMBINED-II

MATCHING SYMPTOMS
1 DECR. MOTOR ACTIVITY
2 ENOPHTHALMOS
3 INCR. PUPIL SIZE
4 INCR. LACRIMATION
5 DIARRHEA
6 ROBICHAUD TEST
7 DECR. BODY WEIGHT
8 ROTAROD FAILURE
9 DECR. BODY TONE

SYMPTOMS OF THE TEST DRUG THAT DID NOT MATCH WITH LIBRARY DRUG
1 INCR. PUPIL SIZE-WL
2 CHROMODACRYORRHEA
3 SALIVATION

4 PILOMOTOR ERECTION
5 INCR. BODY TONE

SYMPTOMS OF THE LIBRARY DRUG THAT DID NOT MATCH WITH THE TEST DRUG
1 DECR. RATE RESP.
2 PALPEBRAL PTOSIS
3 DECR. PUPIL SIZE
4 DECR. PUPIL SIZE-WL

6 65.13 71.43 58.82 COMBINED CNS DRUGS

MATCHING SYMPTOMS
1 DECR. MOTOR ACTIVITY
2 ENOPHTHALMOS
3 INCR. PUPIL SIZE
4 INCR. PUPIL SIZE-WL
5 INCR. LACRIMATION
6 PILOMOTOR ERECTION
7 ROBICHAUD TEST
8 DECR. BODY WEIGHT
9 ROTAROD FAILURE
10 DECR. BODY TONE

SYMPTOMS OF THE TEST DRUG THAT DID NOT MATCH WITH LIBRARY DRUG
1 CHROMODACRYORRHEA
2 SALIVATION
3 DIARRHEA
4 INCR. BODY TONE

SYMPTOMS OF THE LIBRARY DRUG THAT DID NOT MATCH WITH THE TEST DRUG
1 ATAXIA
2 SCREEN GRIP H.L.LOSS
3 SCREEN GRIP F.L.LOSS
4 CLONIC CONVULSIONS
5 PALPEBRAL PTOSIS
6 DECR. PUPIL SIZE
7 DECR. RECTAL TEMP-C

7 64.94 57.14 72.73 CHLORPROMAZINE HCL-STANDARD DRUG

MATCHING SYMPTOMS
1 DECR. MOTOR ACTIVITY
2 ENOPHTHALMOS
3 INCR. PUPIL SIZE
4 INCR. LACRIMATION
5 ROBICHAUD TEST
6 DECR. BODY WEIGHT
7 ROTAROD FAILURE
8 DECR. BODY TONE

SYMPTOMS OF THE TEST DRUG THAT DID NOT MATCH WITH LIBRARY DRUG
1 INCR. PUPIL SIZE-WL
2 CHROMODACRYORRHEA
3 SALIVATION
4 PILOMOTOR ERECTION
5 DIARRHEA
6 INCR. BODY TONE

SYMPTOMS OF THE LIBRARY DRUG THAT DID NOT MATCH WITH THE TEST DRUG
1 INCR. DEPTH RESP.
2 PALPEBRAL PTOSIS
3 DECR. RECTAL TEMP-C

8 64.29 28.57 100.00 IPRONIAZID-STANDARD DRUG

MATCHING SYMPTOMS
1 DECR. MOTOR ACTIVITY
2 ENOPHTHALMOS
3 ROBICHAUD TEST
4 DECR. BODY TONE

SYMPTOMS OF THE TEST DRUG THAT DID NOT MATCH WITH LIBRARY DRUG
1 INCR. PUPIL SIZE
2 INCR. PUPIL SIZE-WL
3 INCR. LACRIMATION
4 CHROMODACRYORRHEA

```
          5   SALIVATION
          6   PILOMOTOR ERECTION
          7   DIARRHEA
          8   DECR. BODY WEIGHT
          9   ROTAROD FAILURE
         10   INCR. BODY TONE

        SYMPTOMS OF THE LIBRARY DRUG THAT DID NOT MATCH WITH THE TEST DRUG
                                  NONE

   9    64.29      64.29      64.29    PROCAINE HCL-STANDARD DRUG

        MATCHING SYMPTOMS
          1   DECR. MOTOR ACTIVITY
          2   ENOPHTHALMOS
          3   INCR. PUPIL SIZE
          4   INCR. PUPIL SIZE-WL
          5   PILOMOTOR ERECTION
          6   ROBICHAUD TEST
          7   DECR. BODY WEIGHT
          8   ROTAROD FAILURE
          9   DECR. BODY TONE

        SYMPTOMS OF THE TEST DRUG THAT DID NOT MATCH WITH LIBRARY DRUG
          1   INCR. LACRIMATION
          2   CHROMODACRYORRHEA
          3   SALIVATION
          4   DIARRHEA
          5   INCR. BODY TONE

        SYMPTOMS OF THE LIBRARY DRUG THAT DID NOT MATCH WITH THE TEST DRUG
          1   ATAXIA
          2   SCREEN GRIP H.L.LOSS
          3   SCREEN GRIP F.L.LOSS
          4   TREMORS
          5   CLONIC CONVULSIONS

  10    63.89      50.00      77.78    FUROSEMIDE-COMBINED-II

        MATCHING SYMPTOMS
          1   DECR. MOTOR ACTIVITY
          2   ENOPHTHALMOS
          3   PILOMOTOR ERECTION
          4   ROBICHAUD TEST
          5   DECR. BODY WEIGHT
          6   ROTAROD FAILURE
          7   DECR. BODY TONE

        SYMPTOMS OF THE TEST DRUG THAT DID NOT MATCH WITH LIBRARY DRUG
          1   INCR. PUPIL SIZE
          2   INCR. PUPIL SIZE-WL
          3   INCR. LACRIMATION
          4   CHROMODACRYORRHEA
          5   SALIVATION
          6   DIARRHEA
          7   INCR. BODY TONE

        SYMPTOMS OF THE LIBRARY DRUG THAT DID NOT MATCH WITH THE TEST DRUG
          1   PALPEBRAL PTOSIS
          2   URINATION

RANK    PHARMACOLOGIC ACTIVITY
  1     PARASYMPATHOMIMETIC
  2     TRANQUILIZER, ANTIHYPERTENSIVE
  3     ANTI-INFLAMMATORY AGENT
  4     TRANQUILIZER, SKELETAL MUSCLE RELAXANT
  5     TRANQUILIZER, ANTIHYPERTENSIVE
  6     AVERAGE CNS
  7     TRANQUILIZER
  8     MAO INHIBITOR
  9     LOCAL ANESTHETIC
 10     DIURETIC

////////////////////////////////////////////////////////////////////
```

RAT SCREEN OUTPUT F

Z11162021 UNKNOWN 680508

SYMPTOMS RANKED IN ORDER OF SEVERITY--EACH SYMPTOM WITH ACTIVITY COMPARED AT EACH TIME PERIOD AGAINST EVERY OTHER SYMPTOM WITH ACTIVITY AND TOTAL NUMBER OF POSITIVE DIFFERENCES RANKED

RANK ORDER OF RESPONSES FOR DOSE 3.00 MG/KG

	NO. OF PLUSES	
1	17	PILOMOTOR ERECTION
2	6	INCR. PUPIL SIZE
3	6	INCR. PUPIL SIZE-WL

RANK ORDER OF RESPONSES FOR DOSE 10.00 MG/KG

	NO. OF PLUSES	
1	38	PILOMOTOR ERECTION
2	25	INCR. PUPIL SIZE
3	25	INCR. PUPIL SIZE-WL
4	6	CHROMODACRYORRHEA
5	2	DECR. MOTOR ACTIVITY
6	2	SALIVATION
7	2	DECR. BODY TONE

RANK ORDER OF RESPONSES FOR DOSE 31.00 MG/KG

	NO. OF PLUSES	
1	69	INCR. PUPIL SIZE-WL
2	57	PILOMOTOR ERECTION
3	55	INCR. PUPIL SIZE
4	54	INCR. LACRIMATION
5	46	DIARRHEA
6	29	SALIVATION
7	23	CHROMODACRYORRHEA
8	15	DECR. BODY WEIGHT
9	13	DECR. BODY TONE
10	10	DECR. MOTOR ACTIVITY
11	7	ROTAROD FAILURE
12	6	INCR. BODY TONE
13	3	ENOPHTHALMOS

RANK ORDER OF RESPONSES FOR DOSE 100.00 MG/KG

	NO. OF PLUSES	
1	68	INCR. PUPIL SIZE
2	64	PILOMOTOR ERECTION
3	58	INCR. PUPIL SIZE-WL
4	55	SALIVATION
5	54	INCR. LACRIMATION
6	43	DIARRHEA
7	42	CHROMODACRYORRHEA
8	26	DECR. BODY WEIGHT
9	24	ROTAROD FAILURE
10	17	INCR. BODY TONE
11	16	DECR. MOTOR ACTIVITY
12	11	ENOPHTHALMOS
13	9	DECR. BODY TONE
14	2	ROBICHAUD TEST

RANK ORDER OF RESPONSES FOR DOSE 316.00 MG/KG

	NO. OF PLUSES	
1	78	PILOMOTOR ERECTION
2	65	INCR. PUPIL SIZE-WL
3	62	DIARRHEA
4	56	INCR. LACRIMATION
5	55	INCR. PUPIL SIZE
6	51	SALIVATION
7	39	DECR. BODY WEIGHT
8	37	DECR. MOTOR ACTIVITY
9	33	ROTAROD FAILURE
10	30	CHROMODACRYORRHEA
11	28	DECR. BODY TONE
12	20	INCR. BODY TONE
13	16	SCREEN GRIP H.L.LOSS
14	11	ENOPHTHALMOS
15	11	ROBICHAUD TEST
16	1	EAR/MUCOSA-HYPEREMIA

//

RAT SCREEN OUTPUT G

Z11162021

RANK ORDER ACCORDING TO THE CUMULATED WEIGHTED SUM OF ADJUSTED TRUE MATCHES CRITERION--USING COMPLETE MATRICIES

RANK	CUM WEIGHTED SUM ADJ TRUE MATCHES	DRUG NAME
1	* 2340	PILOCARPINE HCL-STANDARD DRUG
2	2159	COMBINED ANS DRUGS
3	2144	PROCAINE HCL-STANDARD DRUG
4	2136	EPHEDRINE SULFATE-STANDARD DRUG
5	2129	ATROPINE SULFATE-STANDARD DRUG
6	2125	CYPROHEPTADINE HCL-STANDARD DRUG
7	2124	AMPHETAMINE SULFATE-STANDARD DRUG
8	2123	NEOSTIGMINE BR-STANDARD DRUG
9	2122	PRONETHALOL-STANDARD DRUG
10	2120	DCI-COMBINED-II
11	2114	MECAMYLAMINE HCL-STANDARD DRUG
12	2111	IMIPRAMINE-STANDARD DRUG
13	2110	COMBINED CNS DRUGS
14	2104	COMBINED MISC DRUGS
15	2103	MEPROBAMATE-STANDARD DRUG
16	2101	PHENOBARBITAL SODIUM-STANDARD DRUG
17	2101	IPRONIAZID-STANDARD DRUG
18	2097	LIBRIUM-STANDARD DRUG
19	2095	CHLORPROMAZINE HCL-STANDARD DRUG
20	2092	TOLBUTAMIDE-STANDARD DRUG
21	2092	ACETYLSALICYLIC ACID-STANDARD DRUG
22	2089	FUROSEMIDE-COMBINED-II
23	2084	CHLOROTHIAZIDE-STANDARD DRUG
24	2082	INDOMETHACIN-STANDARD DRUG
25	2081	TOLAZOLINE HCL-STANDARD DRUG
26	2079	DILANTIN SODIUM-STANDARD DRUG
27	2057	HYDRALAZINE-COMBINED-II
28	2047	GUANETHIDINE SULFATE-STANDARD DRUG
29	2012	RESERPINE ACETATE-COMBINED-II
30	1949	RESERPINE-COMBINED-II

* DRUGS ARE THOSE THAT MEET STATISTICAL REQUIREMENTS FOR BEING MORE SIGNIFICANT THAN OTHERS IN THE RANK SERIES

References

Arman, C.G. van, Begany, A.J., Miller, L.M., Pless, H.H.: Some details of the inflammations caused by yeast and carrageenin. J. Pharmacol. Exp. Therap. 150, 328-334 (1965)

Bastian, J.W.: Classification of CNS drugs by a mouse screening battery. Arch. Intern. Pharmacodyn. 133, 347-364 (1961)

Benitz, K.-F., Hall, L.M.: The carrageenin-induced abscess as a new test for anti-inflammatory activity of steroids and nonsteroids. Arch. Intern. Pharmacodyn. 144, 185-195 (1963)

Benoit, P.S., Fong, H.H.S., Svoboda, G.H., Farnsworth, N.R.: Biological and phytochemical evaluation of plants. XIV. Anti-inflammatory evaluation of 163 species of plants. Lloydia 39, 160-171 (1976)

Brady, L.R., Benedict, R.G., Tyler, V.E., Jr., Stuntz, D.E., Malone, M.H.: Identification of *Conocybe filaris* as a toxic basidiomycete. Lloydia 38, 172-173 (1975)

Buckley, J.P., Theobald, R.J., Cavero, I., Krukoff, B.A., Leighton, A.P., Kupchan, S.M.: Preliminary pharmacological evaluation of extracts of "Takini": *Heliostylis tomentosa* and *Heliostylis pedunculata*. Lloydia 36, 341-345 (1973)

Burn, J.H.: Practical Pharmacology, 1st ed. Oxford: Blackwell Sci., 1952

Campbell, D.E.S., Richter, W.: An observational method for estimating toxicity and drug actions in mice applied to 68 reference drugs. Acta Pharmacol. Toxicol. 25, 345-363 (1967)

Carrano, R.A., Malone, M.H.: New pharmacologic aspects of β-diethyl-aminoethyl-2, 2-diphenylpentanoate. J. Pharm. Sci. 55, 563-567 (1966)

Carrano, R.A., Malone, M.H.: Pharmacologic study of norcaperatic and agaricic acids. J. Pharm. Sci. 56, 1611-1614 (1967)

Carrano, R.A., Truax, H.M.: The Rat Screen Computer Analysis -- An In-House Manual. Wilmington: Atlas Chemical Industries Inc., 1968

Chignell, C.F.: Methods in Pharmacology. New York: Appleton-Century-Crofts, 1972, Vol. II

Chilton, W.S., Tsou, G., DeCato, L., Jr., Malone, M.H.: The unsaturated norleucines of *Amanita solitaria*. Chemical and pharmacological studies. Lloydia 36, 169-173 (1973)

Daniel, E.E., Paton, D.M.: Methods in Pharmacology. New York-London: Plenum Press, 1975, Vol. III

Dewey, W.L., Malone, M.H., Harris, L.S., Botton, I.: Pharmacologic and toxicologic evaluation of 2-(*N*-tetradecyl-*N*-ethylamino)-2-methyl-1,3-propanediol hydrochloride, an inhibitor of intestinal absorption. Toxicol. Appl. Pharmacol. 12, 115-131 (1968)

Domer, F.R.: Animal Experiments in Pharmacological Analysis, 1st ed. Springfield: Charles C Thomas, 1971, pp. 61-64

Domer, F.R., Schueler, F.W.: Pharmacological investigations of a series of *p*-xylylene *bis*-ammonium congeners. Arch. Intern. Pharmacodyn. 114, 217-226 (1958)

Farnsworth, N.R., Henry, L.K., Svoboda, G.H., Blomster, R.N., Fong, H.H.S., Quimby, M.W., Yates, M.J.: Biological and phytochemical evaluation of plants. II. Test results from an additional 200 accessions. Lloydia 31, 237-248 (1968)

Farnsworth, N.R., Henry, L.K., Svoboda, G.H., Blomster, R.N., Yates, M.J., Euler, K.L.: Biological and phytochemical evaluation of plants. I. Biological test procedures and results from 200 accessions. Lloydia 29, 101-122 (1966)

Feng, P.C., Haynes, L.J., Magnus, K.E., Plimmer, J.R.: Further pharmacological screening of some West Indian plants. J. Pharm. Pharmacol. 16, 115-117 (1964)

Feng, P.C., Haynes, L.J., Magnus, K.E., Plimmer, J.R., Sherrott, H.S.A.: Pharmacological screening of some West Indian plants. J. Pharm. Pharmacol. 14, 556-561 (1962)

Fong, H.H.S., Farnsworth, N.R., Henry, L.K., Svoboda, G.H., Yates, M.J.: Biological and phytochemical evaluation of plants. X. Test results from a third 200 accessions. Lloydia 35, 35-48 (1972)

Gosselin, R.A.: The status of natural products in the American pharmaceutical market. Lloydia 25, 241-243 (1962)

Hall, C.S.: Emotional behavior in the rat: I. Defecation and urination as measure of individual differences in emotionality. J. Comp. Psychol. 18, 385-403 (1934)

Holck, H.G.O., Miya, T.S., Dunham, N.W., Yim, G.K.W.: Laboratory Guide in Pharmacology, 1st ed. Minneapolis: Burgess, 1959, pp. 78-80

Hooper, P.A., Leonard, B.E.: Pharmacological properties of some West Indian plants. J. Pharm. Pharmacol. 17, 98-107 (1965)

Irwin, S.: Multidimensional screening-evaluative procedures. In: Program Notes. New London: Gordon Research Conference on Medicinal Chemistry, 1959, p. 133

Irwin, S.: Drug screening and evaluative procedures. Science 136, 123-128 (1962)

Irwin, S.: Drug screening and evaluation of new compounds in animals. In: Animal and Clinical Pharmacologic Techniques in Drug Evaluation, 1st ed. Nodine, J.H., Siegler, P.E. (eds.). Chicago: Year Book Medical Publishers Inc., 1964, pp. 36-54

Irwin, S., Slabok, M., Debiase, P.L., Govier, W.M.: Perphenazine (Trilafon), a new potent tranquilizer and antiemetic: I. Behavior profile, acute toxicity, and behavioral mode of action. Arch. Intern. Pharmacodyn. 118, 358-374 (1959)

Janssen, P.A.J.: Screening tests. In: Animal Behavior and Drug Action, 1st ed. Steinberg, H., DeReuck, A.V.S., Knight, J. (eds.). Boston: Little and Brown, 1964, pp. 392-401

Janssen, P.A.J., Niemegeers, C.J.E., Schellekens, K.H.L.: Is it possible to predict the clinical effects of neuroleptic drugs (major tranquilizers) from animal data? Part I: "Neuroleptic activity spectra" for rats. Arzneimittel Forsch. 15, 104-117 (1965a)

Janssen, P.A.J., Niemegeers, C.J.E., Schellekens, K.H.L.: Is it possible to predict the clinical effects of neuroleptic drugs (major tranquilizers) from animal

data? Part II: "Neuroleptic activity spectra" for dogs. Arzneimittel Forsch. 15, 1196-1206 (1965b)
Jiu, J.: A survey of some medicinal plants of Mexico for selected biological activities. Lloydia 29, 250-259 (1966)
Kaplan, H.R., Malone, M.H.: A pharmacologic study of nesodine, cryogenine, and other alkaloids of *Heimia salicifolia*. Lloydia 29, 348-359 (1966)
Khanna, J.M., Malone, M.H., Euler, K.L., Brady, L.R.: Atromentin, anticoagulant from *Hydnellum diabolus*. J. Pharm. Sci. 54, 1016-1020 (1965)
Krider, M.M., Monroe, H.A., Jr., Wall, M.E., Willaman, J.J.: Steroidal sapogenins. XL. Simplified procedure for the qualitative detection of cardiac glycosides. J. Am. Pharm. Assoc. Sci. Ed. 46, 304-307 (1957)
Laurence, D.R., Bacharach, A.L.: Evaluation of Drug Activities: Pharmacometrics, 1st ed. London-New York: Academic Press, 1964
Malone, M.H.: Observational (hippocratic) screening. In: Experiments in the Pharmaceutical Biological Sciences, 1st ed. Malone, M.H., McLaughlin, J.L. (eds.). Bethesda: Biol. Sci. Sect. Am. Assoc. Colleges Pharm., 1973, pp. 120-123
Malone, M.H., Carrano, R.A.: Hippocratic and pharmacodynamic screening. In: Compilation of Symposium Papers Presented at the 5th Nat. Meet. A.Ph.A. Acad. Pharmaceut. Sci. 1st ed. Washington: Am. Pharmaceut. Assoc., 1970, pp. 149-176
Malone, M.H., Robichaud, R.C.: A hippocratic screen for pure or crude drug materials. Lloydia 25, 320-332 (1962)
Malone, M.H., Robichaud, R.C., Tyler, V.E., Jr., Brady, L.R.: A bioassay for muscarine activity and its detection in certain *Inocybe*. Lloydia, 24, 204-210 (1961)
Malone, M.H., Tyler, V.E., Jr., Brady, L.R.: Hippocratic screening of 66 species of higher fungi. Lloydia 30, 250-257 (1967)
Marozzi, F.J., Malone, M.H.: Analgesic and anti-inflammatory evaluation of thymotic acid and certain homologs. J. Pharm. Sci. 57, 989-994 (1968)
McLeod, L.J., Staff: Univ. Edinburgh Dep. Pharmacol.: Pharmacological Experiments on Intact Preparations, 1st ed. Edinburgh-London: E. & S. Livingstone Ltd., 1970
Mileski, D.R., Kaplan, H.R., Malone, M.H., Nieforth, K.A.: Synthesis and preliminary pharmacology of 2-aminophenol derivatives. J. Pharm. Sci. 54, 295-298 (1965)
Miyata, J.T., Tyler, V.E., Jr., Brady, L.R., Malone, M.H.: The occurrence of norcaperatic acid in *Cantharellus floccosus*. Lloydia 29, 43-49 (1966)
Morton, J.J.P., Malone, M.H.: A pharmacodynamic screen in dogs for pure or extracted drug materials. Lloydia 30, 269-279 (1967)
Nieschulz, O., Hoffmann, I., Popendiker, K.: Pharmakologische Untersuchungen über *N*-Alkyl-piperidyl-phenothiazin-Dervate. Arzneimittel Forsch. 6, 651-660 (1956)
Nieschulz, O., Popendiker, K., Hoffmann, I.: Pharmakologische Untersuchungen über *N*-Methyl-piperazinyl-*N*'-aethyl-phenothiazin. Arzneimittel Forsch. 7, 106-112 (1957)
Nodine, J.H., Siegler, P.E.: Animal and Clinical Pharmacologic Techniques in Drug Evaluation, 1st ed. Chicago: Year Book Medical Publishers Inc., 1964
Norton, S., deBeer, E.J.: Effects of drugs on the behavioral patterns of cats. Ann. N.Y. Acad. Sci. 65, 249-257 (1956)
Nucifora, T.L., Malone, M.H.: Comparative psychopharmacologic investigation of cryogenine, certain nonsteroid anti-inflammatroy compounds, lupine alkaloids, and cyproheptadine. Arch. Intern. Pharmacodyn. 191, 345-356 (1971)
Orgell, W.H.: Inhibition of human plasma cholinesterase in vitro by plant extracts. Lloydia 26, 59-66 (1963)
Perry, W.L.M., Staff: Univ. Edinburgh Dep. Pharmacol.: Pharmacological Experiments on Isolated Preparations, 1st ed. Edinburgh-London: E. & S. Livingstone Ltd., 1968
Robichaud, R.C., Malone, M.H., Schwarting, A.E.: Pharmacodynamics of cryogenine, an alkaloid isolated from *Heimia salicifolia* Link and Otto. Part I. Arch. Intern. Pharmacodyn. 150, 220-232 (1964)
Rubin, B., Malone, M.H., Waugh, M.H., Burke, J.C.: Comparative activity of *Rauwolfia serpentina* whole root and reserpine in laboratory animals. Monograph. Therap. 1 (2), 40-44 (1956)
Schwartz, A.: Methods in Pharmacology, 1st ed. New York: Appleton-Century-Crofts, 1971

Sharaf, A.A., Hussein, A.M., Mansour, M.Y.: Studies on the antidiabetic effect of some plants. Planta Medica 11, 159-168 (1963)

Siegler, P.E., Moyer, J.H., III: Animal and Clinical Pharmacologic Techniques in Drug Evaluation. Chicago: Year Book Medical Publishers Inc., 1967, Vol. II

Sklar, S., Nieforth, K.A., Malone, M.H.: Synthesis and preliminary screening of *N*-ethyltryptamine derivatives related to reserpine and lysergic acid. J. Pharm. Sci. 60, 304-306 (1971)

Smith, W.C.: Pharmacological screening tests. In: Progress in Medicinal Chemistry, 1st ed. Ellis, G.P., West, G.B. (eds.). London: Butterworths, 1961

Ther, L.: Pharmakologische Methoden, 1st ed. Stuttgart: Wissenschaftliche Verlagsgesellschaft mbH, 1948

Thorp, R.H.: Pharmacological screening tests and their place in research. Australasian J. Pharm. 32, 791-792 (1951)

Turner, R.A.: Screening Methods in Pharmacology, 1st ed. New York-London: Academic Press, 1965

Turner, R.A., Hebborn, P.: Screening Methods in Pharmacology. New York-London: Academic Press, 1971, Vol. II

Tutupalli, L.V., Chaubal, M.G., Malone, M.H.: Saururaceae. VI. Hippocratic screening of *Anemopsis californica*. Lloydia 38, 352-354 (1975)

Tyler, V.E., Jr., Brady, L.R., Benedict, R.G., Khanna, J.M., Malone, M.H.: Chromatographic and pharmacologic evaluation of some toxic *Galerina* species. Lloydia 26, 154-157 (1963)

Tyler, V.E., Jr., Malone, M.H.: An investigation of the culture, constituents, and physiological activity of *Panaeolus campanulatus*. J. Am. Pharm. Assoc. Sci. Ed. 49, 23-27 (1960)

Winter, C.A., Risley, E.A., Nuss, G.W.: Carrageenin-induced edema in hind paw of the rat as an assay for anti-inflammatory drugs. Proc. Soc. Exp. Biol. Med. 111, 544-547 (1962)

Worthley, E.G., Schott, C.D.: Pharmacotoxic evaluation of nine vehicles administered intraperitoneally to mice. Lloydia 29, 123-129 (1966)

Recent Experimental and Clinical Data Concerning Antitumor and Cytotoxic Agents from Plants

G. A. CORDELL

A. Introduction

Plants have been used in the treatment of cancer for over 3500 years (Hartwell, 1967), but it is only since 1959 that a concerted systematic effort has been made to screen crude plant extracts for their inhibitory activity against animal tumor systems. In this period, in excess of 180,000 plant extracts from 2500 genera of plants have been screened by a program conducted under the auspices of the National Cancer Institute.

These plants have provided a wide range of structures eliciting antitumor activity and this in itself has provided stimulation in two vital areas: in the development organic synthesis for potentially superior agents and in providing more compounds to use as tools in attempting to interpret the biochemical mechanisms involved in the growth and control of tumors.

The recent years have been very exciting, for substantial progress has been made in bringing new compounds to the point of advanced pharmacologic testing. The future must, therefore, be visualized as an optimistic one in which several new agents will be the subject of careful evaluation in the chemotherapy of advanced tumors. This review will attempt to enumerate some of the most recent advances made in the isolation and testing of plant-derived anticancer agents, indicating the current prospects for future clinical entities.

It is well known from previous reviews of this area (Hartwell and Abbott, 1969; Danielli, 1971a, b; Jewers et al., 1973; Strauch and Hiller, 1974) that the natural products which exhibit anticancer activity represent an enormous variety of chemical structures. Indeed there is hardly a chemical class of natural product which does not have a compound showing anticancer activity either in vivo or in vitro.

This is extremely important in attempting to isolate the compound (or compounds) responsible for an observed activity, for the active constituents are isolated by carefully monitoring the biological activity and separating only active fractions. In this way one may isolate almost any class of compound as an active constituent, and it may not be one traditionally associated with a particular plant family. A recent example is a compound isolated from *Allamanda cathartica*, a plant in the family Apocynaceae. Previous phytochemical knowledge would indicate that possibly indole alkaloids or cardenolides might be the active constituent. However, isolation based on such classical phytochemical ideas would not have afforded the active constituent. By following instead the biological activity, Kupchan and co-workers (Kupchan et al., 1974a) isolated an iridoid lactone of novel structure having in vivo P-388 antileukemic (PS activity) to which the name allamandin (1) was given.

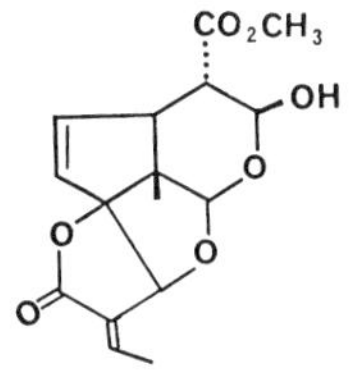

Formula 1. Allamandin

The remainder of this quite brief review of recent work is based approximately on the molecular complexity of the active compound. The terpene derivatives are therefore treated first with the alkaloids, dimeric alkaloids and ansa macrolides considered subsequently.

B. Terpenoids

I. Sesquiterpenes

The sesquiterpenes continue to provide numerous examples of structures exhibiting antitumor and/or cytotoxic activity. Of these the most important are those which exhibit in vivo activity.

Molephantinin (2) from *Elephantopus mollis* (Lee et al., 1975b) shows WM activity, ambrosin (3) from *Hymenoclea salsola* (Torrance et al., 1975) exhibits P-388 activity and eupahyssopin (4) from *Eupatorium hyssopifolium* was active in the WM system (Lee et al., 1976b). All three of the above compounds are germacrenolides isolated from members of the Compositae.

A number of germacrenolides and other sesquiterpene lactones have been correlated with parthenolide. It was only very recently, however, that the stereochemistry of the 4,5-epoxide was confirmed (Quick and Rogers, 1976).

Other sesquiterpene lactone skeleta also exhibit in vivo activity. The guaianolide deoxyelephantopin (5) from *Elephantopus carolinianus* was active in the in vivo WM system (Lee et al., 1975a) and zaluzanin C (6) was active in the P-388 system (Jolad et al., 1974). The pseudoguaianolide, fastigilin C (7) obtained from *Baileya multiradiata* (Pettit et al., 1975) was also active in this system.

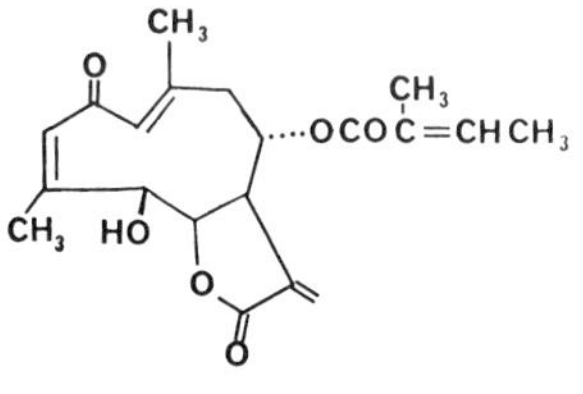

Formula 2. Molephantinin WA
Elephantopus mollis

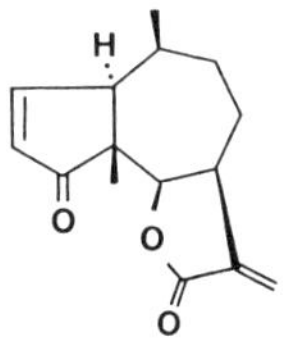

Formula 3. Ambrosin P-388
Hymenoclea salsola

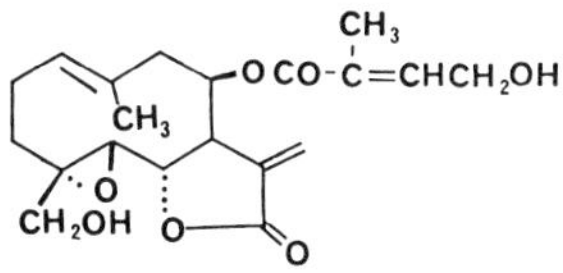

Formula 4. Eupahyssopin WA
Eupatorium hyssopifolium

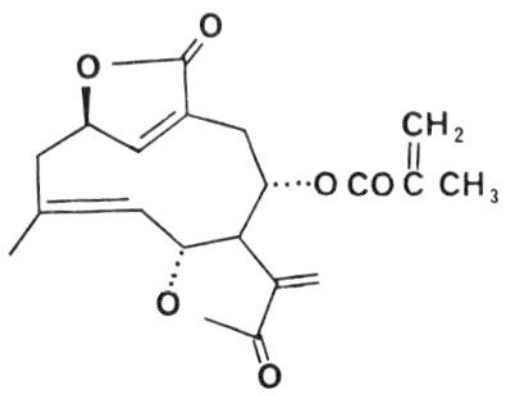

Formula 5. Deoxyelephantopin WA
Elephantopus carolinus

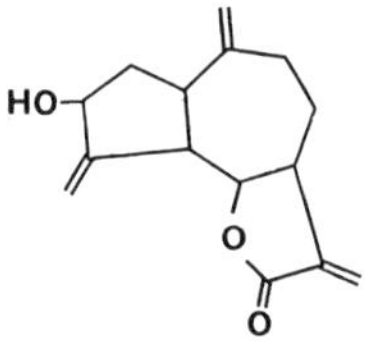

Formula 6. Zaluzanin - C P-388
Zaluzania spp.

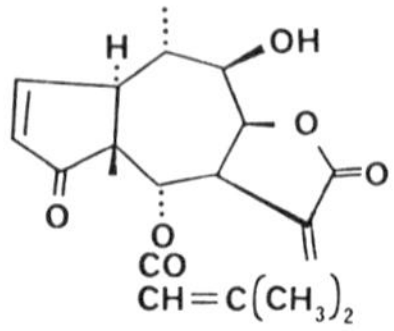

Formula 7. Fastigilin - C P-388
Baileya multiradiata

The common sneezeweed, *Helenium autumnale* var. *montanum* (Compositae) has afforded helenalin (8), a sesquiterpene lactone which shows activity in the PS WM and B-16 melanoma system (Pettit et al., 1974). Helenalin is also cytotoxic and Lee and co-workers (Lee et al., 1975c) have investigated the importance of the cyclopentenone and α-methylene lactone functionalities.

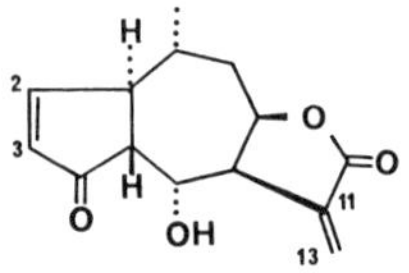

Factors influencing the cytotoxicity of Helenalin and its derivatives

	H.Ep-2 µg/ml
Formula 8. Helenalin	0.1
2,3-Epoxyhelenalin	0.1
2,3,11,13-Diepoxyhelenalin	0.5
2,3-Epoxy-11,13-Dihydrohelenalin	0.3
2,3,11,13-Tetrahydrohelenalin	40.0

The first dimeric sesquiterpene lactone, microlenin (9) was recently obtained from *Helenium microcephalum* (Lee et al., 1976a); it too exhibits marginal activity in the WA test system at low doses.

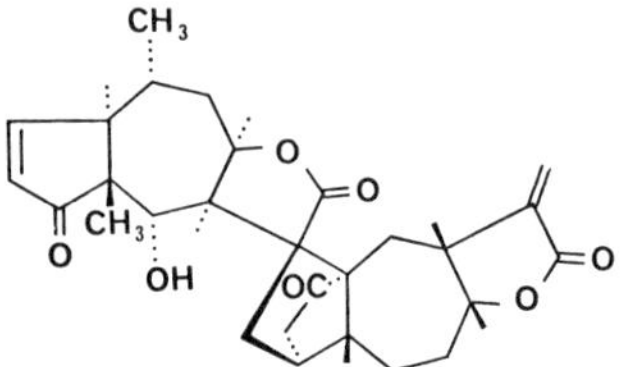

Formula 9. Microlenin WA
Helenium microcephalum

Vernolepin (10) has recently been the subject of considerable interest. Originally isolated by Kupchan and co-workers (Kupchan et al., 1968) from *Vernonia hymenolepsis* and more recently from *Vernonia guineensis* (Toubiana et al., 1975), vernolepin exhibits in vivo WM activity.

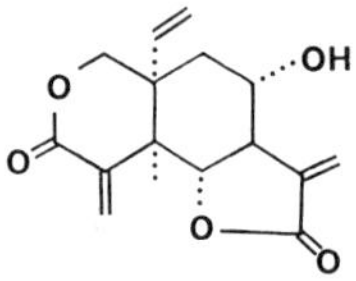

Formula 10. Vernolepin
Vernonia hymenolepis

As with many other tumor inhibitors vernolepin has become a synthetic target. There have been a number of synthetic approaches described to the vernolepin nucleus, but to date only one of these has been carried through to a successful conclusion (Grieco et al., 1976). The overall synthetic route used to vernolepin is shown in Scheme 1. The crucial intermediate in this route is the ester diacetate (11), which has the necessary functionalizations to allow subsequent steps. The synthetic sesquence commences with the decalone (12), which is converted to the α-prenylated α, β-unsaturated ketone (13). The ketone can be converted to the diol (14), which is then acetylated, oxidized, methylated and hydrolyzed to the ester diacetate (11). The enol acetate of (11) gives the diester diacetate (15) after dehydration. Removal of the methyl ether group, hydrolysis and spontaneous lactonization afforded a mixture of bis-nor-sesquiterpene lactones in which bis-nor-vernolepin (16) predominated. Double methylenation of this product gave vernolepin (10) (Grieco et al., 1976). Gossypol (17), a well-known constituent of cottonseed was isolated as the in vivo active constituent of *Montezuma speciosissima* (Malvaceae) (Jolad et al., 1975).

Scheme 1. Synthesis of vernolepin

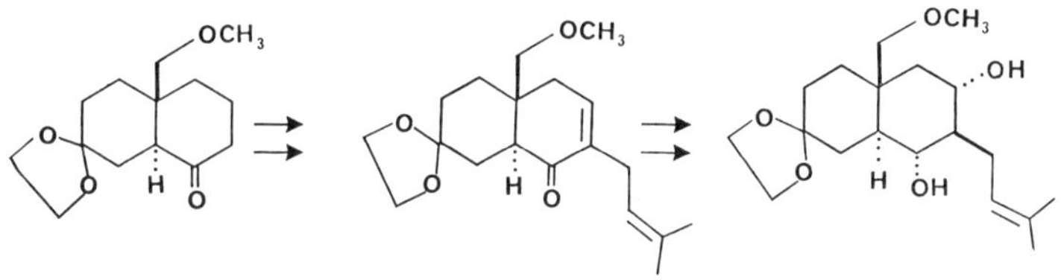

Formula 12 Formula 13 Formula 14

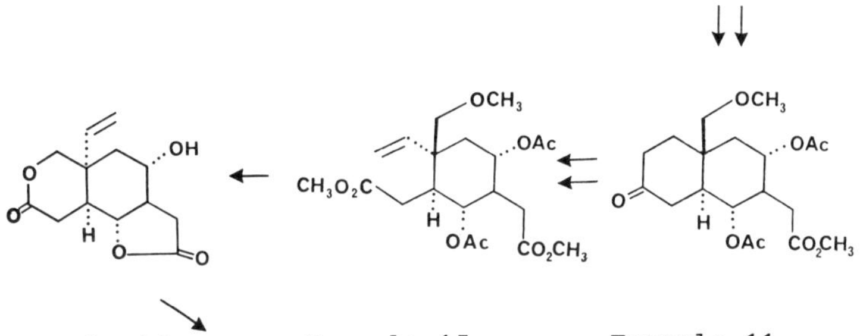

Formula 16 Formula 15 Formula 11

Formula 10. Vernolepin

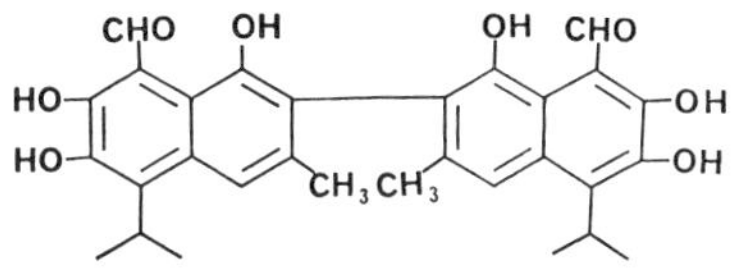

Formula 17. Gossypol

II. Diterpenes

The diterpenes have recently been a very interesting source of structurally new antitumor agents, some of exceptional promise. Tripdiolide (18) and triptolide (19) from the Celastraceous plant *Tripterygium wil-*

fordii (Kupchan et al., 1972a; Kupchan, 1974) are extremely active in the P-388 test system at low doses. Since most of the tumor inhibitors are suggested to act by nucleophilic attack of thiol groups, Kupchan and Schubert (Kupchan and Schubert, 1974) have examined the ability of tripdiolide and triptolide to react with propane thiol. These compounds contain a potentially highly susceptible center at C-9, but it was found that ring-opening by attack at C-9 with cleavage of the 9, 11-epoxy group is very highly dependent on the stereochemistry of the 14-hydroxy group. Whereas the 14β-hydroxy compound was reactive, the corresponding 14α-hydroxy compound was unreactive. It is studies such as these which are extremely important if we are to begin to understand the mechanisms by which antitumor agents operate, and by which their activity can be potentiated.

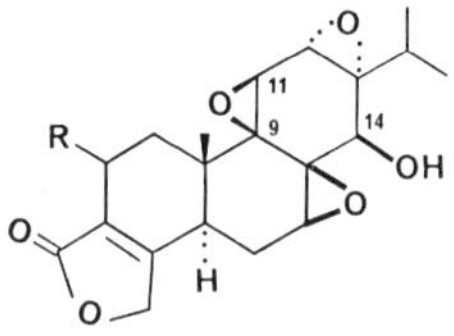

Formula 18. R = OH
Formula 19. R = H

Podocarpus species in the family Taxaceae have also yielded novel diterpenoid tumor inhibitors. Podolide (20), a dilactane from *Podocarpus gracilior* (Kupchan et al., 1975a) and nagilactone C (21) from a number of *Podocarpus* species (Hayashi et al., 1975) exhibit in vivo activity in the PS system. The structures of podolide (Bryan and Smith, 1975) and nagilactone A diacetate (22) (Hirotsu et al., 1975) have been confirmed by single crystal X-ray crystallography.

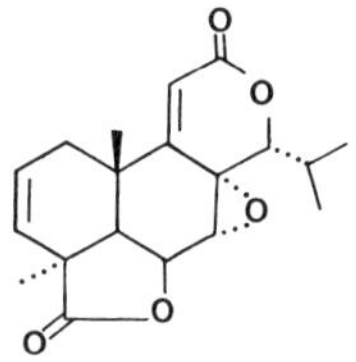

Formula 20. Podolide
Podocarpus gracilor
P-388, 9KB

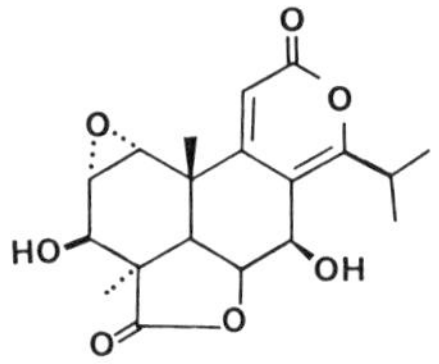

Formula 21. Nagilactone C
Podocarpus spp.
P-388, 9KB

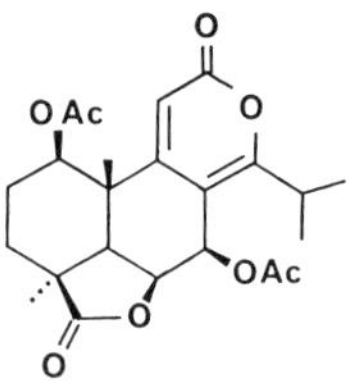

Formula 22

One of the interesting observations made recently is that a number of cocarcinogens may at lower doses elicit antileukemic activity. These plants are in the families Euphorbiaceae and Thymelaeaceae and several interesting compounds have been obtained.

Croton oil from the seeds of *Croton tiglium* contains a number of highly irritant and cocarcinogenic substituents, but Kupchan and co-workers (Kupchan et al., 1976) have isolated a phorbol derivative, phorbol 12-tiglate 13-decanoate (23) exhibiting antileukemic activity. From another member of the Euphorbiaceae, *Euphorbia escula*, the same group isolated ingenol dibenzoate (24) which at the μg/kg level also showed in vivo activity.

Many indigenous populations have used *Daphne* species for the treatment of cancer (Hartwell, 1971). Kupchan and Baxter (Kupchan and Baxter, 1975) have found that the antileukemic principle of *Daphne mezereum* is mezerein (25), which was active at 50 μg/kg dose levels in both the PS and LE in vivo systems.

Another highly toxic genus in the Thymelaeaceae, *Gnidia*, is being studied by several laboratories. From *Gnidia lamprantha* three antileukemic principles have been isolated (Kupchan et al., 1975e). Gnididin (26), gniditrin (27), and gnidicin (28) showed in vivo activity at the μg/kg level.

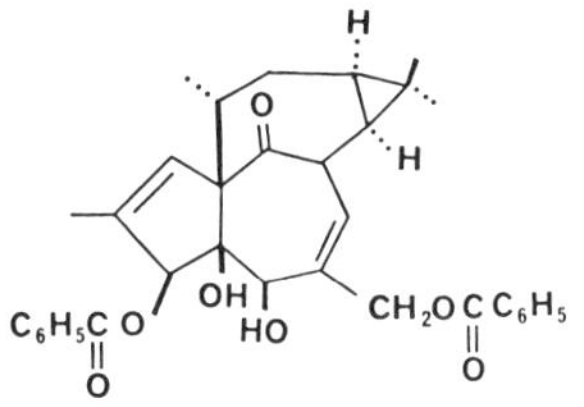

Formula 24. Ingenol dibenzoate
Euphorbia escula

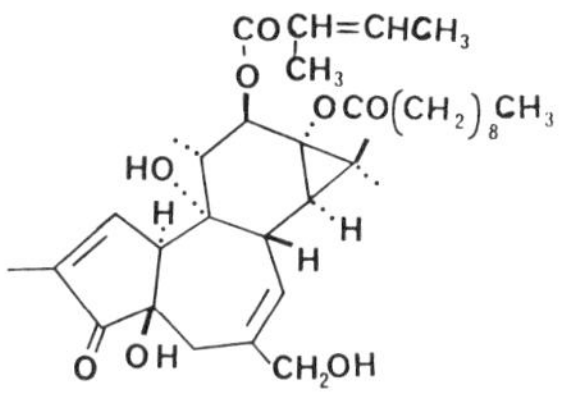

Formula 23. Phorbol 12-Tiglate 13-Decanoate
Croton tiglium oil

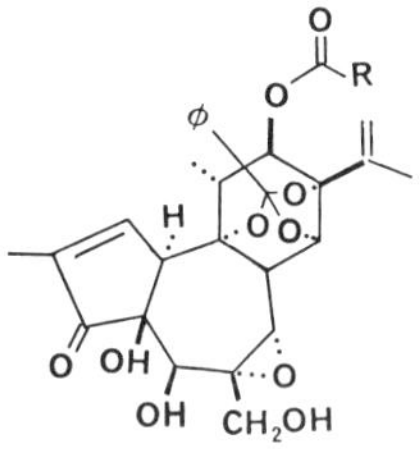

Formula 25.	Mezerein	R = $-(CH{=}CH)_2C_6H_5$	*Daphne mezereum*
Formula 26.	Gnididin	R = $-CH{=}CHCH{=}CH(CH_2)_4CH_3$	
Formula 27.	Gniditrin	R = $-CH{=}CH(CH{=}CH)_2(CH_2)_2CH_3$	
Formula 28.	Gnidicin	R = $CH{=}CHC_6H_5$	*Gnidia lamprantha*

III. Simaroubolides

Quassinoids have been known from plants of the Simaroubaceae for many years and Polonsky has summarized their isolation, chemistry and biosynthesis (Polonsky, 1973). A new development in the pharmacology of these interesting substances has been the observation by several groups that plants in this family exhibit antileukemic activity, and a number of compounds have been isolated.

Kupchan and co-workers (Kupchan et al., 1975c) have examined *Brucea antidysenterica* and obtained bruceantin (29), active in the P-388, LE, LL and B-16 melanoma test systems. Bruceantin is presently at the Decision Network III stage having passed animal toxicology and formu-

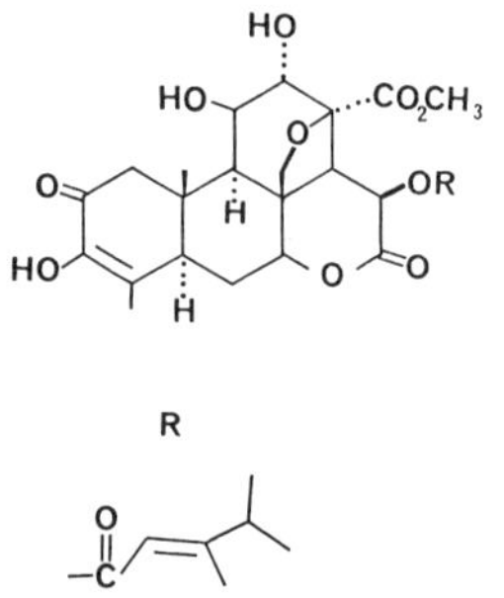

Formula 29. Bruceantin

lation. It is presently being considered for phase I clinical toxicologic evaluation. The same group (Kupchan and Lacadie, 1975) have reported on the isolation of the new simaroubolides dehydroailanthinone (30) and 2'-acetylglaucarubinone (31), in addition to the known compounds glaucarubinone (32) and ailanthinone (33) from the simaroubaceous plant *Pierreodendron kerstingii*. Each of the compounds was active in the P-388 test system and it is expected that compounds in this class will continue to be of interest in an effort to potentiate the very interesting in vivo activity.

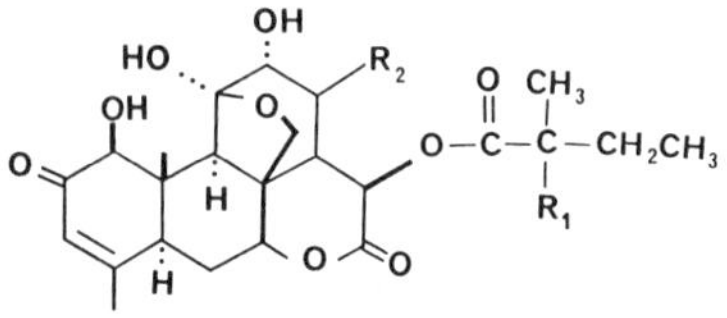

		R_1	R_2
Formula 30.	Dehydroailanthinone	H	$=CH_2$
Formula 31.	2'-Acetylglaucarubinone	-OAc	α-CH_3
Formula 32.	Glaucarubinone	-OH	α-CH_3
Formula 33.	Ailanthinone	-H	α-CH_3

C. Miscellaneous Compounds

A novel type of compound eliciting in vivo activity has been obtained from the euphorbiaceous plant, *Croton macrostachys* (Kupchan et al., 1969) Crotepoxide (34), also obtained from *Piper futokadzura* (Takahashi, 1969) and *Piper attenuatum* (Desai et al., 1975) has been synthesized by two independent routes (Oda et al., 1975; Demuth et al., 1976).

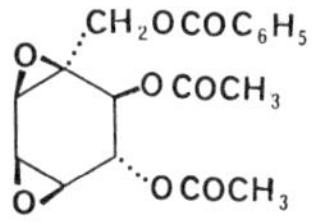

Formula 34. Crotepoxide
Croton macrostachys
Piper spp.

One of the simplest natural products to exhibit antileukemic activity is jacaranone (35), a quinoid derivative from *Jacaranda caucana* (Bignoniaceae) (Ogura et al., 1976).

Lignans have been of interest in the treatment of cancer since 1942 and extensive studies have been made of derivatives of podophyllotoxin, particularly glycosides. The Sandoz Company in Basel, has developed two new derivatives which have been subjected to clinical trial. One

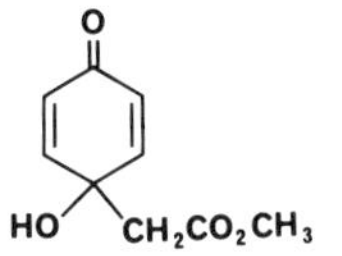

Formula 35

is 4'-demethylepipodophyllotoxin-β-D-thenylidene-glycoside (VM-26) and the other is 4'-demethylepipodo-phyllotoxin-β-D-ethylidene glucoside (VP-213).

VM-26 has been evaluated clinically in both the United States and Europe and has exhibited activity against Hodgkin's disease and non-Hodgkin's lymphomas, especially reticulum cell sarcoma. Some activity was also observed against bladder carcinoma and brain tumors.

VP-213 has received quite reasonable trails both in the United States in Europe. Toxicities normally observed were reversible bone marrow suppression and occasionally nausea and vomiting. As with VM-26, few responses were noted against solid tumors, but significant responses were noted in previously treated Hodgkin's lymphomas and in leukemias notably monocytic leukemia. Several Phase II trials are continuing of this interesting compound.

The antitumor activity of extracts of *Linum album* (Linaceae) was traced to podophyllotxin, α-and β-peltatin, and a new lignan, 3'-demethylpodophyllotoxin (36) (Weiss et al., 1975).

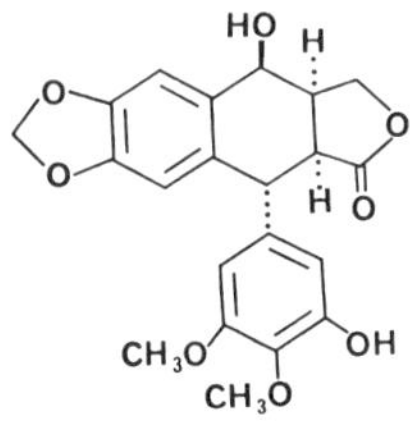

Formula 36. 3'-Demethylpodophyllotoxin
Linum album

Steganotaenia araliacea has afforded the antileukemic lignans stegancin (37) and steganagin (38) (Kupchan et al., 1973a), and two syntheses of steganone (39) have been reported (Kende and Liebeskind, 1976; Hughes and Raphael, 1976). Steganone (39) has been converted to steganacin (37) (Kende and Liebeskind, 1976).

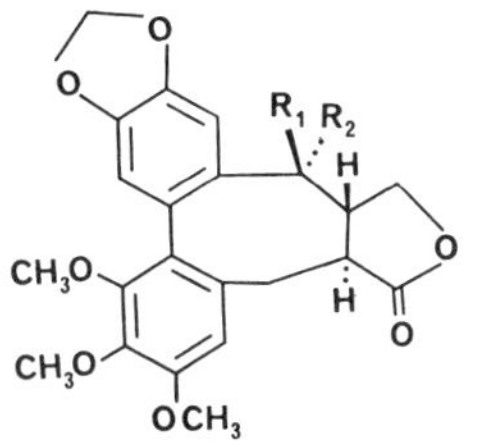

Formula 37. R_1 = OAc, R_2 = H
Formula 38. R_1 = OAng, R_2 = H
Formula 39. R_1, R_2 = =O

D. Alkaloids

The largest and most diverse group of compounds exhibiting anticancer activity are the alkaloids, and this is the area where there is the greatest progress. It is impossible to review all of the efforts which have been made in the recent past, but rather an attempt will be made to examine some of the major alkaloid groups and areas of great current interest.

I. Pyrrolizidine Alkaloids

Alkaloids of the pyrrolizidine type from *Senecio* and *Crotalaria* species are potent hepatotoxins, but, as with the phorbol esters noted previously, at lower doses antileukemic activity was observed. Thus monocrotaline (40) has been obtained as the antitumor principle from *Crotalaria spectabilis* and *Crotalaria assamica* (Anon, 1974a). Its antitumor effects were traced to an inhibition of cell multiplication (Anon, 1973).

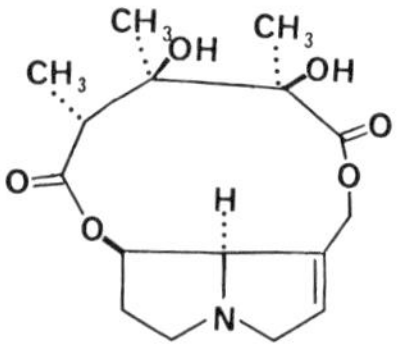

Formula 40. Monocrotaline

II. Isoquinoline Alkaloids

Thalicarpine (41), an aporphine-benzylisoquinoline alkaloid from *Thalictrum minus* subsp. *elatum* (Dutschewska and Mollov, 1966) and *Thalictrum dasycarpum* (Kupchan et al., 1963) is a potent antileukemic agent of substantial interest. Although a number of syntheses of alkaloids of this general type had been reported previously, Kupchan and Liepa (Kupchan and Liepa, 1974a,b, 1975) have described a more efficient synthesis based on hernandaline (42) as the key intermediate.

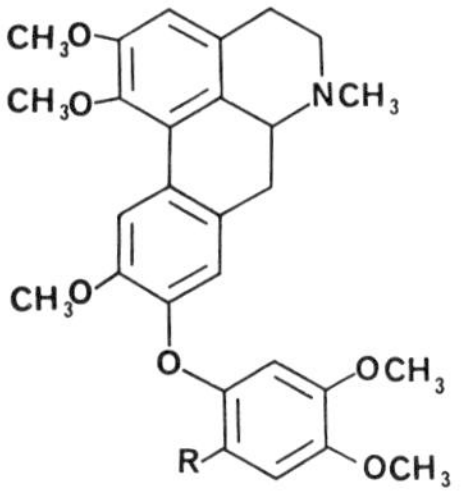

Formula 41. Thalicarpine R =

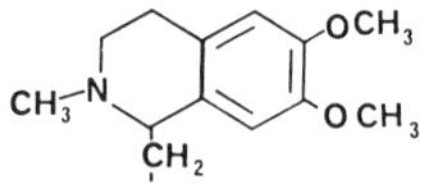

Formula 42. Hernandaline R = CHO

Rapid administration of thalicarpine (41) led to hypotension, bradycardia and inhibition of respiration, but slow i.v. infusion eliminated these effects (Todorov and Damyanova, 1975).

Antitumor activity in vivo was observed against the Yoshida and Jensen sarcomas and Walker carcinosarcoma, but thalicarpine (41) was inactive against the sarcoma 37 and Guerin carcinoma (Maleev et al., 1975).

Tetrandrine (43), a bisbenzylisoquinoline alkaloid from *Cyclea peltata* in the Menispermaceae also exhibits antileukemic activity (Kupchan et al., 1937b) and its crystal structure has been determined (Gilmore et al., 1976). Both the dl and d-isomers of tetrandrine (43) are active in the Walker carcinosarcoma test system and a preclinical toxicological evaluation has been conducted.

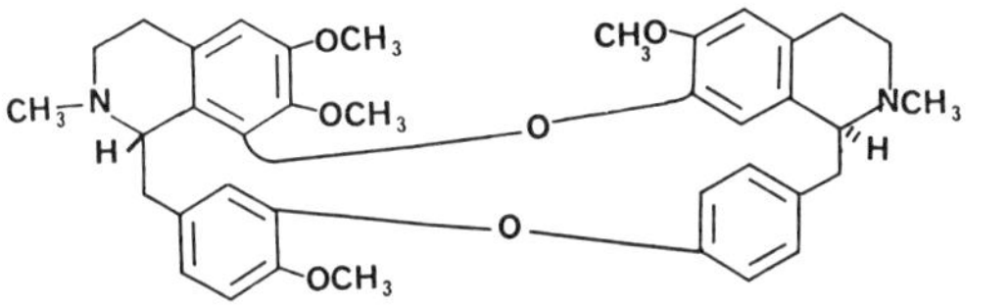

Formula 43. Tetrandrine
Cyclea peltata

Intravenous injection of d-tetrandrine produced hypotension and bradycardia in the anesthetized rhesus monkey and high doses were toxic (Herman and Chadwick, 1974). Hypotensive effects and hepatoxicity were observed upon administration of tetrandrine to dogs (Gralla et al., 1974). Both thalicarpine (41) and tetrandrine (43) are currently in Phase II studies at the M.D. Anderson Hospital in Houston, Texas.

The anticancer activity of emetine (44), an alkaloid of *Cephaelis ipecacuanha* (Rubiaceae) and several other Rubiaceous species, has been suspected for many years (Grollman and Jarkovsky, 1975). However, no clinical efficacy was found against breast, bronchial, gynecologic and genitourinary carcinomas (Siddiqui et al., 1973), or gastrointestinal cancers (Moertel et al., 1974). Dehydroemetine (45) may be a more promising entity (Israel et al., 1974).

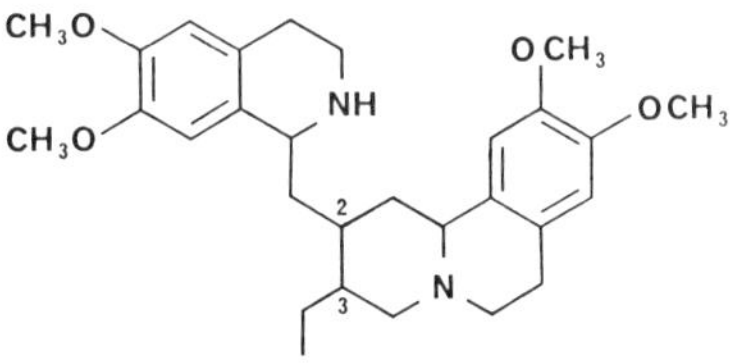

Formula 44. Emetine

Formula 45. $\Delta^{2,3}$

III. Benzophenanthridines

Although known for many years, the benzophenanthridines have only quite recently become of interest for their tumor-inhibitory activity. Two alkaloids have stimulated this interest, nitidine (46) and fagaronine (47). Each of these compounds is isolated from members of the Rutaceae; nitidine (46) from a number of *Zanthoxylum* species and fagaronine (47) from *Fagara zanthoxyloides* (Messmer et al., 1972).

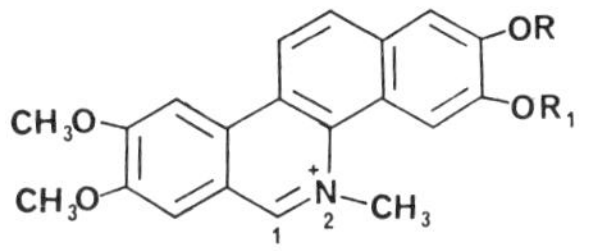

	R	R_1	Other
Formula 46	$-CH_2-$		
Formula 47	H	CH_3	
Formula 50	$-CH_2-$		dihydro 1,2

Evidence confirming the structure of fagaronine has come from several sources. Evaluation of the pmr spectrum of N-demethyl fagaronine under neutral and basic conditions defined the phenolic group at C-2 (Tin-Wa et al., 1974).

Two groups have reported syntheses of fagaronine. The route used by Stermitz and co-workers (Gillespie et al., 1974) is based upon the Kessar phenanthridine synthesis, the key step of which is cyclization of the anil (48) with sodamide in liquid ammonia. Because fagaronine is assymetrically substituted an appropriate protecting group was required. In this case an isopropyl group was used which could be cleaved with dimethyl sulfate, xylene and nitrobenzene at 180°C. The starting point for the synthesis is a nitronaphthalene which following reduction was condensed with *o*-bromoveratraldehyde to give the anil (48). Subsequent cyclization, N-alkylation, removal of the protecting group and anion exchange gave fagaronine (47).

Synthesis of fagaronine

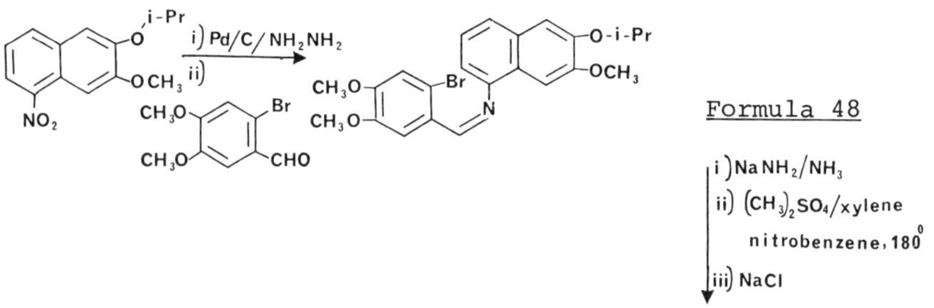

Formula 48

Formula 47. Fagaronine chloride

Ninomiya and co-workers (Ninomiya et al., 1975a) used a somewhat similar route in synthesizing N-demethylfagaronine. An appropriately protected α-naphthylamine was condensed with *o*-bromoveratroyl chloride and the product photocylized to give a lactam (49), which could be easily converted to N-demethyl-fagaronine. The same group has also reported the synthesis of dihydronitidine (50) (Ninomiya et al., 1975b).

Synthesis of N-demethylfagaronine

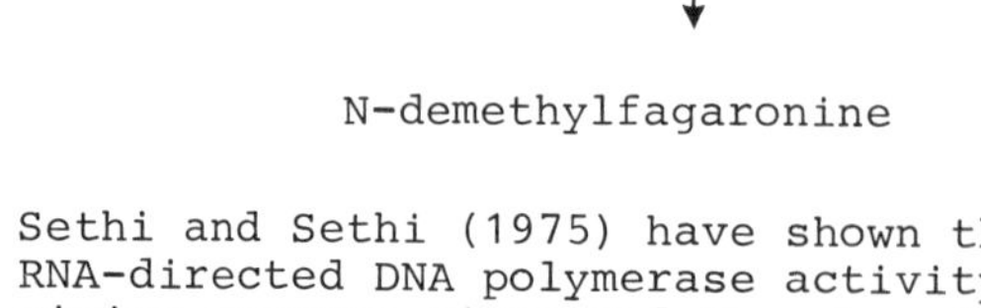

N-demethylfagaronine

Sethi and Sethi (1975) have shown that fagaronine is an inhibitor or RNA-directed DNA polymerase activity from avian myelo-blastosis virus, simian sarcoma virus and Rauscher leukemia virus.

Fagaronine (46) and nitidine (47) are active in both the P-388 and L-1210 test systems but in addition nitidine is cytotoxic. Nitidine has been chosen for preclinical pharmacologic and toxicologic evaluation.

IV. Miscellaneous Alkaloids

A number of minor alkaloid groups exhibit anticancer activity which could potentially be the subject of further study.

Thiophosphamide derivatives of berberine (51) exhibit antitumor activity (Petlichnaya and Turkevich, 1975) and the phosphate of berberoline (52) is also active (Sawa and Ikegawa, 1975).

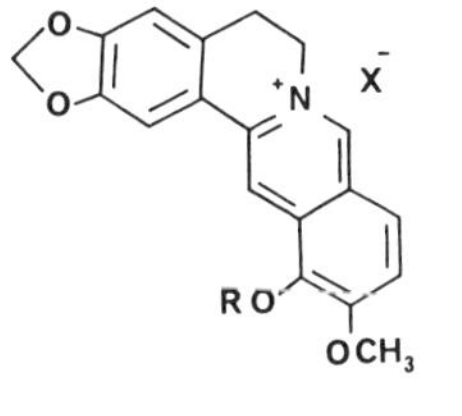

Formula 51. R = CH_3
Formula 52. R = H

Cryptopleurine (53) is highly cytotoxic and has been synthesized in racemic form (Kotani et al., 1974; Tobinaga, 1975).

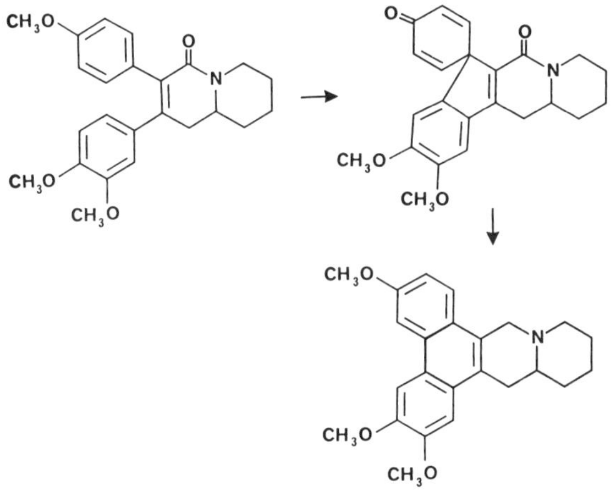

Formula 53

The alkaloid acronycine (54) from *Acronychia baueri*, has the broadest spectrum of in vivo antitumor activity of any natural product.

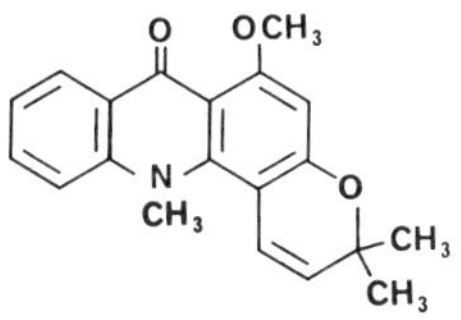

Formula 54

The prodrug acetylacronycinium perchlorate together with a stabilizer sodium gentisate has been formulated as a lyophilized, reconstitutable i.v. solution. The prodrug is claimed to be 1000 times more soluble than the parent compound, and solutions are stable for up to 24 h (Huang et al., 1976). It is encouraging to see that efforts are being made to attack the problem of formulation of highly insoluble species.

V. Monomeric Indole Alkaloids

Olivacine (55) a potent tumor inhibitor in the L-1210 system (Regina et al., 1974) continues to be the subject of synthetic endeavors (Kametani et al., 1975a, b; Kutney and Grierson, 1975).

Synthesis of olivacine

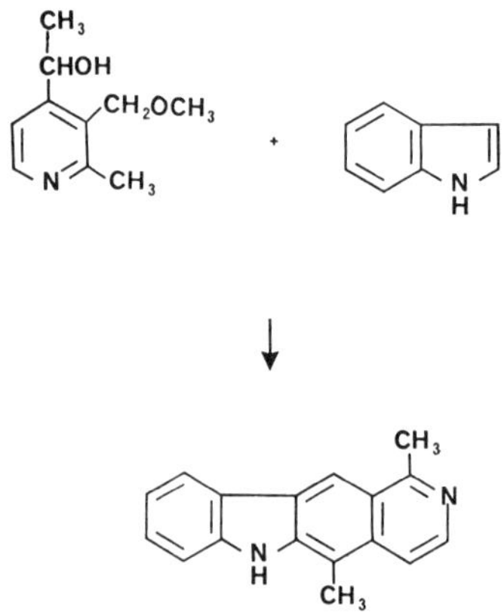

Formula 55. Olivacine

Ellipticine (56) and derivatives are being subjected to careful scrutiny as potential antitumor agents.

9-Methoxyellipticine (57) as the lactate salt, ellipticine (56), 9-hydroxyellipticine (58) and 9-aminoellipticine (59) are all active in the L-1210 system (Hayat et al., 1974). Inhibiting rat liver carcinomas induced by BT6 (Truhaut et al., 1976) ellipticine increases production of cytochrome P450.

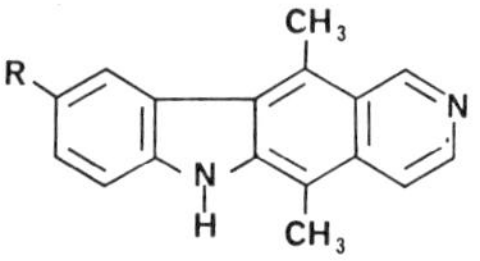

Formula 56. R = H
Formula 57. R = OCH_3
Formula 58. R = OH
Formula 59. R = NH_2

9-Hydroxyellipticine (58), prepared from O-methoxyellipticine (57) (Anon, 1975c; Dat-Xuong et al., 1975), was the most active derivative and the most immunosuppressive. In the mouse, side effects included stimulated respiration and contraction of the heart muscle (Anon, 1975c).

Intravenous injection of ellipticine in anesthetized rhesus monkeys produced immediate hemolysis and a decreased heart rate (Herman et al., 1974a) Hemolysis could be prevented by administration in citrate buffer (Herman et al., 1974b).

A potent inhibitor of respiration in isolated pigeon mitochondria (Gosalvez et al., 1974), ellipticine (Mohn et al., 1975) and 9-methoxyellipticine (Festy et al., 1971) strongly bind, by intercalation to helical DNA.

The possibility of setting up sites of alkylation within a compound was mentioned previously as a possible alternative biochemical mechanism of action, and clearly this possibility was in mind when

2-methyl-9-hydroxyellipticine (60) and 2,6-dimethyl-9-hydroxyellipticine (61) were evaluated in the L-1210 system (Le Pecq et al., 1975). Both compounds were highly active and at lower doses than 9-hydroxyellipticine (58).

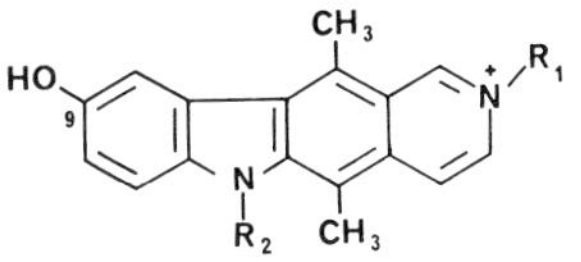

Formula 60. $R_1 = CH_3$, $R_2 = H$

Formula 61. $R_1 = CH_3$, $R_2 = CH_3$

A number of syntheses of ellipticine and related compounds have appeared but two routes developed by Potier and co-workers are of special note.

In one synthetic approach, the Mannich product of dimethylamide and acetaldehyde is reacted with (62) to give a low yield of the tetrahydro-ellipticine (63), which can be dehydrogenated to give ellipticine (56) (Besselievere et al., 1975).

An alternative, more efficient route involves a modified Polonovskii reaction in which the N-oxide (64) on treatment with trifluoroacetic acid affords, in 92 % yield, the enamine (65), which can be dehydrogenated to ellipticine (56) (Langlois et al., 1975).

Synthesis of ellipticine

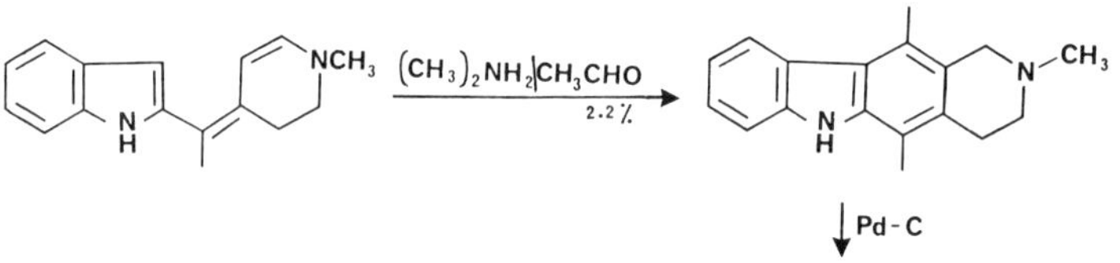

Formula 62

Formula 63

via

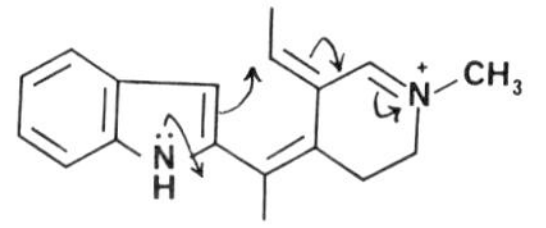

Formula 56. Ellipticine

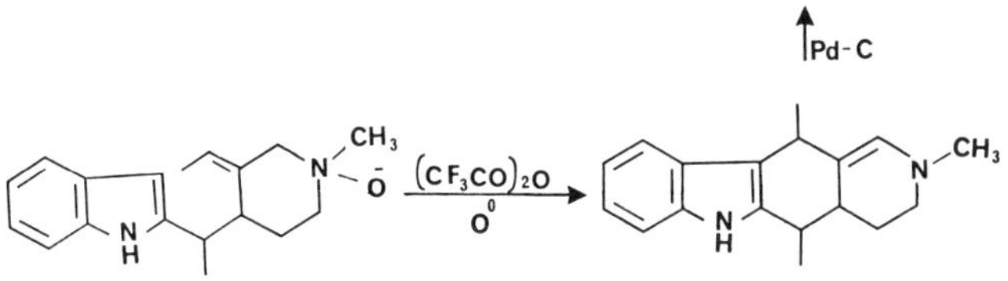

Formula 64

Formula 65

VI. Camptothecine

A number of reviews of the synthesis, pharmacology, antitumor properties and mechanism of action of camptothecine (66) have appeared (Schultz, 1973; Shamma and Georgiev, 1974; Horwitz, 1975; Winterfeldt, 1975).

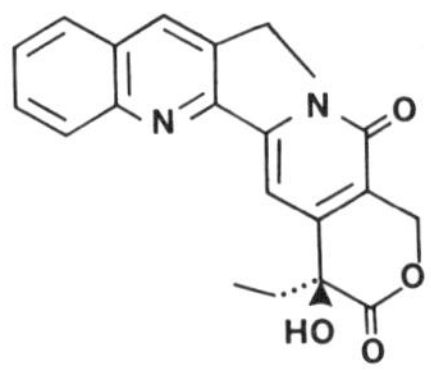

Formula 66. Camptothecine
Camptotheca acuminata
Mappia foetida

Several new syntheses of camptothecine (66) have been reported (Sugasawa et al., 1974; Krohn and Winterfeld, 1975; Richman, 1975; Tang et al., 1975; Corey et al., 1975c; Walraven and Pandit, 1975; Anon, 1976; Bradley and Büchi, 1976). Most of the syntheses show no improvements over the previously published syntheses. The synthesis of Bradley and Büchi is probably the most efficient devised to date.

Previously unpublished work on the preclinical pharmacology of camptothecine in several species has been reported (Schaeppi et al., 1974). The most important effects in the monkey or dog were emesis, dehydration, hemorrhagic diarrhea, hypocellularity of the bone marrow and necrosis of the liver.

Camptothecine is widely used in China in the treatment of various forms of cancer. The failure of camptothecine to proceed through to an objective, extensive clinical evaluation must now be revaluated. Alternative formulations with the aim of increasing drug availability appear to be appropriate, and the previously described efforts with salts of acronycine may well be relevant in this case as well.

VII. *Cephalotaxus* Alkaloids

Cephalotaxus harringtonia in the family Cephalotaxaceae produces several alkaloid esters exhibiting substantial in vivo activity in a variety of experimental leukemia systems (Powell et al., 1972; Mikolajczak et al., 1972).

The most important active alkaloid is harringtonine (67) and removal of the ester group leads to cephalotaxine (68) which is inactive. Powell and co-workers (Mikolajczak et al., 1974a) have prepared a number of ester analogs of harringtonine (Fig. 1), but these were inactive. The α-hydroxy group is therefore essential for antileukemic activity. The "rearranged" ester (69) was also inactive (Mikolajczak et al., 1975).

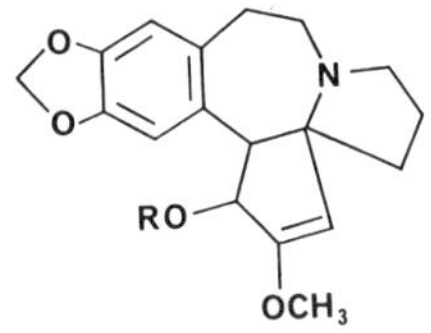

Formula 67. Harringtonine $R = CO\,C(OH)(CH_2CO_2CH_3)\,CH_2CH_2C(CH_3)_2$

Formula 68. Cephalotaxine R = H

Fig. 1. Harringtonine and synthetic derivatives

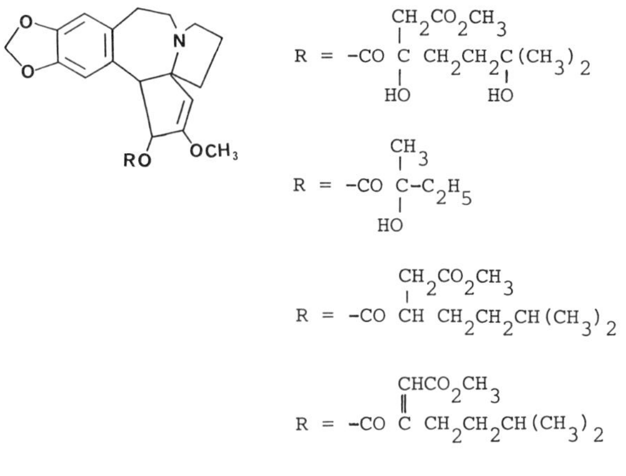

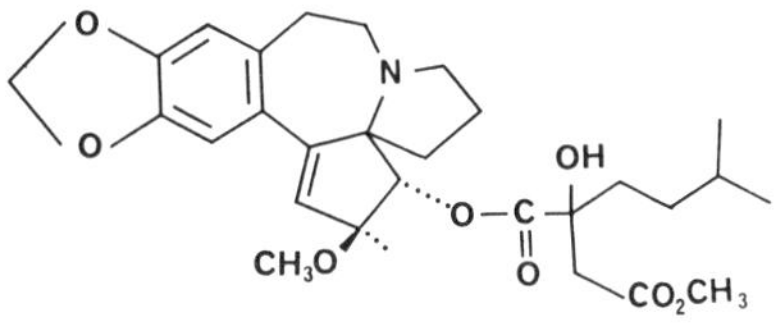

Formula 69. "Rearranged" cephalotaxine ester

The esters of cephalotaxine are not crystalline so that X-ray structural analysis has been restricted to the methioiodide of cephalotaxine (Abraham et al., 1969), the p-bromobenzoate of cephalotaxine (Arora et al., 1974) and cephalotaxine (Arora et al., 1976). The absolute configuration of the important ester moiety has been determined separately (Brandange et al., 1974).

The *Cephalotaxus* alkaloids which exhibit antitumor activity are only available in minute quantities. It therefore became important to evolve synthetic strategies which might make available increased quantities of compound for more substantial evaluation. Two groups have been successful in their synthetic endeavors of cephalotaxine (Weinreb and Semmelhack, 1975). In addition, syntheses of deoxyharringtorine (Mikolajczak et al., 1974b; Li and Dai, 1975) and a partial synthesis of harringtonine (Anon, 1975a) have appeared.

The two main synthetic routes are worthy of special mention. The Weinreb and Auerbach synthesis (Weinreb and Auerbach, 1975) (Scheme 2) proceeds in eight steps from 1-prolinol (70) and 3,4-methylenedioxyphenyl acetyl chloride (71). The key steps are the cyclization of an amidealdehyde with BF_3-etherate, acylation and cyclization of an enamine to give an α-diketone and isomerization and reduction to afford cephalotaxine (68).

The Semmelhack synthesis (Semmelhack et al., 1975) follows a quite different synthetic strategy. Here it is envisioned that the C and D rings can be produced as a spiro intermediate which can subsequently be united with an appropriately functionalized aromatic derivative.

Scheme 2. Synthesis of cephalotaxine

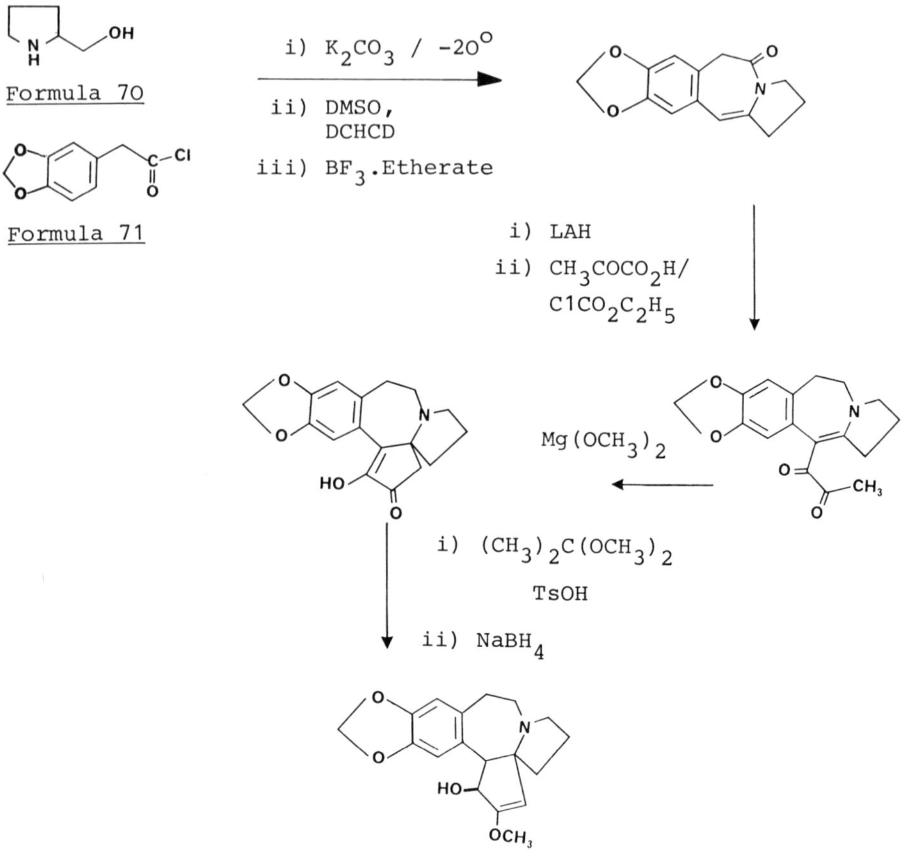

Formula 68

In Scheme 3 the principal steps of this procedure are shown. The first cruciol step is the alkylation of the spiropyrrolidine (72) with the indonitrobenzene sulfonate ester (73). Cyclization of the product could be carried out in a number of alternative ways (Semmelhack et al., 1972, 1973), but the most successful was to photolyze (74) under basic conditions to afford an intermediate anion radical (75) which cyclized to cephalotaxinone (76) in 94 % yield.

An interesting development in the chemistry of these alkaloids has been the biosynthetic proposal of Parry and Schwab (1975).

VIII. Dimeric Indole Alkaloids

Leurocristine (vincristine, VCR) (77) and vincaleukoblastine (vinblastine, VLB) (78) continue to be the two most important plant antitumor agents in the clinicians armamentarium. The only structural difference between these two compounds is the replacement of the vindoline N-methyl group by an N-formyl group.

Leurocristine is of greater clinical importance than vincaleukoblastine but is obtained in considerably lower yield from the plant source, *Catharanthus roseus*. It was, therefore, important to develop routes to VCR from VLB.

Scheme 3. Synthesis of cephalotaxinone

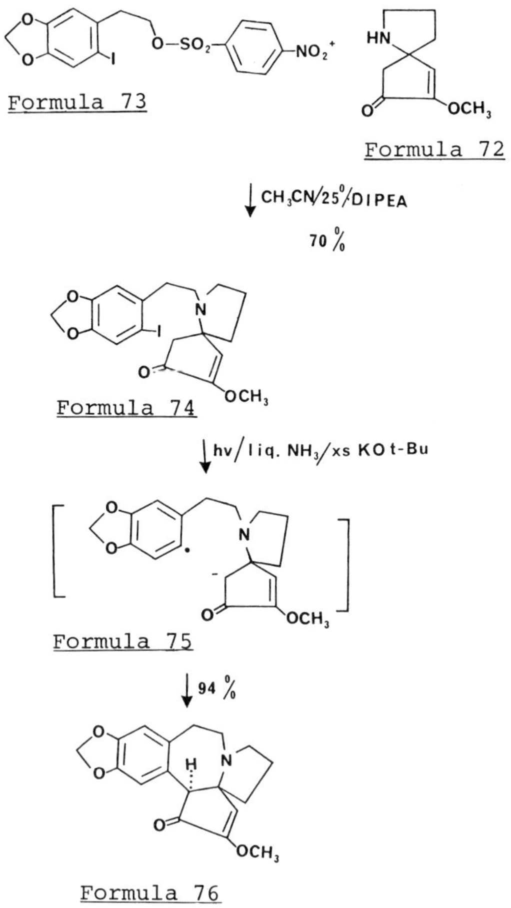

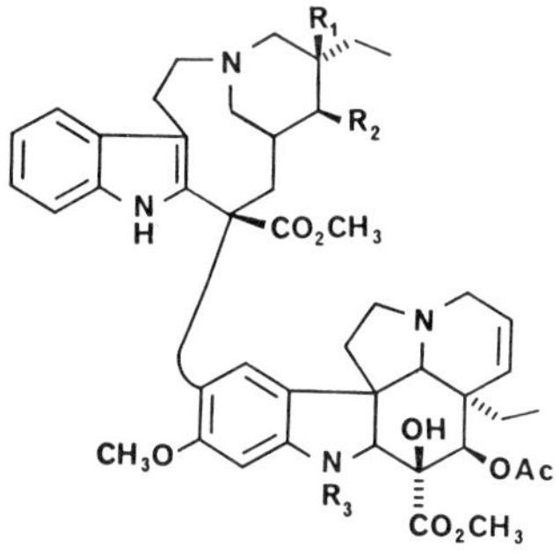

Formula 77.	VCR	OH	H	CHO
Formula 78.	VLB	OH	H	CH_3
Formula 82		Δ		CH_3
Formula 83		H	H	CH_3
Formula 84.	Leurosidine	H	OH	CH_3
Formula 85.	Leurosine	—O—		CH_3
Formula 86		OH	OH	CH_3

An approach developed by the Lilly group involves the N-demethylation of VLB (Neuss et al., 1974; Brannon and Neuss, 1975) by *Streptomyces albogriseolus*, followed by N-formylation.

Chemical approaches have also been successful in carrying out this conversion, and two procedures have been described recently. The first method involves a low temperature (-60°C) chromic acid oxidation (Anon, 1974b; Jovanovics et al., 1975) followed by formylation. The second technique utilizes Pd/C and formic acid in an oxygen atmosphere (Anon, 1975b).

The most dramatic developments in the recent past have been in the area of synthesis of the dimeric indole alkaloids. Before describing some of the work relating to the linking of the two monomeric units, it is appropriate to consider some of the synthetic work and the component halves.

Vincaleucoblastine (78) is comprised of two units, an indole half, 16β-carbomethoxyvelbanamine (79) and an indoline half, vindoline (80). The linking of the two units joins the C-10 of vindoline with C-16 of the velbanamine derivative, with the 16-carbomethoxyl group of the indole unit assuming a β-configuration.

In the synthesis of the dimeric species it became essential to distinguish between compounds having the two possible configuration at C-16. An extremely effective method was discovered by the groups of Kutney and Scott (Kutney et al., 1975c). The method relies on a study of the circular dichroism absorption in the region 200 - 350 nm where two absorptions are observed at 207 and 224 nm. The magnitude and sign of these bands is reversed in going from the natural (16'β) to the unnatural (16'α) configurations. This observation proved crucial in determining the efficiency of the synthesis with respect to the natural isomer. The 16'α configuration gives rise to compounds devoid of antileukemic activity.

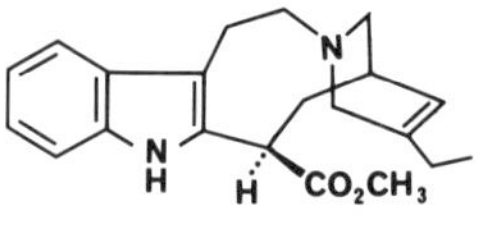

Formula 79

Each of the "halves" of the dimeric alkaloids have been synthesized. The upper portion of the molecule 16β-carbomethxycleavamine (79) and related compounds have been synthesized by both Büchi's (Büchi et al., 1968, 1970) and Kutney's (Kutney and Bylsma, 1970, 1975) groups. The lower portion, vindoline (80) has also recently been synthesized and two independent routes have been reported. Vindorosine (81), demethoxyvindoline, had been synthesized by Büchi (Büchi et al., 1971), but efforts to use an analogous sequence in the methoxylated series failed at any early point. The successful synthetic route involved the tosylate of 5-hydroxytryptamine as a starting material. The protecting group is replaced at an intermediate stage and the remainder of the route follows closely that developed previously (Büchi, 1975; Ando et al., 1975). Kutney has reported on a quite different approach to vindoline (80) (Kutney, 1976). Initial attempts to link the two monomeric units gave the 16'-epi series of dimers which were inactive (Potier et al., 1975, Kutney et al., 1975a, b). Subsequently,

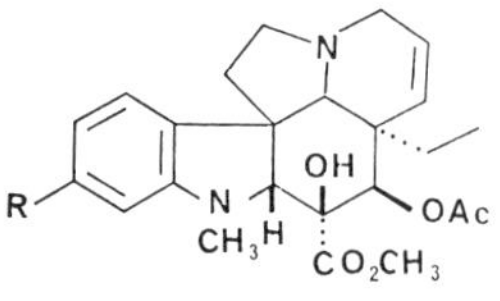

Formula 80. Vindoline R = OCH_3

Formula 81. Vindorosine R = H

the thermal and solvent factors required to carry out the synthesis of the "natural" dimeric alkaloids were deduced (Potier et al., 1975; Kutney et al., 1975d) and this has permitted the recent synthetic advances which have included the synthesis of 15',20'-dehydrovinblastine (82), 20'deoxyvinblastine (83) (Kutney et al., 1975d), (82) (Potier et al., 1975), leurosidine (84) (Langlois and Potier, 1976), leurosine (85) and 20'-hydroxyvinblastine (86) (Kutney et al., 1976) and vincaleukoblastine (78) (Atta-ur-Rahman et al., 1976).

Space does not permit extensive discussion of the intimate details of these reactions but it is appropriate to mention the important effect of temperature. Given that a compound such as catharanthine N-oxide (87) is used as one substrate molecule and vindoline as the other molecule, and that TFAA/methylene chloride is used under reflux, a mixture of isomers consisting mainly of the natural isomer is produced. At -50° only the natural isomer is obtained.

Synthesis of natural dimeric alkaloids

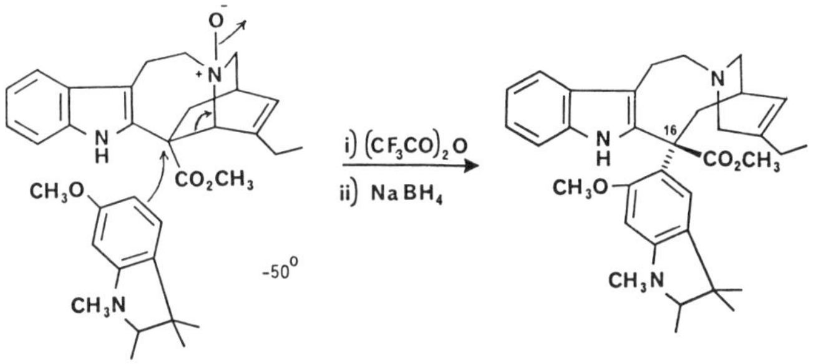

Concerted 50% Formula 87

The reason for this is that two separate mechanisms were operating, one is a concerted reaction operating at low temperatures which is both regio and stereoselective, and the second is an elimination within the catharanthine N-oxide prior to attack by vindoline. The subsequent condensation of the iminium species with vindoline although regioselective is not particularly stereoselective.

It is worthwhile to briefly summarize the clinical usefulness of VLB and VCR. VLB is for the most part only useful in the treatment of Hodgkin's disease where the overall response rate is 68 % and the complete response rate is 30 %. In combination with bleomycin, VLB is also effective in the treatment of testicular cancer.

Vincristine is a more useful agent and neurotoxicity is the most common side effect. Although now rarely used alone, VCR is highly active in the treatment of childhood leukemia where a 41 % complete remission rate has been observed. It is the main component of the several highly effective combination regimens. VCR is also of significant usefulness in the treatment of Wilm's tumor, and has proved useful in the treatment of embryonal rhabdomyosarcoma. It is among the most active drugs in the treatment of nonHodgkin's lymphomas being a critical component of all the major combinations. VCR has also produced tumor regression in patients with breast cancer.

IX. Maytansinoids

Maytansine (88) (Kupchan et al., 1972b) and the related maytanoid esters (89-91) (Kupchan et al., 1972c; Wani et al., 1973) are potent antileukemic agents obtained from *Maytenus ovatus* and *Maytenus buchananii* in the Celastraceae (Kupchan et al., 1972b, c, 1975d), and *Colubrina texensis* in the Rhamnaceae (Wani et al., 1973).

Kupchan's group has continued to develop the chemistry of the ester side chain, in particular its significance for the antileukemic activity (Kupchan et al., 1974b, 1975b). The presence of an ester moiety on the C-3 hydroxy group is essential for the in vivo activity. Thus maytansinol (92) is inactive, but when the 3-hydroxy group is acylated as in maytanacine (93) and the other natural esters, antileukemic activity is restored. The synthetic compounds (94, 95 and 96) produced from maytansinol (92) by esterification were also active.

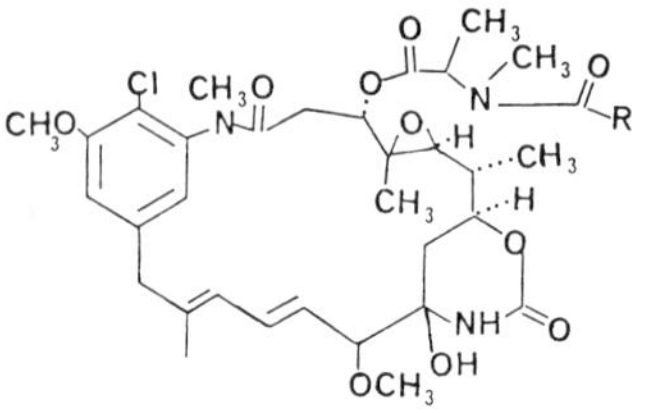

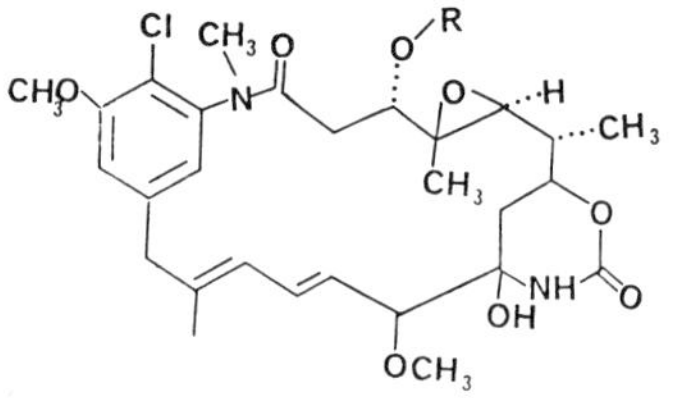

Compound		R
Formula 88.	Maytansine	CH_3
Formula 89.	Maytanprine	CH_2CH_3
Formula 90.	Maytanbutine	$CH(CH_3)_2$
Formula 91.	Maytanvaline	$CH_2CH(CH_3)_2$

Compound		R
Formula 93.	Maytanacine	$COCH_3$
Formula 92.	Maytansinol	H
Formula 94.	Synthetic esters	$COCH_2CH_3$
Formula 95.	Synthetic esters	$COCH_2Br$
Formula 96.	Synthetic esters	$COCH = CHCH_3$

Maytansinol (92) and maytanacine (93) occur in *Putterlickia verrucosa* seeds (Kupchan et al., 1975b), but more importantly the seeds are a rich source of maytansine (88), where the level is 12 mg/kg. Unfortunately *P. verrucosa* is a poor producer of seeds but it is hoped that the seeds of *M. buchananii* may be an improved source of maytansine.

Maytansine is a potent inhibitor of cell division (Remillard et al., 1975; Wolpert-Defilippes et al., 1975). At 6 x 10^{-8}M, it irreversibly inhibits cell division in the eggs of clams and sea urchins. The compound is also a potent inhibitor of murine sarcoma virus in mice (O'Connor et al., 1975).

Three groups have reported preliminary results on the synthesis of maytansine (Meyers and Shaw, 1974; Meyers et al., 1975; Meyers and Brinkmeyer, 1975; Corey and Bock, 1975; Elliott and Fried, 1976). The published data describe very early approaches to some of the "zones" of maytansine, but will not be discussed in detail at this time.

Maytansine is currently in a Phase I clinical study for toxicologic evaluation. It appears to be an agent of exceptional promise and its progress must be watched by all with great interest.

E. Summary

The previous discussion has covered some of the recent studies in the area of antitumor agents from plants. It has attempted to demonstrate that in the recent past substantical advances have been made in this area. Particularly interesting are the terpene esters of the Euphorbiaceae, Simaroubaceae and Thymelaceaceae, the synthesis of the dimeric indole alkaloids and in the isolation and chemistry of the maytanoid esters.

References

Abraham, D.J., Rosenstein, R.D., McCandy, E.L.: Single crystal X-ray structures of chemotherapeutic agents. II. The structure of cephalotaxine methiodide. Tetrahedron Lett. 4085-4086 (1969)

Ando, M., Büchi, G., Ohnuma, T.: The total synthesis of vindoline. J. Am. Chem. Soc. 97, 6880-6881 (1975)

Anon: Antitumor effect and toxicity of the alkaloid of *Crotalaria assamica*. Chung-Hua I Hsueh Tsa Chih 104, 472-477 (1973). Through Chem. Abstr. 83, 11176f

Anon: *Crotalaria assamica*. Resource plant of monocrotaline. Chih. Wu Hsueh Pao 16, 380-381 (1974a). Through Chem. Abstr. 83, 25024

Anon: Semisynthetic preparation of vincristine. Fr. Demande 2,210,393 (1974b). Through Chem. Abstr. 82, 73294b

Anon: Partial synthesis of harringtonine. K'O Hsueh T'ung Pao 20, 437 (1975a). Through Chem. Abstr. 84, 105859z

Anon: N-Formyl bisindole alkaloids. Belg. Pat. 823,560 (1975b). Through Chem. Abstr. 84, 59835p

Anon: 9-Hydroxyellipticine. Ger. Offen. 2,451,360 (1975c). Through Chem. Abstr. 83, 126493y

Anon: Total synthesis of dl-camptothecine. K'O Hsueh T'ung Pao 21, 40-44 (1976). Through Chem. Abstr. 84, 122100n

Arora, S.K., Bates, R.B., Grady, R.A., Germain, G., Declerco, J.P., Powell, R.G.: Crystal and molecular structure of cephalotaxine. J. Org. Chem. 41, 551-554 (1976)

Arora, S.K., Bates, R.B., Grady, R.A., Powell, R.G.: Crystal and molecular structure of cephalotaxine *p*-bromo benzoate. J. Org. Chem. 39, 1269-1271 (1974)

Atta-ur-Rahman, Basha, A., Ghazala, M.: Synthetic studies of antileukemic alkaloids. VII. The partial synthesis of vinblastine. Tetrahedron Lett. 2351-2354 (1976)

Besselievere, R., Thal, C., Husson, H.-P., Potier, P.: Novel synthesis of the indole alkaloid ellipticine. J. Chem. Soc., Chem. Commun. 90-91 (1975)

Bradley, J.C., Büchi, G.: A short synthesis of camptothecin. J. Org. Chem. 41, 699-701 (1976)

Brändange, S., Josephson, S., Vallén, S., Powell, R.G.: Absolute configuration of 2,3-dihydroxy-2-isopentylbutanedioic acid, a component of the alkaloid isoharringtonine. Acta Chem. Scand. 28B, 1237-1248 (1974)

Brannon, D.R., Neuss, N.: Microbial N-demethylation of vindoline and vinblastine. Ger. Offen. 2,440,931 (1975). Through Chem. Abstr. 83, 7184k

Bryan, R.F., Smith, P.M.: X-Ray determination of the structure of podolide, an antileukemic norditerpene dilactone. J. Chem. Soc. Perkin Trans. II. 1482-1486 (1975)

Büchi, G.H.: Synthesis of naturally occuring indole derivatives. Chimia 29, 172-173 (1975)

Büchi, G.H., Kulsa, P., Ogasawara, K., Rosati, R.L.: Synthesis of velbanamine and catharanthine. J. Am. Chem. Soc. 92, 999-1005 (1970)

Büchi, G.H., Kulsa, P., Rosati, R.L.: The total synthesis of velbanamine. J. Am. Chem. Soc. 90, 2448-2449 (1968)

Büchi, G.H., Matsumoto, K.E., Nishimura, H.: Total synthesis of vindorosine. J. Am. Chem. Soc. 93, 3299-3301 (1971)

Corey, E.J., Bock, M.G.: Stereocontrolled route to a key intermediate for the synthesis of maytansine. Tetrahedron Lett. 2643-2646 (1975)

Corey, E.J., Crouse, D.N., Anderson, J.E.: A total synthesis of natural 20 (S)-camptothecin. J. Org. Chem. 40, 2140-2141 (1975)

Danielli, B.: Recenti acquisizioni nel campo degli antitumorali di origine vegetale. Parte I. Fitoterapia 42, 11-39 (1971a)

Danielli, B.: Recenti acquisizioni nel campo degli antitumorali di origine vegetale. Parte II. Fitoterapia 42, 94-120 (1971b)

Dat-Xuong, N., Adeline, M.-T., Lecointe, P., Janot, M.-M.: L'hydroxy-9-ellipticine et quelques uns de ses derives. C.R. Acad. Sci., Paris, Ser. D. 281, 623-626 (1975)

Demuth, M.R., Garrett, P.E., White, J.D.: Synthesis of (±)-crotepoxide, (±)-epi-crotepoxide, and (±)-isocrotepoxide. J. Am. Chem. Soc. 98, 634-635 (1976)

Desai, H.K., Gawad, D.H., Govindachari, T.R., Joshi, B.S., Kamat, V.N., Parthasarathy, P.C., Ramachandran, K.S., Shanbhag, M.N., Sidhaye, A.R., Viswanathan, N.: Chemical investigation of some Indian plants. Part VIII. Indian J. Chem. 13, 97-98 (1975)

Dutschewska, H.B., Mollov, N.M.: Structure of dehydrothalicarpine, a new aporphine benzylisoquinoline alkaloid from *Thalictrum minus* spp. *elatum*. Chem. Ind. (London) 770-771 (1966)

Elliot, W.J., Fried, J.: Maytansinoids. Synthesis of a fragment of known absolute configuration involving chiral centers C-6 and C-7. J. Org. Chem. 41, 2469-2475 (1976)

Festy, B., Poisson, J., Paoletti, C.: A new intercalating drug: 9-methoxyellipticine. FEBS Lett. 17, 321-323 (1971)

Gillespie, J.P., Amoros, L.G., Stermitz, F.R.: Synthesis of fagaronine. An anticancer benzophenanthridine alkaloid. J. Org. Chem. 39, 3239-3241 (1974)

Gilmore, C.J., Bryan, R.F., Kupchan, S.M.: Conformation and reactivity of the macrocyclic tumor-inhibitory alkaloid tetrandrine. J. Am. Chem. Soc. 98, 1947-1952 (1976)

Gosalvez, M., Blanco, M., Hunter, J., Miko, M., Chance, B.: Effects of anticancer agents on the respiration of isolated mitochondria and tumor cells. Europ. J. Cancer 10, 567-574 (1974)

Gralla, E.J., Coleman, G.L., Jonas, A.M.: Toxicology studies with d-tetrandrine (NSC-77037), a plant alkaloid with vascular and lymphotoxic effects in dogs and monkeys. Cancer Chemother. Repts. Pt. 3 5, 79-85 (1974)

Grieco, P.A., Nishizawa, M., Burke, S.D., Marinovic, N.: Total synthesis of (±)-vernolepin and (±)-vernomenin. J. Am. Chem. Soc. 98, 1612-1613 (1976)

Grollman, A.P., Jarkovsky, Z.: Emetine and related alkaloids. In: Antibiotics. Mechanism of Action of Antimicrobial and Antitumor Agents. Corcoran, J.W., Hahn, F.E. (eds.). New York: Springer, 1975, Vol. III, pp. 420-435

Hartwell, J.L.: Plants used against Cancer. A survey. Lloydia 30, 379-436 (1967)

Hartwell, J.L.: Plants used against Cancer. A survey. Lloydia 32, 204-255 (1971)

Hartwell, J.L., Abbott, B.J.: Antineoplastic principles in plants: Recent developments in the field. Advan. Pharmacol. Chemother. 7, 117-209 (1969)

Hayashi, Y., Sakan, T., Sakurai, Y., Tashiro, T.: Antitumor activity of naglactones. Gann 66, 587-588 (1975)

Hayat, M., Mathe, G., Janot, M.-M., Potier, P., Dat-Xuong, N., Cave, A., Sevenet, T., Kan-Fan, C., Poisson, J., Miet, J., Le Men, J., Le Goffic, F., Gouyette, A., Ahond, A., Dalton, L.K., Connors, T.A.: Experimental screening of three

forms and nineteen derivatives or analogs of ellipticine: Oncostatic effect on L-1210 leukemia and immunosuppressive effect of four of them. Biomedicine 21, 101-106 (1974)
Herman, E.H., Chadwick, D.P.: Cardiovascular effects of d-tetrandrine. Pharmacology 12, 97-109 (1974)
Herman, E.H., Chadwick, D.P., Mhatre, R.M.: Comparison of the acute hemolytic and cardiovascular actions of ellipticine (NSC-71795) and some ellipticine analogs. Cancer Chemother. Repts. Pt. 1 58, 637-643 (1974a)
Herman, E.H., Lee, I.P., Mhatre, R.M., Chadwick, D.P.: Prevention of hemolysis induced by ellipticine (NSC-71795) in rhesus monkeys. Cancer Chemother Repts. Pt. 1 58, 171-9 (1974b)
Hirotsu, K., Higuchi, T., Shimada, A., Hayashi, Y., Sakan, T.: Crystal and molecular structure of nagilactone. A diacetate. Bull. Chem. Soc. Japan 48, 1157-1162 (1975)
Horwitz, S.B.: Camptothecin. Antibiotics 3, 48-57 (1975)
Huang, C.H., Kreilgard, B., Repta, A.J.: Formulation of a parenteral solution of acetylacronycinium perchlorate a soluble prodrug of the antitumor agent acronycine. Bull. Parenter. Drug Assoc. 30, 1-12 (1976)
Hughes, L.R., Raphael, R.A.: Synthesis of the antileukemic lignan precursor (±)-steganone. Tetrahedron Lett. 1543-1546 (1976)
Israel, L., Depierre, A., Chahinian, P.: Dehydroemetine in 50 disseminated carcinomas unresponsive to other drugs. Proc. Am. Assoc. Cancer Res. 15, 11 (1974)
Jewers, K., Manchanda, A.H., Rose, H.M.: Naturally-occurring antitumor agents. Progr. Med. Chem. 9, 1-63 (1973)
Jolad, S.D., Wiedhopf, R.M., Cole, J.R.: Tumor-inhibitory agent from *Zaluzania robinsonii* (Compositae). J. Pharm. Sci. 63, 1321-1322 (1974)
Jolad, S.D., Wiedhopf, R.M., Cole, J.R.: Tumor-inhibitory agent from *Montezuma speciosissima* (Malvaceae). J. Pharm. Sci. 64, 1889-1890 (1975)
Jovanovics, K., Szasz, K., Fekete, G., Bittner, E., Dezberi, E., Eles, J.: Chromic acid oxidation of vinblastine sulfate to form vincristine. U.S. Patent 3,899, 493 (1975. Through Chem. Abstr. 83, 179360f
Kametani, T., Ichikawa, Y., Suzuki, T., Fukumoto, K.: Fascinating synthesis of olivacine. Heterocycles 3, 401 (1975a)
Kametani, T., Suzuki, T., Ichikawa, Y., Fukumoto, K.: Studies on the synthesis of heterocyclic compounds. Part CDXXXIV. A novel total synthesis of olivacine. (1,5-Dimethyl-6H-pyridol[4,3-b-]carbazole). J. Chem. Soc. Perkin Trans. I 2102-2104 (1975b)
Kende, A.S., Liebeskind, L.S.: Total synthesis of steganacin. J. Am. Chem. Soc. 98, 267-268 (1976)
Kotani, E., Kitazawa, M., Tobinaga, S.X.: New synthesis of the alkaloid (±)-cryptopleurine by anodic oxidation. Tetrahedron Lett. 30, 3027-3030 (1974)
Krohn, K., Winterfeldt, E.: Alkylierung von Camptothecinvorstufen - ein neuer Weg zum Camptothecin. Chem. Ber. 108, 3030-3042 (1975)
Kupchan, S.M.: Antileukemic triepoxyditerpenes from *Tripterygium wilfordii*. Ger. Offen. Patent 2,316,916 (1974). Through Chem. Abstr. 82, 77095k
Kupchan, S.M., Baxter, R.L.: Mezerein: Antileukemic principle isolated from *Daphne mezereum* L. Science 187, 652-653 (1975)
Kupchan, S.M., Baxter, R.L., Ziegler, M.F., Smith, P.M., Bryan, R.F.: Podolide, a new antileukemic norditerpene dilactone from *Podocarpus gracilior*. Experientia 31, 137-138 (1975a)
Kupchan, S.M., Branfman, A.R., Sneden, A.T., Verma, A.K., Dailey, R.G., Jr., Komoda, Y., Nagao, Y.: Novel maytansinoids. Naturally occurring and synthetic antileukemic esters and maytansinol. J. Am. Chem. Soc. 97, 5294-5295 (1975b)
Kupchan, S.M., Britton, R.W., Lacadie, J.A., Ziegler, M.F., Sigel, S.W.: The isolation and structure elucidation of bruceantin and bruceantinol, new potent antileukemic quassinoids from *Brucea antidysenterica*. J. Org. Chem. 40, 648-656 (1975c)
Kupchan, S.M., Britton, R.W., Ziegler, M.F., Gilmore, C.J., Restivo, R.J., Bryan, R.F.: Steganacin and steganangin, novel antileukemic lignan lactones from *Steganotaenia araliacea*. J. Am. Chem. Soc. 95, 1335-1336 (1973a)

Kupchan, S.M., Chakravarti, K.K., Yokoryama, N.: Thalictrum Alkaloids I. Thalicarpine, a new hypotensive alkaloid from *Thalictrum dasycarpum*. J. Pharm. Sci. 52, 985-988 (1963)
Kupchan, S.M., Court, W.A., Dailey, R.G., Jr., Gilmore, C.J., Bryan, F.F.: Triptolide and tripdiolide, novel antileukemic diterpenoid triepoxides from *Tripterygium wilfordii*. J. Am. Chem. Soc. 94, 7194-7195 (1972a)
Kupchan, S.M., Dessertine, A.L., Blaylock, B.T., Bryan, R.R.: Isolation and structure elucidation of allamandin, an antileukemic iridoid lactone from *Allamanda cathartica*. J. Org. Chem. 39, 2477-2482 (1974a)
Kupchan, S.M., Hemingway, R.J., Smith, R.M.: Tumor inhibitors. XLV. Crotepoxide, a novel cyclohexane diepoxide tumor inhibitor from *Croton macrostachys*. J. Org. Chem. 34, 3898-3902 (1969)
Kupchan, S.M., Hemingway, R.J., Werner, D., Karin, A., McPhail, A.T., Sim, G.A.: Tumor inhibitors XXXI. Vernolepin, a novel elemanolide dilactone tumor inhibitor from *Verononia hymenolepis*. J. Am. Chem. Soc. 90, 3596-3597 (1968)
Kupchan, S.M., Komoda, Y., Branfman, A.R., Dailey, R.G., Jr., Zimmerly, V.A.: Novel maytansinoids. Structural interrelations and requirements for antileukemic activity. J. Am. Chem. Soc. 96, 3706-3708 (1974b)
Kupchan, S.M., Komoda, Y., Court, W.A., Thomas, G.J., Smith, R.M., Karim, A., Gilmore, C.J., Haltiwanger, R.C., Bryan, R.F.: Maytansine, a novel antileukemic ansa macrolide from *Maytenus ovatus*. J. Am. Chem. Soc. 94, 1354-1356 (1972b)
Kupchan, S.M., Komoda, Y., Thomas, G.J., Court, W.A.: Ansa macrolides. U.S. Pat. 3,896,111 (1975d). Through Chem. Abstr. 83, 209396s
Kupchan, S.M., Komoda, Y., Thomas, G.J., Hintz, H.P.J.: Maytanprine and maytanbutine, new antileukemic ansa macrolides from *Maytenus buchananii*. J. Chem. Soc., Chem. Commun. 1065 (1972c)
Kupchan, S.M., Lacadie, J.A.: Dehydroailanthinone, a new antileukemic quassinoid from *Pierreodendron kerstingii*. J. Org. Chem. 40, 654-655 (1975)
Kupchan, S.M., Liepa, A.J.: Tumor-inhibiting thalicarpines. Brit. Pat. 1,373,399. (1974a). Through Chem. Abstr. 83, 59135q
Kupchan, S.M., Liepa, A.J.: Cytotoxic hernandaline. Brit. Pat. 1,373,400 (1974b). Through Chem. Abstr. 83, 79456y
Kupchan, S.M., Liepa, A.J.: Synthesis of thalicarpine. U.S. Pat. 3,875,167 (1975). Through Chem. Abstr. 83, 28433f
Kupchan, S.M., Liepa, A.J., Baxter, R.L., Hintz, H.P.J.: New alkaloids and related artifacts from *Cyclea peltata*. J. Org. Chem. 38, 1846-1852 (1973b)
Kupchan, S.M., Schubert, R.M.: Selective alkylation. A biomimetic reaction of the antileukemic triptolides. Science 185, 791-793 (1974)
Kupchan, S.M., Sweeny, J.G., Baxter, R.L., Murae, T., Zimmerly, V.A., Sickles, B.: Gnididin, gniditrin, and gnidicin, novel potent antileukemic diterpenoid esters from *Gnidia lamprantha*. J. Am. Chem. Soc. 97, 672-673 (1975e)
Kupchan, S.M., Uchida, I., Branfman, A.R., Dailey, R.G., Jr., Fei, B.Y.: Antileukemic principles isolated from Euphorbiaceae plants. Science 191, 571-572 (1976)
Kutney, J.P.: Studies on the total synthesis of bisindole alkaloids in the vinblastine-vincristine series. American Society of Pharmacognosy Meeting, Cable, Wisconsin, July 11-16th, 1976
Kutney, J.P., Balsevich, J., Bokelman, G.H., Hibino, T., Itoh, I., Ratcliffe, A.H.: Studies on the synthesis of bisindole alkaloids. III. The synthesis of leurosine and 3'-hydroxyvinblastine. Heterocycles 4, 997-1005 (1976)
Kutney, J.P., Beck, J., Bylsma, F., Cook, J., Cretney, W.J., Fuji, K., Imhof, R., Treasurywala, A.M.: Total synthesis of indole and dihydroindole alkaloids. VIII. Studies on the synthesis of bisindole alkaloids in the vinblastine-vincristine series. The chloroindolenine approach. Helv. Chem. Acta 58, 1690-1719 (1975a)
Kutney, J.P., Bylsma, F.: Studies on the synthesis of monomeric and dimeric *Vinca* alkaloids. The total synthesis of isovelbanamine, velbanamine, cleavamine, 18β-carbomethoxycleavamine and catharanthine. J. Am. Chem. Soc. 92, 6090-6092 (1970)
Kutney, J.P., Bylsma, F.: Total synthesis of indole and dihydroindole alkaloids. VII. The total synthesis of isovelbanamine, velbanamine, cleavamine, 18β-carbomethoxylcleavamine and catharanthine. Helv. Chim. Acta 58, 1672-1689 (1975)

Kutney, J.P., Cook, J., Fuji, K., Treasurywala, A.M., Clardy, J., Fayos, J., Wright, H.: Synthesis of bisindole alkaloids. Synthesis, structure, and absolute configuration of 18'-epi-4'-deoxo-4'-epivinblastine, 18'-decarbomethoxy-18'-epi-4-epivinblastine, and 18'-epi-3',4'-dehydrovinblastine. Heterocycles 3, 205-212 (1975b)

Kutney, J.P., Gregonis, D.E., Imhof, R., Itoh, I., Jahngen, E., Scott, A.I., Chan, W.K.: Absolute stereochemistry of the bisindole alkaloids of the vinblastine type. Circular dichroism studies. J. Am. Chem. Soc. 97, 5013-5015 (1975c)

Kutney, J.P., Grierson, D.S.: Improved synthesis of the pyrido-carbazole indole alkaloid olivacine. Heterocycles 3, 171-177 (1975)

Kutney, J.P., Ratcliffe, A.H., Treasurywala, A.M., Wunderly, S.: Synthesis of bisindole alkaloids. II. Synthesis of 3'4'-dehydrovinblastine, 4'-deoxyvinblastine, and related analogs. Biogenetic approach. Heterocyles 3, 639-649 (1975d)

Langlois, Y., Langlois, N., Potier, P.: Application d'un schéma biogénétique en synthèse totale: l'ellipticine. Tetrahedron Lett. 955-958 (1975)

Langlois, N., Potier, P.: Hemisynthese de la leurosidine, alkaloide antitumoral isolé de *Catharanthus roseus* G. Don (Apocynacées) Tetrahedron Lett. 1099-1102 (1976)

Lee, K.-H., Cowherd, C.M., Wolo, M.T.: Antitumor agents XV: Deoxyelephantopin, an antitumor principle from *Elephantopus carolinianus* Willd. J. Pharm. Sci. 64, 1572-1573 (1975a)

Lee, K.-H., Ibuka, T., Huang, H.-C., Harris, D.L.: Antitumor agents XIV: Molephantinin, a new potent antitumor sesquiterpene lactone from *Elephantopus mollis*. J. Pharm. Sci. 64, 1077-1078 (1975b)

Lee, K.-H., Imakura, Y., Sims, D., McPhail, A.T., Onan, K.D.: Structure and stereochemistry of microlenin, a novel antitumor dimeric sesquiterpene lactone from *Helenium microcephalum*; X-Ray crystal structure. Chem. Commun. 341-342 (1976a)

Lee, K.-H., Kim, S.-H., Furukawa, H., Pianthdosi, C., Huang, E.-S.: Antitumor agents. II. Synthesis and cytotoxic activity of helenalin related derivatives. J. Med. Chem. 18, 59-63 (1975c)

Lee, L.-H., Kimura, T., Okamoto, M., Cowherd, C.M., McPhail, A.T., Onan, K.D.: The structure and stereochemistry of eupahyssopin, a new antitumor germacranolide from *Eupatorium hyssopifolium*. Tetrahedron Lett. 1051-1054 (1976b)

LePecq, J.B., Gosse, C., Dat-Xuong, N., Paoletti, C.: Two new antitumoral compounds: 9-hydroxy-2-methyl ellipticinium and 9-hydroxy-2,6-dimethyl ellipticinium. Action on L1210 mouse leukemia. C.R. Acad. Sci., Paris, Ser. D. 281, 1365-1367 (1975)

Li, S.-W., Dai, J.-Y.: A study on deoxyharringtonine and its analogs. Hua Hsueh Hsueh Pao 33, 75-78 (1975)

Maleev, A., Stoichkov, J., Todorov, D., Mikhalaeva, K., Mollov, N.M., Duchevska, Kh.: Antitumor effect of the alkaloid thalibalstine. Dokl. Bolg. Akad. Nauk 28, 713-715 (1975). Through Chem. Abstr. 83. 172576x

Messmer, W.M., Tin-Wa, M., Fong, H.H.S., Bevelle, C., Farnsworth, N.R., Abraham, D.J., Trojánek, J.: Fargaronine, a new tumor inhibitor isolated from *Fagara zanthoxyloides* Lam. (Rutaceae). J. Pharm. Sci. 61, 1858 (1972)

Meyers, A.I., Brinkmeyer, R.S.: Progress toward the total synthesis of maytansine. A model system containing the C-7 to C-16 moiety (southern and eastern zone). Tetrahedron Lett. 1749-1752 (1975)

Meyers, A.I., Horne, D., Shaw, C.C., Trefonas, L.M., Majeste, R.J.: Progress toward the total synthesis of maytansine. A stereoselective synthesis of the C-1 to C-7 moiety (northern zone). Tetrahedron Lett. 1745-1748 (1975)

Meyers, A.I., Shaw, C.-C.: Studies directed toward the total synthesis of maytansine. The preparation and properties of the carbinolamide moiety. Tetrahedron Lett. 717-720 (1974)

Mikolajczak, K.L., Powell, R.G., Smith, C.R., Jr.: Deoxyharringtonine, a new antitumor alkaloid from *Cephalotaxus*: structure and synthetic studies. Tetrahedron Lett. 28, 1995-2001 (1972)

Mikolajczak, K.L., Powell, R.G., Smith, C.R., Jr.: Preparation and antitumor activity of a rearranged ester of cephalotaxine. J. Med. Chem. 18, 63-66 (1975)

Mikolajczak, K.L., Smith, C.R., Jr., Powell, R.G.: Partial synthesis of harringtonine analogs. J. Pharm. Sci. 63, 1280-1283 (1974a)

Mikolajczak, K.L., Smith, C.R., Jr., Weisleder, D., Kelly, T.R., McKenna, J.C., Christenson, P.A.: Synthesis of Deoxyharringtonine. Tetrahedron Lett. 283-286 (1974b)

Moertel, C.G., Schutt, A.J., Hahn, R.G., Reitemeier, R.J.: Treatment of advanced gastrointestinal cancer with emetine (NSC-33669). Cancer Chemother. Rep., Pt. 1 58, 229-232 (1974)

Mohn, K.W., Waring, M.J., Glaubiger, D., Friedman, C.A.: Intercalative binding of ellipticine to DNA. Cancer Res. 35, 71-76 (1975)

Neuss, N., Mallett, G.E., Brannon, D.R., Mabe, J.A., Horton, H.R., Huckstep, L.L.: *Vinca* Alkaloids. XXXIII. Microbiological conversions of vincaleukoblastine, an antitumor alkaloid from *Vinca rosea*. L. Helv. Chim. Acta 57, 1886-1890 (1974)

Ninomiya, I., Naito, T., Ishii, H.: Synthesis of N-demethylfagaronine, Heterocyles 3, 307-309 (1975a)

Ninomiya, I., Naito, T., Ishii, H., Ishida, T., Ueda, M., Harada, K.: Syntheses of dihydroderivatives of the benzo[c]phenanthridine alkaloids avicine and nitidine by enamide photocyclization. J. Chem. Soc. Perkin Trans. 1, 762-764 (1975b)

O'Connor, T.E., Aldrich, C., Haddi, A., Lomax, N., Okano, P., Sethi, S., Wood, H.B.: Proc. 66th Ann. Mett. Am. Assoc. Cancer Res. 16, 29 (1975)

Oda, K., Ichihara, A., Sakamura, S.: Total synthesis of DL-crotepoxide. Tetrahedron Lett. 3187-3190 (1975)

Ogura, M., Cordell, G.A., Farnsworth, N.R.: Potential Anticancer agents. III. Jacaranone, a novel phytoquinoid from *Jacaranda caucana*. Lloydia 39, 255-257 (1976)

Parry, R.J., Schwab, J.M.: Biosynthesis of *Cephalotaxus* alkaloids. I. Novel mode of tyrosine incorporation into cephalotaxine. J. Am. Chem. Soc. 97, 2555-2557 (1975)

Petlichnaya, L.I., Turkevich, N.M.: Some thiophosphamide derivatives of berberine and their interaction with hydrogen chloride. Farm. Zh. (Kiev) 30, 40-43 (1975)

Pettit, G.R., Budzinski, J.C., Cragg, G.M., Brown, P., Johnston, L.D.: Antineoplastic agents 34. *Helenium autumnale* L. J. Med. Chem. 17, 1013-1016 (1974)

Pettit, G.R., Herald, C.L., Judd, G.F., Bolliger, G., Thayer, P.S.: Antineoplastic and cytotoxic components of desert *Baileya*. J. Pharm. Sci. 64, 2023-2024 (1975)

Polonsky, J.: Quassinoid bitter principles. Fortschr. Chem. Org. Naturst. 30, 101-150 (1973)

Potier, P., Langlois, N., Langlos, Y., Gueritte, F.: Partial synthesis of vinblastine-type alkaloids. J. Chem. Soc. Chem. Commun. 670-671 (1975)

Powell, R.G., Weisleder, D., Smith, C.R., Jr.: Antitumor alkaloids from *Cephalotaxus harringtonia*: structure and activity. J. Pharm. Sci. 61, 1227-1230 (1972)

Quick, A., Rogers, D.: Crystal and molecular structure of parthenolide. J. Chem. Soc. Perkin Trans. 2, 465-469 (1976)

Regina, M., Sampaio, P., De Oliveira, M.M., Gilbert, B.: Antineoplastic activity of olivacine. Cien. Cult. (Sao Paulo) 26, 517 (1974)

Remillard, S., Rebun, L.I., Howe, G.A., Kupchan, S.M.: Antimitotic activity of the potent tumor inhibitor maytansine. Science 189, 1002-1004 (1975)

Richman, J.E.: Total synthesis of camptothecine. Diss. Abstr. Int. 36B, 243 (1975)

Sawa, Y., Ikegawa, T.: 2,3-Substituted-9-hydroxy-10-methoxy-berberinium phosphates. Japan Pat. 75,19,914 (1975). Through Chem. Abstr. 83. 114717h

Schaeppi, U., Fleischman, R.W., Cooney, D.A.: Toxicity of camptothecine (NSC-100880). Cancer Chemother. Rep. Pt. 3 5, 25-36 (1974)

Schultz, A.G.: Camptothecin. Chem. Rev. 73, 385-405 (1973)

Semmelhack, M.F., Chong, B.P., Jones. L.D.: Total synthesis of *Cephalotanus* alkaloids. J. Am. Chem. Soc. 94, 8629-8630 (1972)

Semmelhack, M.F., Chong, B.P., Stauffer, R.D., Rogerson, T.D., Chong, A., Jones, L.D.: Total synthesis of the *Cephalotaxus* alkaloids. A problem in nucleophilic aromatic substitution. J. Am. Chem. Soc. 97, 2507-2516 (1975)

Semmelhack, M.F., Stauffer, R.D., Rogerson, T.D.: Nucleophilic aromatic substition via a new nickel-catalyzed process and via the $S_{RN}1$ reaction. Improved synthesis of cephalotaxinone. Tetrahedron Lett. 4519-4522 (1973)

Sethi, V.S., Sethi, M.L.: Inhibition of reverse transcripterase activity of RNA-tumor viruses by fagaronine. Biochem. Biophys. Res. Commun. 63, 1070-1076 (1975)

Shamma, M., Georgiev, V.St.: Camptothecine. J. Pharm. Sci. 63, 163-183 (1974)

Siddiqui, S., Firat, D., Olshin, S.: Phase II study of emetine (NSC-33669) in the treatment of solid tumors. Cancer Chemother. Rep., Pt. 1 57, 423-428 (1973)

Strauch, R., Hiller, K.: Cancerostatisch wirksame Naturstoffe. Pharmazie 29, 656-670 (1974)

Sugasawa, T., Toyoda, T., Sasakura, K.: Camptothecine. Japan. Koaki 74,117,499 (1974). Through Chem. Abst. 82. 125513u

Takahashi, S.: The presence of the tumor inhibitor crotepoxide (futoxide) in *Piper futokadzura*. Phytochemistry 8, 321-322 (1969)

Tang, C.S.F., Morrow, C.J., Rapoport, H.: A total synthesis of dl-camptothecine. J. Am. Chem. Soc. 97, 159-167 (1975)

Tin-Wa, M., Bell, C.L., Bevelle, C., Fong, H.H.S., Farnsworth, N.R.: Potential anticancer agents I: Confirming evidence for the structure of fagaronine. J. Pharm. Sci. 63, 1476-1477 (1974)

Tobinaga, S.: Cryptopleurine. Japan. Koaki Patent 75,59,398 (1975). Through Chem. Abstr. 83, 131809g

Todorov, D., Damyanova, M.: Acute toxicity of the antitumor alkaloid thaliblastine. Dokl. Bolg. Akad. Nauk 28, 709-711 (1975)

Torrance, S.J., Wiedhopf, R.M., Cole, J.R.: Ambrosin, tumor inhibitory agent from *Hymenoclea salsola* (Asteraceae). J. Pharm. Sci. 64, 887-888 (1975)

Toubiana, R., Mompon, B., Ho, C.M., Toubiana, M.-J.: Isolement du vernodalin et du vernolepin a partir de *Vernonia guineensis*: authenticite du squellette elemane. Phytochemistry 14, 775-778 (1975)

Truhaut, R., Dophuoc, H., Cao, T.D., Gak, J.-C., Jacquignon, P., Ba, G.N.: Inhibitory effect of ellipticine on the cancerization of the rat liver induced by BT6: its incidence on the levels of cytochrome P450 and on arginase activity. C. R. Acad. Sci., Paris, Ser. D. 282, 1219-1224 (1976)

Walraven, H.G.M., Pandit, U.K.: A facile two synthon approach to deethyldeoxycamptothecine. Tetrahedron Lett. 4507-4510 (1975)

Wani, M.C., Taylor, H.L., Wall, M.E.: Plant antitumor agents: colubrinol acetate and colubrinol, antileukemic ansa macrolides from *Colubrina texensis*. J. Chem. Soc., Chem. Commun. 390 (1973)

Weinreb, S.M., Auerbach, J.: Total synthesis of the *Cephalotaxus* Alkaloids. Cephalotaxine, cephaloxtaxinone and demethycephalotaxinone. J. Am. Chem. Soc. 97, 2503-2506 (1975)

Weinreb, S.M., Semmelhack, M.F.: Synthesis of the *Cephalotaxus* alkaloids. Acc. Chem. Res. 8, 158-164 (1975)

Weiss, S.G., Tin-Wa, M., Perdue, R.E., Jr., Farnsworth, N.R.: Potential anticancer agents. II.: Antitumor and cytotoxic lignans from *Linum album* (Linaceae). J. Pharm. Sci. 64, 95-98 (1975)

Winterfeldt, E.: Approaches to camptothecine. Recent Dev. Chem. Nat. Carbon Compd. 6, 9-34 (1975)

Wolpert-Defilippes, M.K., Adamson, R.H., Cysyk, R.L., Johns, D.G.: Initial studies on the cytotoxic action of maytansine, a novel ansa macrolide. Biochem. Pharmaco. 24, 751-754 (1975)

Recent Advances in the Field of Antibiotics

CH. TAMM

A. Introduction

Antibiotics are secondary metabolites of microorganisms. Therefore, they are defined as compounds which are not involved in the growth of the producing microorganisms. They take part neither in the formation of cell walls nor contribute to the energy balance of the organism. One can designate an antibiotic as a secondary microbial metabolite which is capable of inhibiting the growth of another microorganism or even destroying it (cf. Waksman, 1945). The discovery of the penicillins and shortly thereafter the streptomycins, before and during the second world war, initiated the aera of "chemical microbiology" and, as a logical consequence, the development of the new field of "microbial technology." As a result of worldwide efforts on both basic research and technical development a great variety of new substances have been produced, which proved useful for human and veterinary medicine. For details reference is made to some selected monographs which describe the development of the past decade (Evans, 1965; Vaněk and Hošťálek, 1965; Korzybski et al., 1967; Gottlieb and Shaw, 1967a,b; Kadis et al., 1971a,b,c; Reiner, 1974; Corcoran and Hahn, 1975).

I am trying to review and to analyze the present situation of this important field of natural product and bioorganic chemistry. The origin of the secondary microbial metabolites is summarized very briefly in Table 1.

Table 1. Origin of secondary microbial metabolites

1. Bacteria
   - Eubacteriales
     - *Bacillus*
     - *Pseudomonas*
   - Actinomycetales
     - *Streptomyces*
     - *Nocardia*
2. Fungi imperfecti
   - *Aspergillus*
   - *Cephalosporium*
   - *Penicillium*
   - *Fusarium*
3. Basidiomycetes and ascomycetes

Some of the numerous secondary metabolites isolated exhibit interesting biological activities. These activities can be classified roughly as shown in Table 2.

Table 2. Biological activity of secondary microbial metabolites

Antibacterial	(Gram-positive, Gram-negative)
Antifungal	
Antiviral	(Plant and animal viruses)
Protozoa	
Cytostatic	
Other toxic and pharmacological effects	

The secondary microbial metabolites do not belong to a single specific class of chemical compounds. On the contrary, they are characterized by the enormous variety of chemical structures encountered, a fact which is most attractive for chemical research because they very often are unusual. However, a crude classification of the microbial metabolites has become possible on the basis of their biogenetic origin. Three major classes are recognized. First, there are compounds, which are derived from acetyl- and or propionyl-coenzyme A. Although compounds, which are designated as isoprenoids, are derived from acetyl-coenzyme as well, they are treated separately because of their specific features. They are found in the second class. The third group contains substances, which originate from amino acids. This classification refers to the main structural features of the mould metabolite, but overlapping occurs quite frequently. Finally, some of the compounds, which are clearly of mixed biogenetic origin, are classified in the fourth group. The classes are listed in Table 3, which in addition, provides further subdivisions and selected examples.

In order to demonstrate recent advances in the field, some selected examples of each class of compounds will be discussed including some results of our own investigations[1]. Each example is used to demonstrate a different new aspect, such as

1. Novel chemical structures with special emphasis on stereochemical principles, and their elucidation by new chemical and physical methods
2. Interesting biological activities
3. Structure-activity relationships
4. Biosynthetic studies

B. Acetate/Propionate-Derived Metabolites

I. Tetracyclines

A relatively "old" group of useful acetate derived antibiotics are the tetracyclines (cf. Dürckheimer, 1975).

As shown in Figure 1, four natural compounds are known, aureomycin isolated 1948 from cultures of *Streptomyces aureofaciens*, terramcycin isolated two years later from *Streptomyces rimosus*, tetracyclin, which

---

[1]The bibliography does not contain a complete list of the original papers. Emphasis is put on the citation of more recent reviews, articles containing leading references and papers reporting very recent results.

Table 3. Classification of secondary microbial metabolites by biogenetic origin

1. Acetate/propionate	
Polyenes, polyines	Amphothericin B
Condensed ring systems	Tetracycline Daunomycin Aflatoxin
Macrolides	Erythromycin Cytochalasin
Polyethers	Nigericin
Macrotetrolides	Nonactin
Nonadrides	Rubratoxin
Ansamycins	Rifamycin
Mixed type	Pseurotin
2. Isoprenoids	
Sesquiterpenes	Trichothecin Verrucarin Roridin
Diterpenes	Gibberellin
Sesterterpenes	Ophiobolin Fusicoccin
Triterpenes/steroids	Ergosterol Fusidic acid
3. Amino acids	
One amino acid	Cycloserine Chloramphenicol
Several amino acids	Penicillin Cephalosporin
Polypeptides	Bacitracin Gramicidin Cyclosporin
4. Mixed precursors	
Aminoglycosides	Streptomycin Kanamycin
Nucleosides	Puromycin

was prepared from aureomycin by catalytic hydrogenation before it was recognized also as natural product, and desmethylchlorotetracyclin. The latter compound was produced by a mutant of *S. aureofaciens* in 1957. Typical for the tetracyclines is their chemical polyfunctionality. Two chromophoric systems are present which are separated by the 12a-hydroxyl group. Many interesting derivatives have been prepared, which have yielded for instance vibramycin. Useful compounds were prepared by the Mannich aminoalkylation of the carboxamido group. The structures are shown in Figure 1.

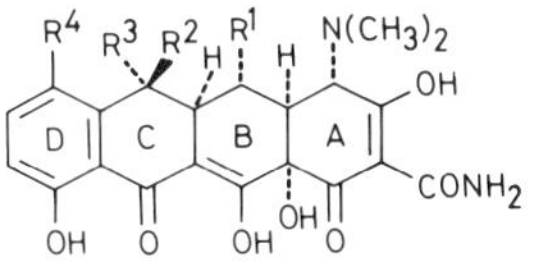

	R^1	R^2	R^3	R^4	
1. Natural antibiotics	H	OH	CH_3	Cl	: Aureomycin
	OH	OH	CH_3	H	: Terramycin
	H	OH	CH_3	H	: Tetracyclin (Achromycin)
	H	OH	H	Cl	: Desmethylchlortetracyclin (Ledermycin)
2. Modified antibiotics (Selected examples)	OH	H	CH_3	H	: Vibramycin
3. Synthetic compounds	H	H	H	H	: 6-Desmethyl-6-desoxytetracyclin

Fig. 1. Tetracyclines: structural types

The manifold structural modifications of tetracyclines have led to a relatively clear understanding of the relationship between chemical structure and biological activity. The results of these studies were compounds possessing better solubility and stability, with faster and more complete resorption, higher antibacterial activity but change of the basic bacteriostatic pattern. However, no extension of the activity spectrum has been achieved. The problem of resistance remains unsolved. Figure 2 summarizes the structural requirements for full biological activity. It also shows which structural modifications are allowed without concurrent loss of activity.

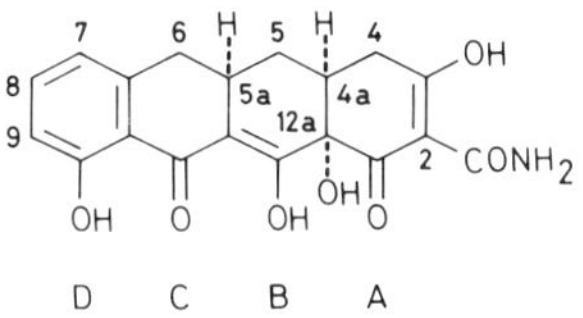

Requirements: Tetracyclin skeleton with chromophoric keto-enol-system of A and B/C/D

Basic group in A

Configuration of C-4; C-4a; C-12a

Modifications: Configuration of C-5; C-5a; C-6

$2\text{-}CON(CH_3)_2$

$4\text{-}NH_2$

C-5 to C-9 (hydrophobic), especially of C-6 and C-7

Fig. 2. Tetracyclines: structure-activity

The mode of action of the tetracyclines is known; they are inhibitors of the protein synthesis. However, the exact molecular mechanism is still uncertain.

II. Anthracyclines

Closely related to the tetracyclines are the anthracyclines.

They are derivatives of a hydroxylated anthraquinone system with an additional cyclohexane ring, fused in a linear manner to the tricyclic skeleton. One of the hydroxyl groups of the cyclohexane ring forms a glycosidic linkage to the new sugar daunosamine. Figure 3 represents the structural formulae of carminomycin, daunomycin and adriamycin,

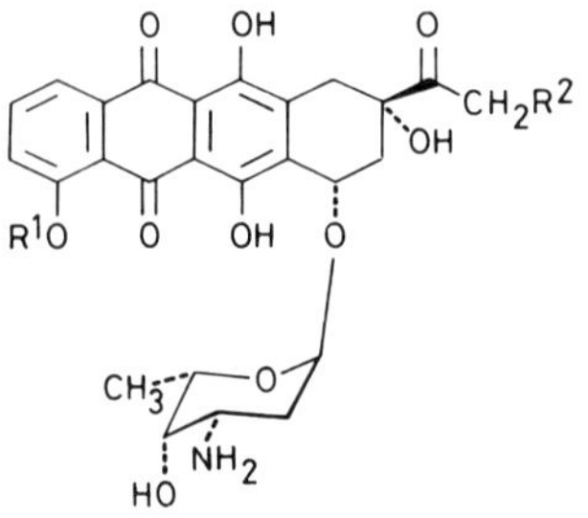

$R^1 = R^2 = H$: Carminomycin

$R^1 = CH_3$; $R^2 = H$: Daunomycin (Daunorubicin)

$R^1 = CH_2$; $R^2 = OH$: Adriamycin (Doxorubicin)

Fig. 3. Other tetracyclines

which are the three known examples of this class. Adriamycin has recently received much attention because of its clinical effectiveness against leukemia, breast cancer, cancer of the bladder, lung and thyroid. N-trifluoroacetyl-adriamycin-14-valerate is reported to be even more specific and faster for the treatment of leukemias and solid tumors. A synthesis of daunorubicin (Wong et al., 1973) and effective total syntheses of the aglycones (+)-daunomycinone and (+)-carminomycinone (Kende et al., 1976; Smith et al., 1976) have been reported.

III. Aflatoxins

The aflatoxins and sterigmatocystins (cf. Roberts, 1974) represent a further group of mould metabolites of the polyketide type.

They belong to the mycotoxins. Mycotoxicosis can be defined as poisoning man or animals by ingestion of foodstuffs contaminated with certain moulds and/or with their metabolic products (mycotoxins). The aflatoxins have been discovered in connection with the turkey X disease in England in the latter part of 1960. It is a mycotoxicosis by ingestion of peanut meal, which is infected by the mould *Aspergillus flavus*. At present, eight aflatoxins are known. Chemically, they are characterized by a bisfurane system which is attached to a coumarin moiety. Aflatoxin B_1, whose structure is shown in Figure 4, is the most active and most toxic member of the family. It is a potent

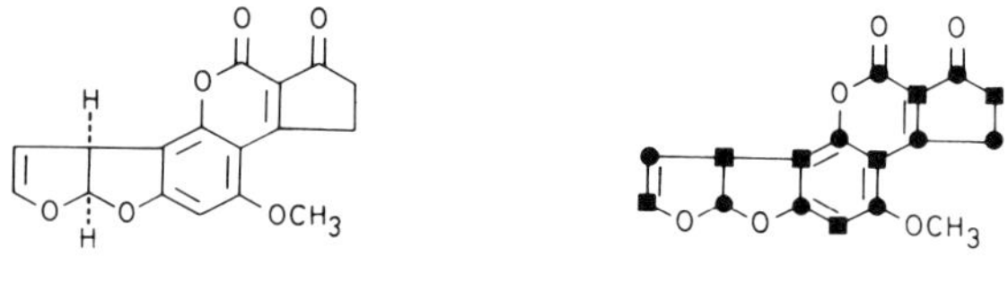

Aflatoxin B_1
(Aspergillus flavus)

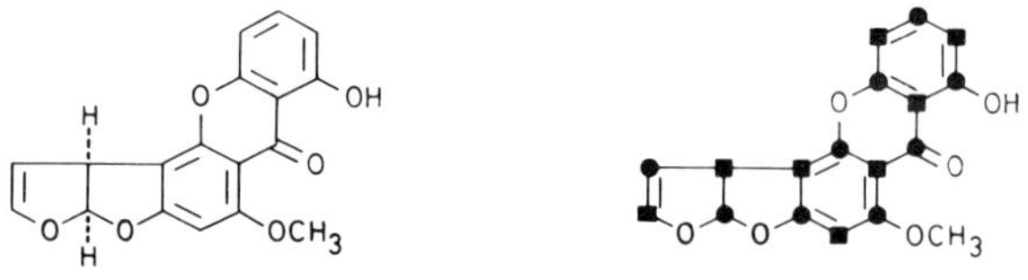

Sterigmatocystin
(Aspergillus versicolor)

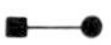

CH_3-COOH

Fig. 4. Aflatoxins and sterigmatocystins

hepatocarcinogen. Incorporation experiments with ^{13}C- and ^{14}C-labeled acetate as precursors established a C_{20}-polyketide as biogenetic intermediate. The distribution pattern of the incorporated acetate units as determined by degradation of the radioactive specimens and by ^{13}C-NMR-spectroscopy is demonstrated in Figure 4 (cf. Pachler et al., 1976). An analogous alternative distribution of the acetate units has been demonstrated also for the closely related sterigmatocystin (cf. Pachler et al., 1976), which has been isolated from *Aspergillus versicolor*.

IV. Macrolides

So far condensed ring systems have been discussed.

But a variety of interesting macrocyclic acetate/propionate derived secondary metabolites have been isolated from various microbial sources. In the first place the macrocyclic lactones or macrolide *antibiotics* (cf. Keller-Schierlein, 1973) should be mentioned. The macrocyclic ring system contains either a polyene system, which is derived from acetate units, or oxygen functions often combined with methyl groups. The latter usually originate from the incorporation of propionate units. Some of the hydroxyl groups are used to form glycosidic linkages with sugar units. Most of these carbohydrates had been unknown before. Typical examples of macrolide antibiotics are the erythromycins. The structures of the naturally occurring substances are shown in Figure 5. They consist of a multibranched,

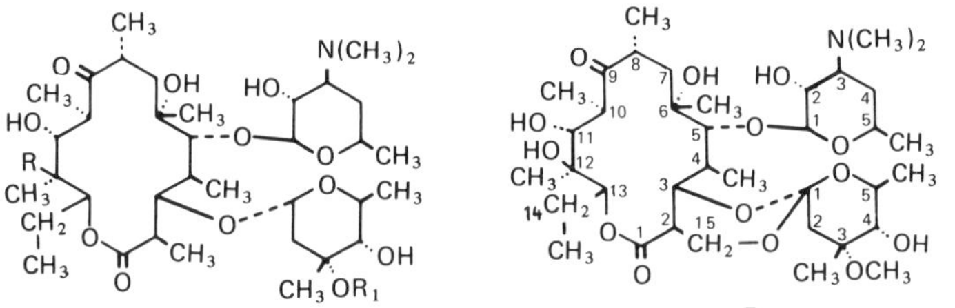

5

	R	R_1
1	OH	CH_3
2	H	CH_3
3	OH	H
4	H	H

Fig. 5. Erythromycins

polyfunctional, 14-membered lactone ring to which the amino sugar desosamine and the nitrogen-free 6-deoxy sugar cladinose are attached by a glycosidic linkage. The erythromycins are mentioned not only because they are of medicinal importance but because one of them, compound 5 (erythromycin E), is the first example of a macrolide having a sugar attached via an ortho ester linkage (Martin et al., 1975). Erythromycin E is formed from erythromycin A (compound 1). The latter is slowly metabolized to compound 5 when incubated with fermentations of certain strains of the producting organism *Streptomyces eryhtreus*. By the isolation of erythromycin E it has been possible to extend and to delineate the later stages of the erythromycin biogenetic pathway. Accordingly, the aglycone erythronolide is synthesized at first. The next step is the attachment of mycarose, followed by the formation of a glycosidic linkage with desosamine. Hydroxylation leads to erythromycin A, which finally is transformed to erythromycin E.

The first total synthesis of a macrolide antibiotic, methymycin, was reported in 1975 (Masamune et al., 1975a,b). The total synthesis of an erythromycin antibiotic has not been achieved yet. The conformational flexibility of erythronolide B, the 14-membered aglycone of the erythromycins has been studied by ^{1}H-NMR-spectroscopy, circular dichroism (Egan et al., 1975) and by ^{13}C-NMR-spectra (Nourse and Roberts, 1975).

V. Cytochalasans

The cytochalasans represent a novel type of mould metabolites of the macrolide series.

The isolation of these compounds resulted from the observation that culture filtrates of certain microorganisms produced morphological changes in the hyphae of test fungi and unusual effects in mammalian cells in tissue cultures. Reversible inhibition of cytoplasmic cleavage resulting in polynucleate cells, inhibition of cell movement, and nuclear extrusion are among a few of the most striking characteristics (Rothweiler and Tamm, 1966; Carter, 1967, 1972). The twenty-two known cytochalasans (phomins, cytochalasins, zygosporins, chaetoglobosins; cf. Fig. 6) are characterized by a highly substitued hydrogenated isoindole group, of known absolute configuration, to

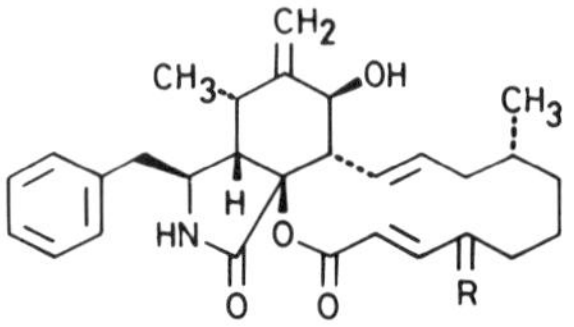

R = O : Cytochalasin A (20-Dehydrophomin)

R = <(OH, H) : Cytochalasin B (Phomin)

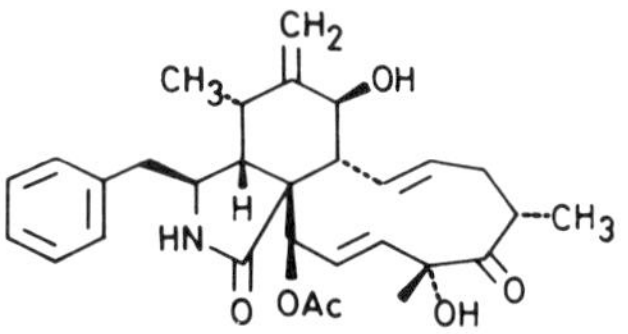

Cytochalasin D (Zygosporin A)

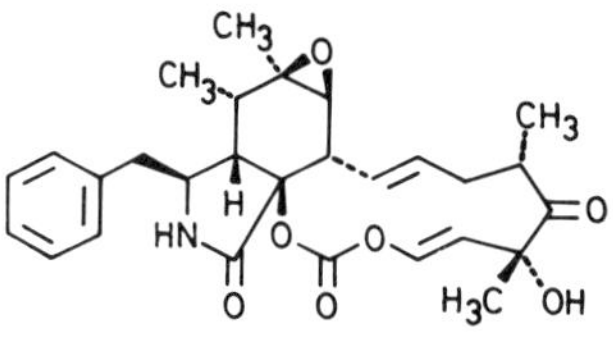

Cytochalasin E

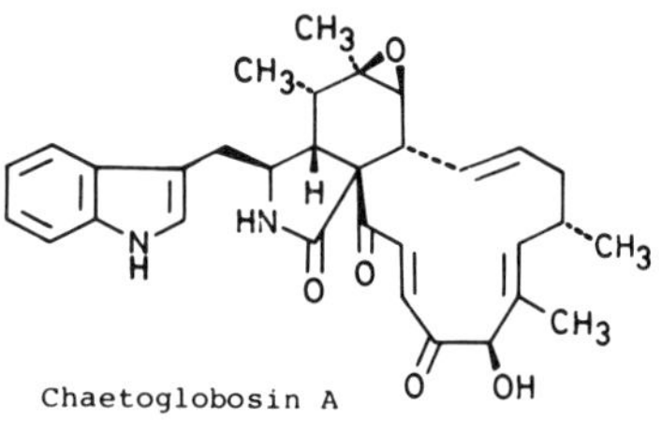

Chaetoglobosin A

Fig. 6. Cytochalasans (phomins, cytochalasins, zygosporins, chaetoglobosins)

which is fused a macrocyclic ring, which is either carbocyclic [e.g. cytochalasin D (zygosporin A)], a lactone [e.g. cytochalasin A (20-dehydrophomin), cytochalasin B (phomin)], or a cyclic carbonate (cytochalasin E) (cf. Binder and Tamm, 1973a; Binder et al., 1973). In 1973 the chaetoglobosins (e.g. chaetoglobosin A), a novel group of cytochalasans containing an indole in the place of the phenyl group, were discovered (Sekita et al., 1973, 1976; Silverton et al., 1976).

The relative and absolute configuration of cytochalasins B and D being established, a study of the biosynthesis of these two representative members of the family was undertaken in our laboratoy. Incorporation experiments with biogenetic precursors radioactively labeled (^{3}H, ^{14}C) or labeled with radioinactive isotopes (^{13}C, ^{15}N) have demonstrated that cytochalasin B (phomin) is formed from one unit of phenylalanine, two C_1-units from the methyl of methionine and nine acetate units (Binder et al., 1970; Graf et al., 1974). The biosynthesis of cytochalasin D involves connection of phenylalanine, three units of methionine and nine acetate entities (Lebet and Tamm, 1974; Graf et al., 1974; Vederas et al., 1975). The incorporation and distribution pattern of the precursors in the mould metabolite was determined by degradation of the radioactive specimens or by partially relaxed Fouriertransform (PRFT)-^{13}C-NMR spectroscopy. The results for cytochalasin D are shown by Figure 7. Analogous distributions were

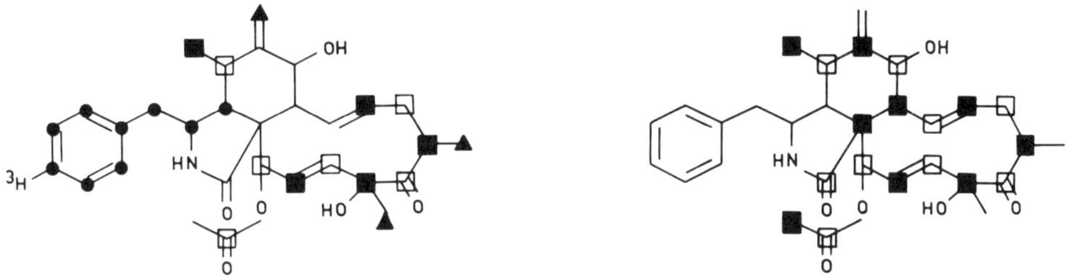

□ = [1-^{14}C]-Acetate; [2-^{14}C]-Propionate
■ = [2-^{14}C]-Acetate
▲ = [CH_3-^{14}C]-L-Methionine
● = [4'-^{3}H][U-^{14}C]-L-Phenylalanine

[1-^{14}C]-Malonate	:	±
[1-^{14}C]-Diethyl Malonate	:	+
[2-^{14}C]-Malonate	:	±
[1-^{14}C]-Propionate	:	±
[1-^{14}C]-Butyrate	:	+
[1-^{14}C]-Myristate	:	+
[1-^{14}C]-Palmitate	:	±
[1-^{14}C]-Formate	:	-

□ = [1-^{13}C]-Acetate } [1,2-^{13}C]-Acetate
■ = [2-^{13}C]-Acetate }

[1-^{13}C]-Propionate	:	+	(Lactam)
[1-^{13}C]-Myristate	:	+	(as Acetate)
[1-^{13}C]-Palmitate	:	+	(as Acetate)

Fig. 7. Atoms in cytochalasin D detected by degradation of ^{14}C- and ^{3}H-labeled specimens and by PRFT-^{13}C-NMR-spectroscopy

determined for cytochalasin B. As shown by ^{13}C-NMR-spectroscopy of specimens obtained after administration of [1,2-^{13}C]-acetate, intact acetate entities are coupled in a head to tail fashion as normally observed in polyketide biogenesis (Vederas et al., 1975). These findings correspond to a combination according to scheme A, cf. Figure 8, and preclude combinations B and C. Figure 8 also shows how the precursors are assembled in order to form cytochalasin D. Analogous results were obtained for cytochalasin B. The mode of incorporation of phenylalanine into cytochalasin D was examined in detail by Vederas and Tamm (1976) because L-phenylalanine (2S-configuration) and the D,L-amino acids appeared to be equally good precursors although cytochalasin D possesses the (S)-configuration at the corresponding

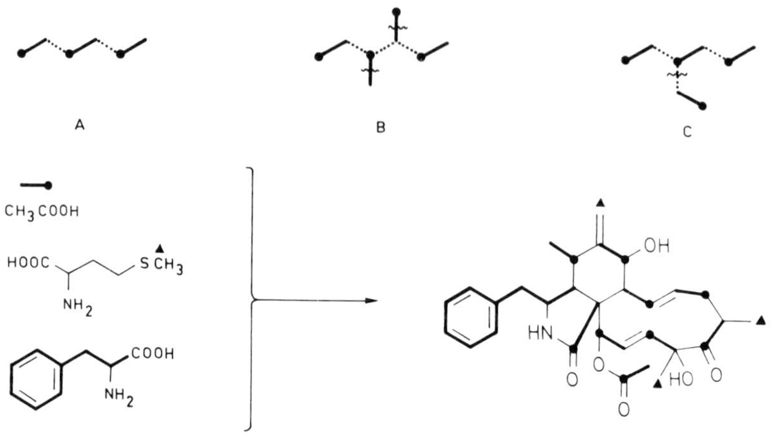

Fig. 8. Assembly of the building blocs in cytochalasin D

C-atom. Rapid equilibration of D- and L-phenylalanine with phenylpyruvic acid was shown to be an explanation for these observations (cf. Fig. 9). Transamination of phenylalanines stereospecifically labeled with tritium at C-2 and C-3 proceeded with complete loss of hydrogen at the α-position and extensive loss at the β-position. Con-

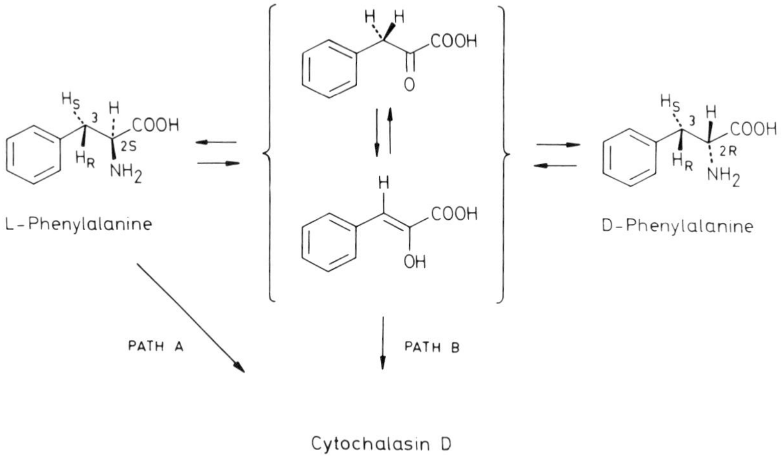

Fig. 9. Mode of incorporation of phenylalanine into cytochalasin D

siderable suppression of the incorporation of the D-amino acid by phenylpyruvic acid indicated that L-enantiomer is the primary precursor of cytochalasin D. Thus, path A is probably the main biosynthetic route, and not path B.

The results of the incorporation experiments carried out with cytochalasin B and D, the isolation of the minor metabolites deoxaphomin, proxiphomin and protophomin by Binder and Tamm (1973b,c), and the incorporation of deoxaphomin into cytochalasin B (phomin) demonstrating the latter compound being an immediate biogenetic precursor of cytochalasin B (Robert and Tamm, 1975), allowed to propose a general scheme of the biosynthesis of cytochalasans as shown in Figure 10.

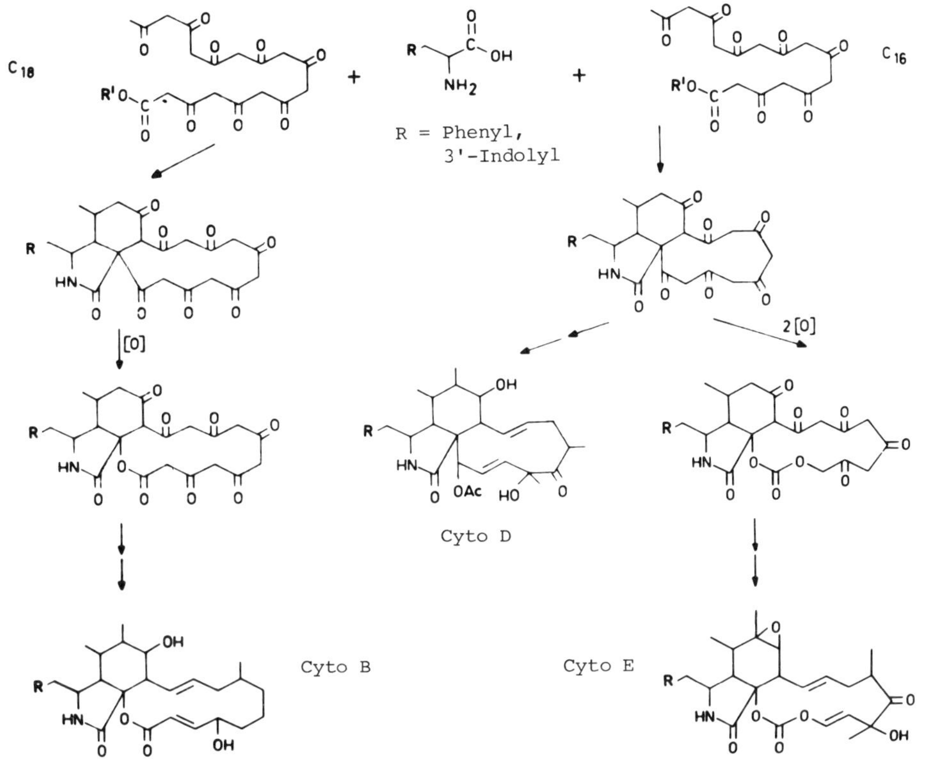

Fig. 10. Scheme of the biogenesis of cytochalasans

The amide linkage of an octa- or nonaketide to phenylalanine or tryptophane is regarded as the initial step. Subsequent condensations with partial reductions and water elimination lead, via a tetramic acid derivative and bicyclic intermediates, to the tricyclic systems which are carbocyclic. After structural modifications (introduction of the C_1-units, reductions, oxidations), a Baeyer-Villiger oxidation converts the carbocyclic intermediate to the lactone system (e.g. cytochalasin B). The carbonate group of cytochalasin E would result from a second insertion of oxygen into a lactone ring. It is obvious that a lot of work has still to be carried out for the verification of the hypothetical scheme of the biogenesis. In conclusion, the cytochalasins represent also from a chemical and biosynthetic point of view a most fascinating class of natural products.

VI. Polyethers

During the past years the polyethers have been isolated as a new type of mould metabolites from streptomyces species.

They exhibit most remarkable ionophoric properties, i.e. they form neutral complexes with monovalent cations such as sodium ions. The polyethers are monocarboxylic acids, which, biogenetically, are formed from acetate and propionate units. It is interesting to note that very soon after the discovery of the natural polyethers the first synthetic crown ethers have been prepared by Pedersen in 1967. The latter were shown to dissolve sodium ions by complexation. The first natural polyether is monensin (cf. Fig. 11). Today it is used as food

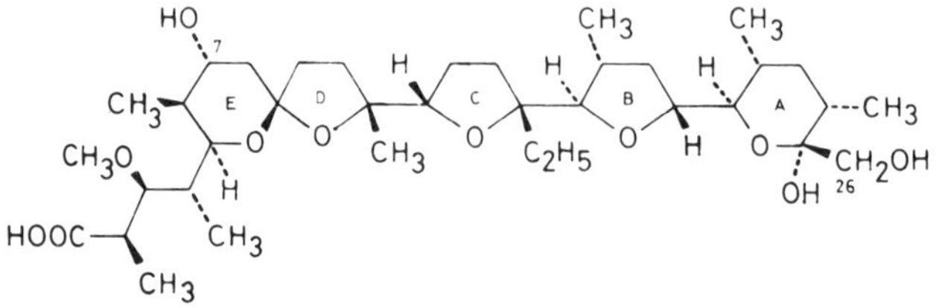

Monensin

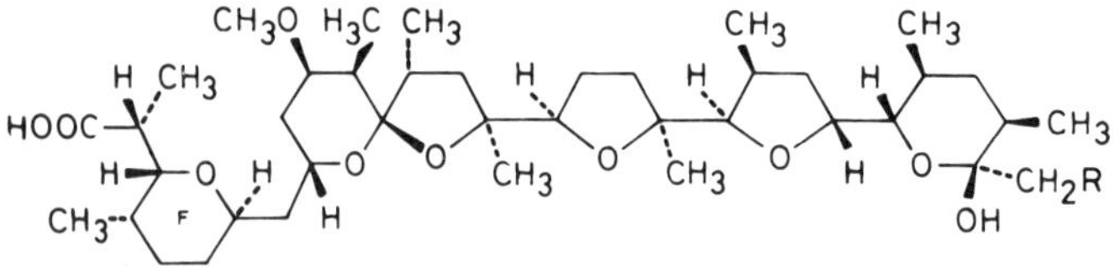

R = OH : Nigericin
R = H : Grisorixin

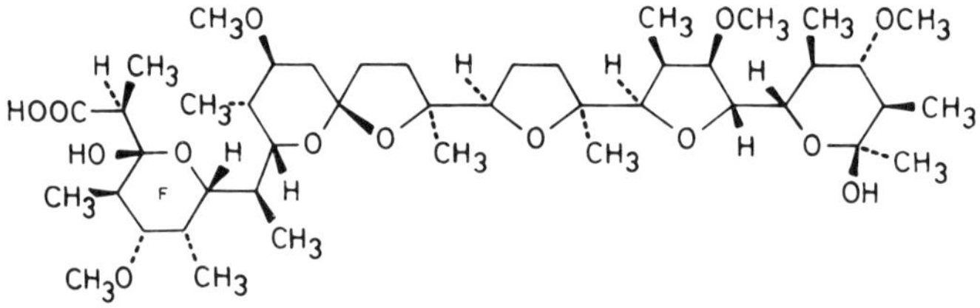

Lonomycin = Emericid = Antibiotic DE-3936

Fig. 11. Polyethers

supplement for poultry as prophylaxis of chicken coccidiosis. The compound is too toxic for humans. Monensin as well as nigericin reverse the action of nonactin and valinomycin. Other examples for polyethers are grisorixin, salinomycin and septamycin. Recently in several laboratories compounds were isolated from *Streptomyces hygroscopicus*, i.e. lonomycin, emericid and antibiotic DE-3936, which proved to be identical. The first polyether possessing an aromatic ring is lasalocid. It binds mono- and divalent cations. It is used as food additive (cf. Schmidt et al., 1974). A numbering system for polyether antibiotics has been proposed (Westley, 1976).

VII. Macrotetrolides

A group of cyclic esters possessing tetrahydrofuraning has been discovered during the last decade, which were named as macrotetrolides (cf. Keller-Schierlein and Gerlach, 1968).

The compounds are most remarkable not only for their antibacterial and cytostatic activity and for their ionophoric properties but also for their stereochemistry. For instance nonactin, which enhances the potassium ion transport through membranes, as valinomycin, is optically inactive although it contains sixteen chiral carbon atoms. The hydrolysis yields four equivalents of nonactinic acid, a C_{10}-hydroxycarboxylic acid. Also the mixture does not exhibit any optical activity. The following four structural possibilities, which are shown schematically in Figure 12, can account for these findings:

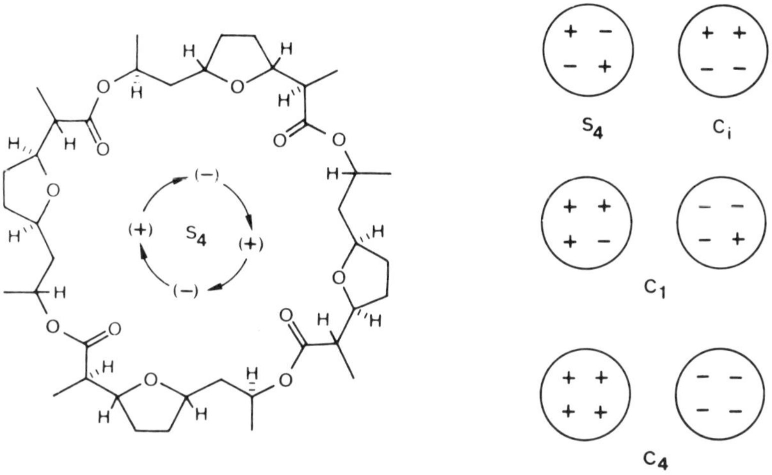

Fig. 12. Macrotetrolides

(1) Structure with S_4-symmetry possesses a fourfold rotatory axis. The result is a reflexion symmetric configuration; (2) Meso-form with a centre of symmetry C_i; (3) Racemate with C_1-symmetry; (4) Racemate with C_4-symmetry. It was shown by total synthesis that nonactin possesses S_4-symmetry (Gerlach et al., 1975; Schmidt et al., 1976). The homologous antibiotic, monactin, presents an additional stereochemical aspect, cyclodiastereoisomerism, which has to be taken in account.

VIII. Nonadrides

A nine-membered ring, which is constructed by two maleic acid anhydride moieties, is found in the nonadrides, a group consisting of seven known mould metabolites (cf. Sutherland, 1967).

The most interesting compound is rubratoxin B, a toxin isolated from *Penicillium rubrum*, which causes animal disease by meal infected by this mould. The structures of the rubratoxins and the related glauconic and byssochlamic acids are shown in Figure 13. The biogenetic precursors of glauconic and byssochlamic acid are six acetate/malonate units and two oxaloacetate units, which are coupled to form a derivative of maleic acid anhydride. The two latter combine either in a head to head or a head to tail fashion. In own experiments, which were designed to elucidate the biosynthesis of the rubratoxins the incorporation of acetate, malonate and of radioactive 2-(E)-(1'-octenyl)-3-methyl-maleinate was observed. These results seem to indicate a head to tail combination of the two units as anticipated (Senn and Tamm, unpubl.).

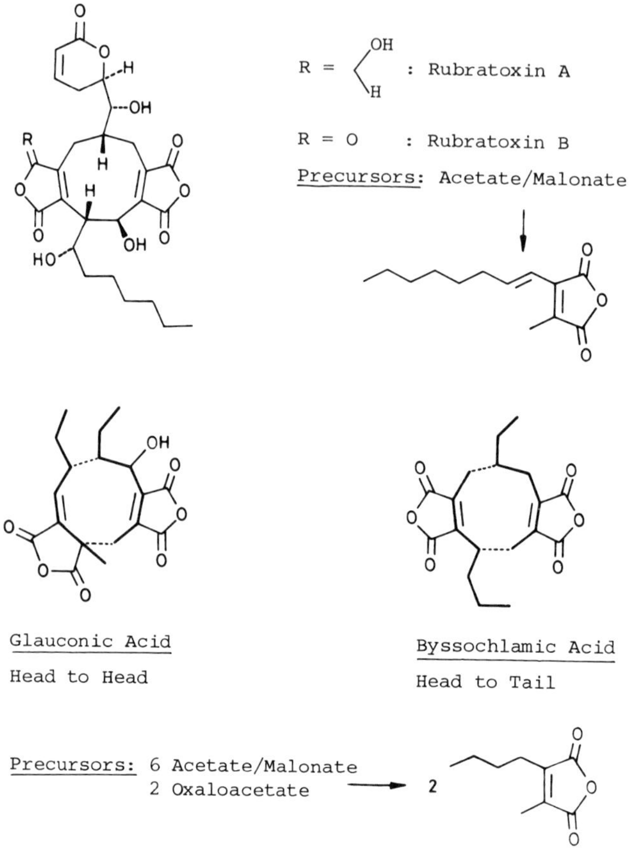

Fig. 13. Nonadrides

IX. Ansamycins

The ansamycins constitute a class of antibiotics characterized by an aliphatic bridge linking two nonadjacent positions of an aromatic nucleus (cf. Rinehart, 1972, 1976) (cf. Fig. 14).

The name is derived from ansa compounds (german "Henkel-Verbindungen"). A derivative of one of the rifamycins, rifamypicin, is marked widely for treatment of tuberculosis and other infections caused by gram-positive organisms, while other derivatives of rifamycin and streptovaricin bind to DNA-dependent RNA-polymerase and inhibit reverse transcriptases. If R_1 of rifamycin S (see Fig. 15) is a negative group, enhancement of this activity is observed (Dampier and Whitlock, 1975). It is interesting to note that maytansine, an ansa macrolide isolated from the plant *Maytenus ovatus*, is a powerful antitumor agent (Kupchan et al., 1972). Very recently, Lancini and Sartori (1976) have isolated rifamycin G, in which a γ-pyrone ring is found in the place of the p-benzoquinone ring. Rifamycin G, which is a metabolic derivative of rifamycin S, rises an interesting biogenetic problem.

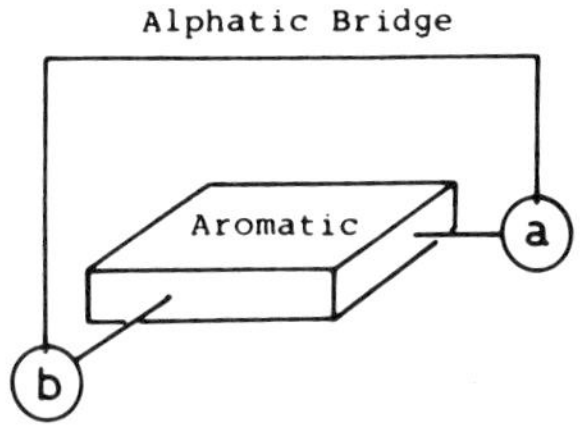

Rifamycins
Streptovaricins
Tolypomycin
Geldanamycin

Maytansine

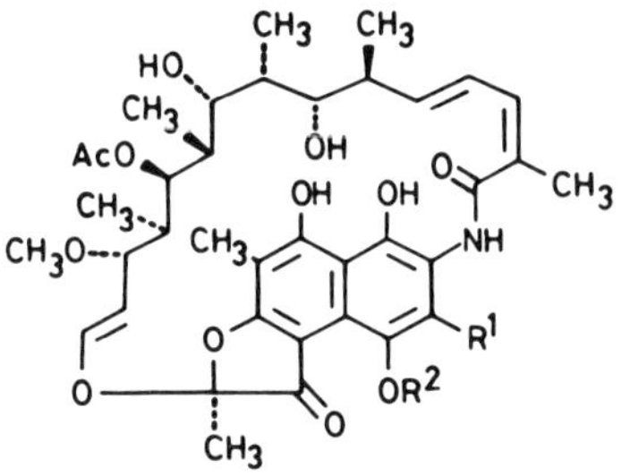

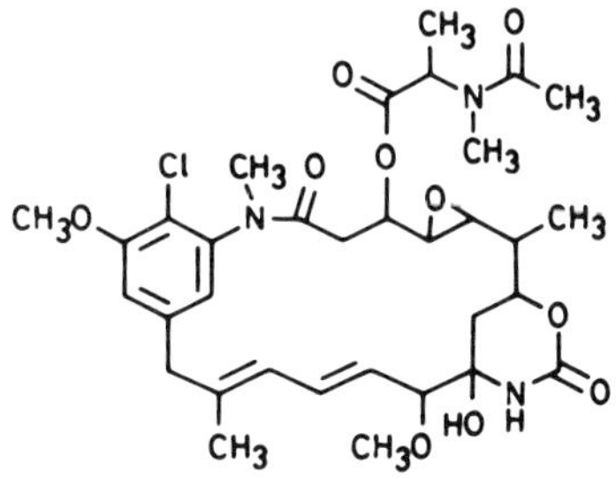

R^1 = H; R^2 = CH_2-COOH : Rifamycin B

R^1 = R^2 = H : Rifamycin SV

R^1 = CH=N-N(piperazine)N-CH_3; R^2 = H : Rifampicin

Maytansine

Fig. 14. Ansamycins

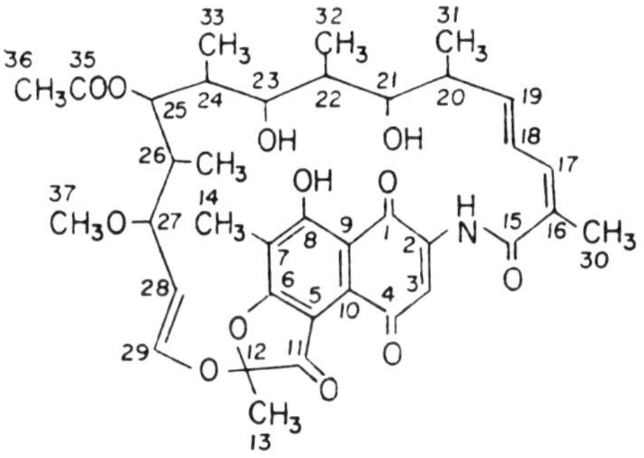

Rifamycin S

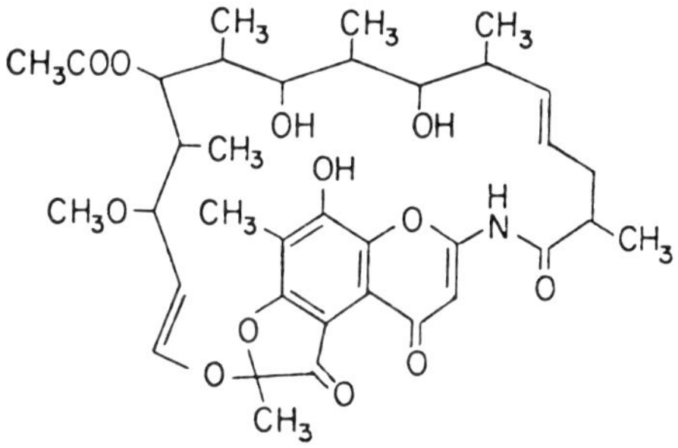

Rifamycin G

Fig. 15. Rifamycins S and G

X. Ovalicin and Pseurotins

Some years ago ovalicin, the main metabolite with immunosuppressive activity of cultures of *Pseudeurotium ovalis* was isolated (Sigg and Weber, 1968)

From the same microorganism we recently have isolated two further minor metabolites, which were named pseurotins A and B. The pseurotins are characterized by a novel, highly substituted and functionalized spirocyclic system containing oxygen and nitrogen atoms (cf. Fig. 16). The

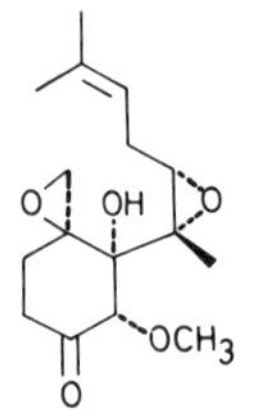

Ovalicin

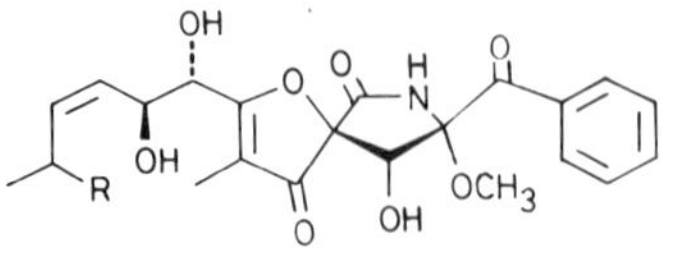

R = H : Pseurotin A

R = OH : Pseurotin B

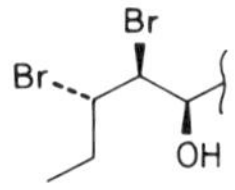

12,13-Dibromopseurotin A

Fig. 16. Ovalicin, pseurotins *(Pseudeurotium ovalis)*

structure and absolute configuration were elucidated by spectral data and chemical transformations, and by X-ray analysis of the dibromo derivative of pseurotin A (Bloch et al., 1976; Weber et al., 1976). Biogenetically, the pseurotins seem to belong to a mixed type.

C. Isoprenoid Metabolites

Examples in which the isoprenoid origin prevails, are the verrucarins and roridins, which have been isolated in Basel from cultures of *Myrothecium verrucaria* and *Myrothecium roridum*. Some are highly toxic substances possessing high cytostatic activity. They are macrocyclic di- and triesters of verrucarol, a trichothecane derivative of sesquiterpenoid nature (cf. Kadis et al., 1971b; Tamm, 1974). The structures of the main metabolites are shown in Figure 17. The acidic hydrolysis

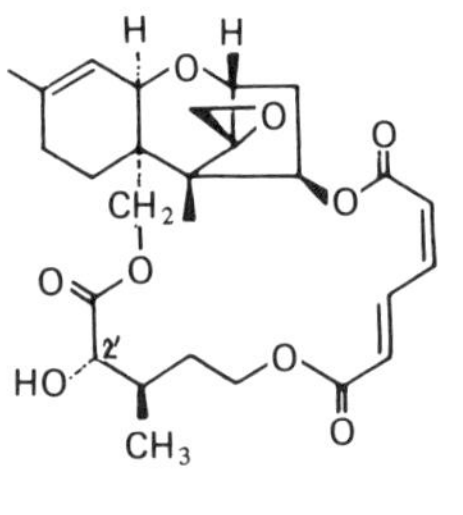

Verrucarin A

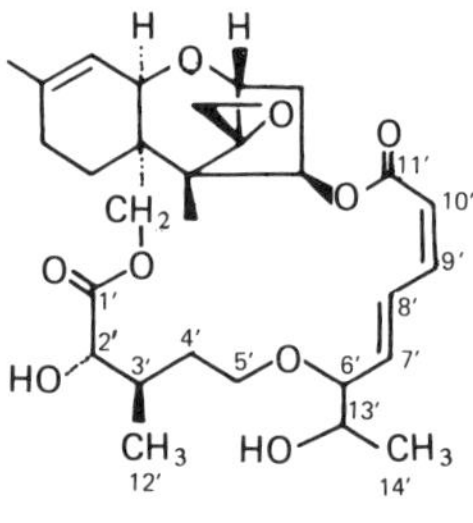

Roridin A

Fig. 17. Structure of verrucarin A and roridin A

products are cis,trans-muconic acid and verrucarinic acid in the case of verrucarin A. Roridin A yields a single C_{14}-dicarboxylic acid, roridinic acid. Verrucarinic acid, which readily lactonizes to verrucarinolactone, is a natural isomer of mevalonic acid (see Fig. 18).

Incorporation experiments with ^{14}C-mevalonates and with mevalonates tritiated stereospecifically at C-2 in our laboratory demonstrated the transformation of mevalonic into verrucarinic acid. Degradation experiments showed that this transformation occurs with a hydrogen 1,2-shift of the pro-2R hydrogen atom of mevalonate to C-3 of ver-

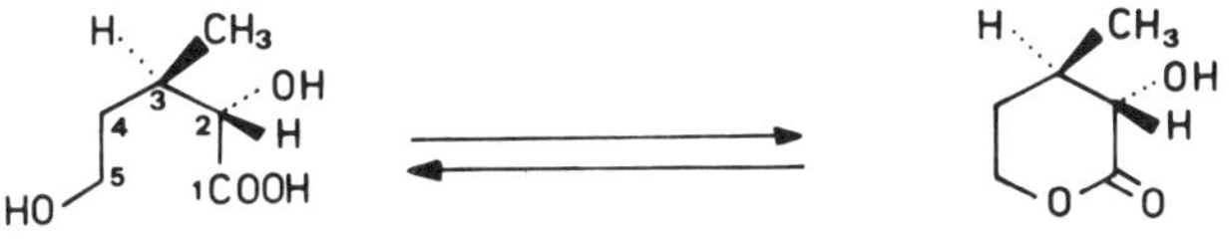

(2S,3R)-Verrucarinic acid   (2S,3R)-Verrucarino-lactone

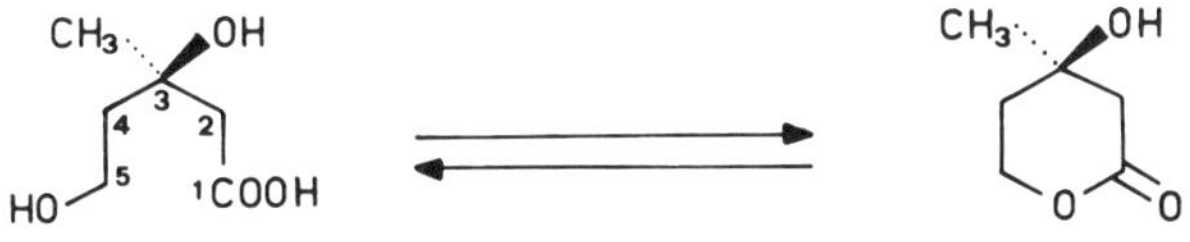

(3R)-Mevalonic acid   (3R)-Mevalolactone

Fig. 18. Structure of verrucarinic acid

rucarinate (Achini et al., 1974). A possible mechanistic pathway is outlined in Figure 19. Cis,trans-muconic acid was shown to be formed from three acetate units. The structural moiety of roridinic acid

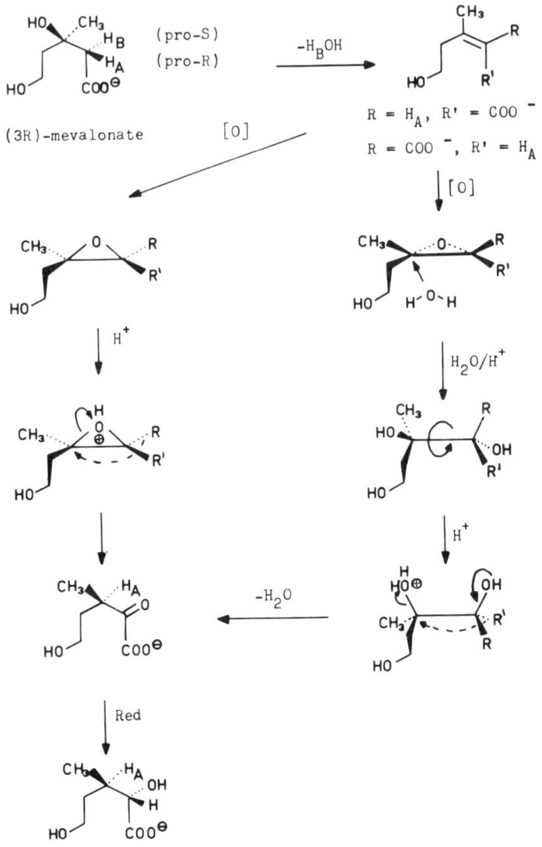

Fig. 19. Mechanism of the biogenetic formation of verrucarinate from mevalonate

corresponding to verrucarinic acid originates from mevalonate and the cis,trans-muconic acid and C_2-side chain structural elements are built up from four acetate units (Müller et al., 1975a).

The sesquiterpenoid nature of verrucarol was established by Achini et al. (1971), who observed the incorporation of three molecules of mevalonic acid into verrucarol. Müller et al. (1975b) demonstrated that it is the natural (3R)-enantiomer, which is the biogenetic active unit. Mevalonate is transformed to farnesyl pyrophosphate. It has been shown by feeding experiments that this acyclic sesquiterpene acts as precursor of verrucarol (Arigoni et al., 1973). However, it is neither the all-trans, nor the cis,cis-form of farnesol, but the cis,trans-isomer, which undergoes cyclization to form the trichothecane skeleton as outlined in the biogenetic scheme of verrucarol in Figure 20. The evidence of a hydrogen 1,5-shift has ruled out

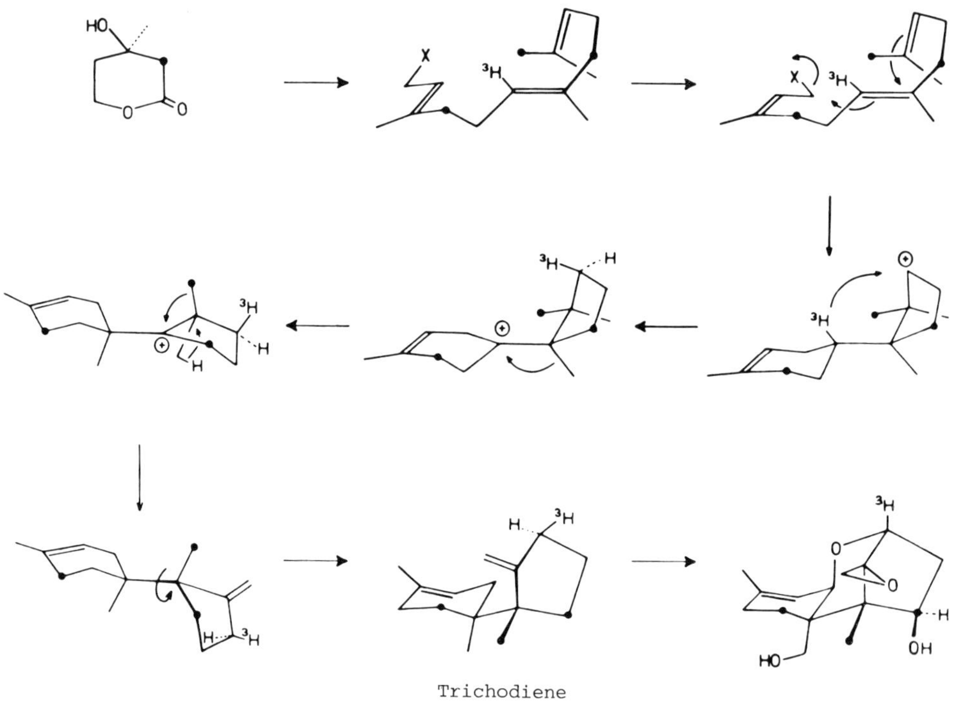

Fig. 20. Biogenetic scheme for verrucarol and related trichothecanes

bisabolene as an intermediate and has shown that farnesol cyclizes directly. This conclusion was confirmed by the negative incorporation results obtained with α-bisabolols and γ-bisabolenes (Knöll and Tamm, 1975).

The cyclization of cis,trans-farnesyl pyrophosphate requires specific folding of the chain (Achini et al., 1971; Müller et al., 1975b).

The next step of the biogenetic sequence is the cyclization, which is followed by various rearrangements. The cyclization is accompanied by an intramolecular 1,5-hydride shift from the central double bond of the precursor to C-2 of the product, as demonstrated by the mode of incorporation of [6-^{3}H-12,13-$^{14}C_2$]-farnesyl pyrophosphate into verrucarol (Arigoni et al., 1973). The double addition to the central double bond of the immediate aliphatic precursor occurs in an overall cis-fashion. The next step is anticipated to be a 1,2-shift of a methyl group followed by the abstraction of a proton, in order to form trichodiene. The cyclization of trichodiene, i.e. the insertion of the oxygen function at C-2, takes place with retention of configuration. To cast additional light on the mechanism of this cyclization, i.e. on the origin of the hydrogen atom at C-11 of the trichothecane skeleton, the incorporation of the stereospecifically tritiated precursor (3R)-[(5R)-5-^{3}H]-mevalonate into verrucarol was investigated (Müller and Tamm, 1975c). The identity of the 11-hydrogen of the trichothecane skeleton with the 5-pro-R hydrogen H_B of (3R)-mevalonate was proven by unambiguous chemical degradation. The 5-pro-S hydrogen atom H_A is eliminated. In addition, in the course of the transformation of trichodiene to trichodiol, which represents a next step, it is again the 11-hydrogen atom H_B, which is retained. If the isomerization of all-trans-farnesol to cis,trans-farnesol occurs via the aldehydes as an oxidation-reduction reaction (Müller and Tamm, 1975c), as outlined in Figure 21, it is again the 11-hydrogen atom H_B, which is retained. The

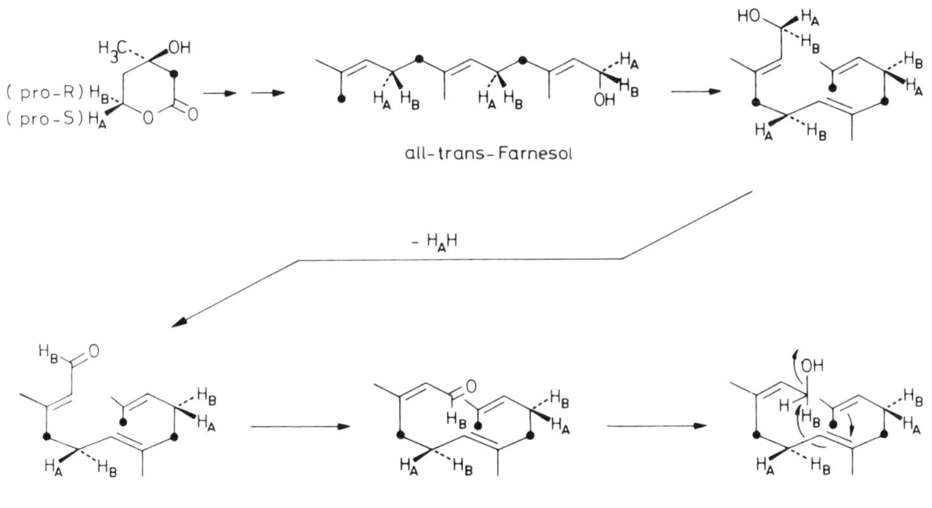

Fig. 21. Detailed biogenetic scheme I

same hydrogen atom, which is added in the course of.the oxidation-reduction process, is removed in this later stage of the biosynthetic pathway. The proposed formation of trichodiol would require an intramolecular hydride shift (cf. Fig. 22).

The 12,13-epoxy-trichoethec-9-ene system formed is modified by various hydroxylations in order to form the naturally occurring derivatives. These hydroxylations proceed with retention of configuration as demonstrated for C-4 of verrucarol (Achini et al., 1971; Müller et al., 1975b) and of other trichothecenes.

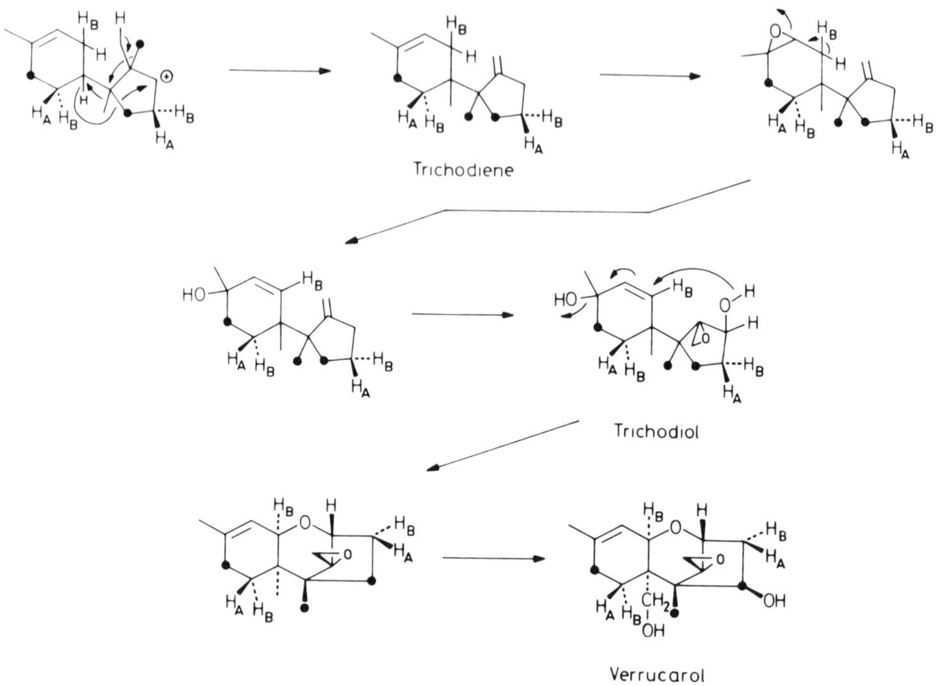

Fig. 22. Detailed biogenetic scheme II

The macrocyclic di- and triesters, the verrucarins and roridins represent a biogenetic combination of an isoprenoid moiety with a polyketide or its biogenetic equivalents. The isoprenoid part containing twenty-one carbon atoms is built up from a C_{15}-unit (trichothecane) and by a C_6-unit (verrucarinate). It is unknown whether the trichothecane moiety and the acids are constructed separately, simultaneously or in subsequent steps before they are joined together. At what stage and by which sequence the ester linkages are formed is another unresolved problem.

Very recently the structural elucidation of baccharin, a very potent antileukemic trichothecene-triepoxide, which was isolated from *Baccharis megapotamica* (Asteraceae), was reported (Kupchan et al., 1976). The isolation of baccharin constitutes the first known case of the appearance of a 12,13-epoxytrichothecene in higher plants.

D. Amino Acid-Derived Metabolites

I. Penicillins and Cephalosporins

The final section of this lecture deals with some recent results concerning mould metabolites, which are exclusively derived from amino acids.

The development of the semisynthetic penicillins and cephalosporins has intensified both synthetic approaches and biosynthetic investigations of the pename- and cephame systems (cf. Morin and Jackson, 1970; Cooper, 1973; McGregor, 1974; Sammes, 1976). Figure 23 represents the structural formulas of the most important natural penicillins and cephalosporins.

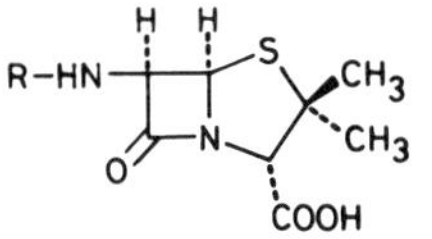

R = H : 6-Aminopenicillanic Acid
R = C_6H_5-CH_2-CO : Penicillin G
R = C_6H_5-O-CH_2-CO : Penicillin V
R = HOOC-$\overset{D}{C}$H-$(CH_2)_3$-CO : Cephalosporin N (with NH_2 on the CH)

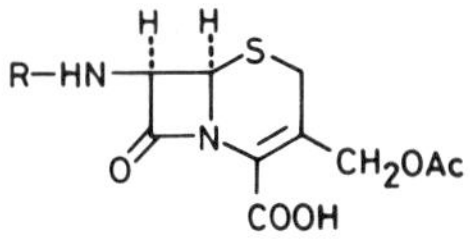

R = H : 7-Aminocephalosporanic Acid
R = HOOC-$\overset{D}{C}$H-$(CH_2)_3$-CO : Cephalosporin C (with NH_2 on the CH)

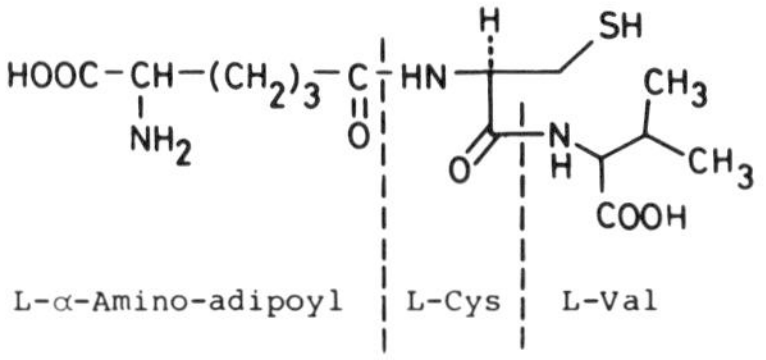

Tripeptide <u>not</u> incorporated

Fig. 23. Penicillins and cephalosporins

The penicillins prevent cell wall formation in bacteria. Specifically they are thought to prevent cross-linking of peptido-glycan peptide chains, the terminal reaction of cell wall biosynthesis. Some semi-synthetic analogs, which have been prepared from 6-amino-penicillanic acid and 7-amino-cephalosporanic acid proved to be active against the so-called penicillin-resistent strains. The isolation of modified β-lactams from *Streptomyces lipmanii* and *Streptomyces clavuligerus*, the cephamycins, which possess a 7-methoxy group (Nagarajan et al., 1971; Fukase et al., 1976) and the preparation of 6-methoxy-penicillins, has stimulated research in this field. Both series of compounds contain an α-aminoadipoyl side chain, which is also characteristic for the cephalosporins C and N. Penicillamine (β,β-dimethyl-cysteine), which is obtained from the natural penicillins with dilute acids, has been recommended for the treatment of rheumatic arthritis for longer periods of time.

Inspite of a lot of efforts, total synthesis in the penicillin series has been so far little successful, probably because of the coincidence of ring strain and high concentration of functionality. However, for the cephalosporins two stereocontrolled total syntheses have been published.

The biosynthesis of the penicillins and cephalosporins has been elucidated yet completely. The Arnstein-hypothesis, which postulates a tripeptide consisting of L-α-aminoadipic acid, L-cysteine and L-valine as intermediate, proved to be untenable. L-cysteine and L-valine have been incorporated stereospecifically. L-α-aminoadipic acid was found to be a precursor. But it requires inversion of configuration.

II. Other Natural β-Lactams

Recently, various other natural β-lactams have been discovered in nature. Interesting examples are shown in Figure 24.

Some are reminiscent of the wildfire toxin whose structure has been proven in 1971 by Stewart. Wildfire is a highly infectious leafspot disease of tobacco plants. The disease gained its name from its rapid and destructive spread through tobacco fields (first reported 1917 in North Carolina, U.S.A.). Now it is under control and no longer an economic problem. *Pseudomonas tabaci* is the responsible microorganism. In plants affected, the leaves are covered with circular yellow lesions.

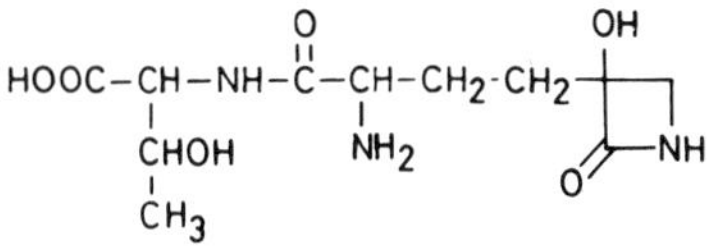

Wildfire toxin

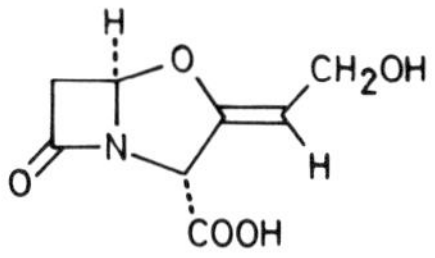

Clavulanic acid

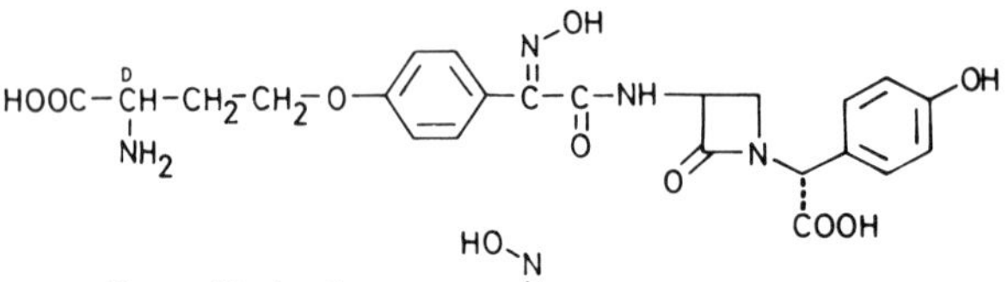

Nocardicin A

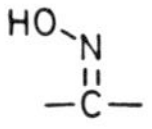

B

Fig. 24. Other natural β-lactams

Clavulanic acid, which contains an oxazolidine ring in place of the thiazolidine ring of the penicillins has been isolated from *Streptomyces clavuligerus* (Howarth et al., 1976).

Finally, the nocardicins, which have been isolated from cultures of *Nocardia uniformis* represent chemically and biologically most fascinating β-lactam derivatives (Hashimoto et al., 1976). As shown in Figure 24, nocardicins A and B are isomers differing from each other only with respect to the orientation of the oxime group. Nocardicin A is active against a variety of gram-negative bacteria and shows an especially high antimicrobial activity against *Pseudomonas*, while the activity of nocardicin B is weaker. Thus, these antibiotics are unique in several respects: they are the first examples of monocyclic β-lactam antibiotics possessing relatively high potency. The syn relation of the oxime function to the acylamino group is favored for antimicrobial activity. The p-hydroxyphenylglycine units are found rarely in nature. The structures of the nocardicins are stereochemically related to the penicillin molecule. They proved to be enzyme inhibitors in the cell wall biosynthesis of bacteria.

III. Cyclic Polypeptides

Among the polypeptides found as secondary microbial metabolites, those with cyclic structures have focussed a lot of attention.

A typical, very recent example is cyclosporin A, which is produced by the fungus *Cylindrocarpon lucidum* and *Trichoderma polysporum* (Rüegger et al., 1976). It is a cyclic undecapeptide, whose structure is

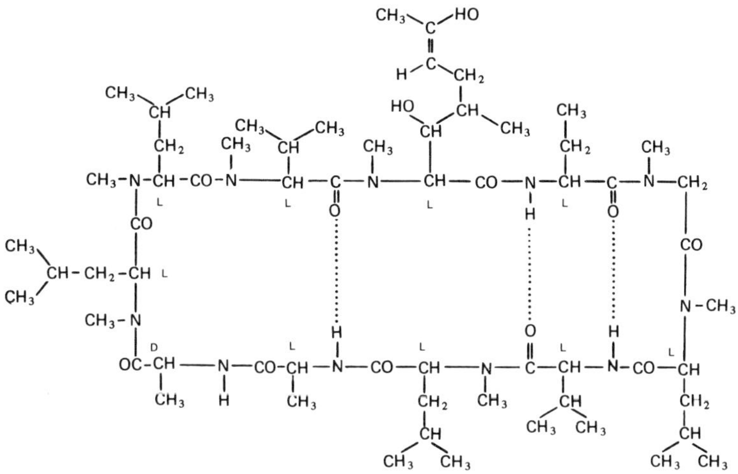

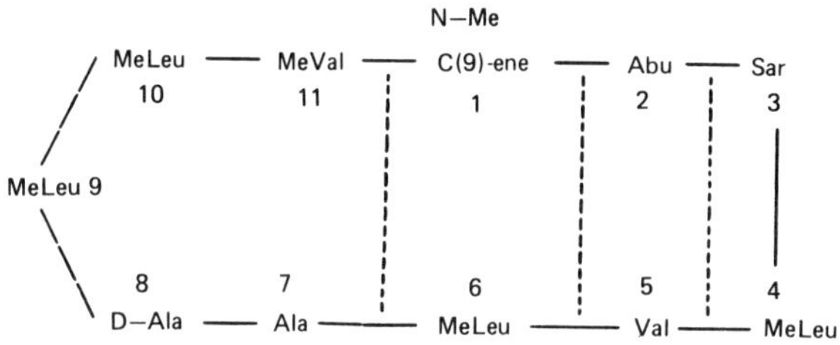

N-CH$_3$ C(9)-ene : 2S-Methylamino-3R-hydroxy-4R-methyl-oct-6-en-1-oic Acid

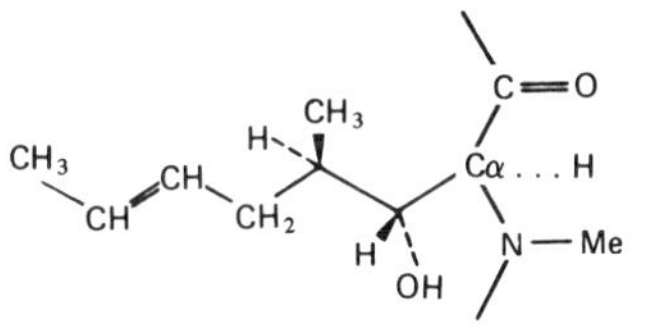

Fig. 25. Cyclosporin A *(Trichoderma polysporum)*

shown in Figure 25, neutral and rich in hydrophobic amino acids, insoluble in water and n-hexane, but soluble in other organic solvents. Cyclosporin A contains a new C_9-amino acid of unusual structure, which, however, has not been isolated in pure form. The reaction of cyclosporin A with iodine and thallium acetate formed a derivative suitable for an X-ray analysis (Petcher et al., 1976). This analysis permitted to draw conclusions concerning the conformation of the ring. It contributes to the problem of the relationship between conformation and biological activity (cf. Ovchinnikov and Ivanov, 1975). Cyclosporin A exhibits immunosuppressive and antiphlogistic activities in several pharmacological models. Experimental evidence suggests that cyclosporin A rather than being cytostatic or lympholytic, affects an early stage of mitogenic triggering of the immunocompetent lymphoid cell (cf. Borel et al., 1976).

E. Conclusion

I have presented numerous examples of interesting novel chemical structures and discussed biosynthetic problems and biological activities. Microorganisms still offer many surprises! It can be predicted that this development has not reached yet the end. New compounds with unusual chemical and stereochemical features will be found. But even in the region of known substances a tremendous amount of research remains to be done in order to establish complete biosynthetic pathways, to flash more light into structure-activity relationships and to design potent partial and total syntheses in vitro.

Acknowledgement. Our own investigations have been supported generously by the Schweizerischer Nationalfonds zur Förderung der wissenschaftlichen Forschung and by Sandoz, A.G., Basel.

References

Achini, R., Müller, B., Tamm, Ch.: Biosynthesis of the verrucarins and roridins. Part 1. The transformation of mevalonic acid into verrucarinic acid. Evidence for a hydrogen 1,2-shift. Helv. Chim. Acta 57, 1442-1459 (1974)
Achini, R., Müller, B., Tamm, Ch.: Biosynthesis of verrucarol, the sesquiterpene moiety of the verrucarins and roridins. Chem. Commun. 1971, 404-405
Arigoni, D., Cane, D.E., Müller, B., Tamm, Ch.: The mode of incorporation of farnesyl pyrophosphate into verrucarol. Helv. Chim. Acta 56, 2946-2949 (1973)
Binder, M., Kiechel, J.R., Tamm, Ch.: Zur Biogenese des Antibioticums Phomin. 1. Teil: Die Grundbausteine. Helv. Chim. Acta 53, 1797-1812 (1970)
Binder, M., Tamm, Ch.: The cytochalasans: A new class of biologically active microbial metabolites. Angew. Chemie, Intern. Ed. 12, 370-380 or: Die Cytochalasane, eine neue Klasse biologisch aktiver Metabolite aus Mikroorganismen. Angew. Chemie 85, 369-381 (1973a)
Binder, M., Tamm, Ch., Turner, W.B., Minato, H.: Nomenclature of a class of biologically active mould metabolites: the cytochalasins, phomins, and zygosporins. J. Chem. Soc. Perkin I 1973, 1146-1147
Binder, M., Tamm, Ch.: Desoxaphomin, das erste [13]Cytochalasan, ein möglicher biogenetischer Vorläufer der 24-Oxa-[14]Cytochalasane. Helv. Chim. Acta 56, 966-976 (1973b)
Binder, M., Tamm, Ch.: Proxiphomin and Protophomin, zwei neue Cytochalasane. Helv. Chim. Acta 56, 2387-2396 (1973c)
Bloch, P., Tamm, Ch., Bollinger, P., Petcher, T.J., Weber, H.P.: Pseurotin, a new metabolite of *Pseudeurotium ovalis Stolk* having an unusual hetero-spirocyclic system. Helv. Chim. Acta 59, 133-137 (1976)
Borel, J.F., Feuer, C., Gubler, H.U., Stähelin, H.: Biological effects of cyclosporin A: A new antilymphocytic agent. Agents and Actions 6, 468-475 (1976)
Carter, S.B.: Effects of cytochalasins on mammalian cells. Nature (London) 213, 261-264 (1967)
Carter, S.B.: The cytochalasins as research tools in cytology. Endeavour 31, 77-82 (1972)
Cooper, R.D.G., Hatfield, L.D., Spry, O.D.: Chemical interconversion of the β-lactam antibiotics. Accounts Chem. Res. 6, 32-40 (1973)
Corcoran, J.W., Hahn, F.E. (eds.): Antibiotics. Mechanism of Action of antimicrobial and Antitumor Agents. Berlin-Heidelberg-New York: Springer 1975, Vol. III

Dampier, M.F., Whitlock, H.W.Jr.: Electronegative Groups at C-3 of Rifamycin S Enhance its Activity toward DNA-dependent RNA-polymerase. J. Am. Chem. Soc. 97, 6254-6256 (1975)

Dürckheimer, W.: Tetracycline: Chemie, Biochemie and Struktur-Wirkungs-Beziehungen. Angew. Chemie 87, 751-784 (1975)

Egan, R.S., Martin, J.R., Perun, T.J., Mitcher, L.A.: Conformational flexibility of erythronolide B, the 14-membered aglycon ring of the erythromycins. J. Am. Chem. Soc. 97, 4578-4583 (1975)

Evans, R.M.: The Chemistry of Antibiotics Used in Medicine. Oxford-London-Edinburgh-New York-Paris-Frankfurt: Pergamon Press,1965

Fukase, H., Hasegawa, T., Hatano, K., Iwasaki, H., Yoneda, M.: C-2801X, a new cephamycin-type antibiotic. J. Antibiotics 29, 113-120 (1976)

Gerlach, H., Oertle, K., Thalmann, A., Servi, S.: Synthese des Nonactins. Helv. Chim. Acta 58, 2036-2043 (1975)

Gottlieb, D., Shaw, P.D. (eds.): Antibiotics. Mechanism of Action. Berlin-Heidelberg-New York: Springer, 1967a, Vol. I

Gottlieb, D., Shaw, P.D.: Antibiotics. Biosynthesis. Berlin-Heidelberg-New York: Springer, 1967b, Vol. II

Graf, W., Robert, J.-L., Vederas, J.C., Tamm, Ch., Solomon, P.H., Miura, I., Nakanishi, K.: Biosynthesis of cytochalasans. Part III. ^{13}C-NMR of cytochalasin B (Phomin) and cytochalasin D. Incorporation of [1-^{13}C]- and [2-^{13}C]-sodium acetate. Helv. Chim. Acta 57, 1801-1815 (1974)

Hashimoto, M., Komori, T., Kamiya, T.: Nocardicin A and B, novel monocyclic β-lactam antibiotics from *Nocardia* species. J. Am. Chem. Soc. 98, 3023-3025 (1976)

Howarth, T.T., Brown, A.G.: Clavulanic acid, a novel β-lactam isolated from *Streptomyces clavuligerus*; X-ray crystal structure analysis. J. Chem. Soc. Chem. Commun. 266-267 (1976)

Kadis, S., Ciegler, A., Ajl, S.J.: Microbial Toxins. Fungal Toxins. New York-London: Academic Press, 1971a, Vol. VI

Kadis, S., Ciegler, A., Ajl, S.J.: Microbial Toxins. Algal and Fungal Toxins. New York-London: Academic Press, 1971b, Vol. VII

Kadis, S., Ciegler, A., Ajl, S.J.: Microbial Toxins. Fungal Toxins. New York-London: Academic Press, 1971c, Vol. VIII

Keller-Schierlein, W.: Chemie der Makrolid-Antibiotica. In: Progress in the Chemistry of Organic Natural Products. Herz, W., Grisebach, H., Kirby, G.W. (eds.). Vienna-New York: Springer, 1973, Vol. XXX, pp. 313-460

Keller-Schierlein, W., Gerlach, H.: Macrotetrolides. In: Progress in the Chemistry of Organic Natural Products. Zechmeister, L. (ed.). Vienna-New York: Springer, 1968, Vol. XXVI, pp. 161-189

Kende, A.S., Tsay, Y., Mills, J.E.: Total synthesis of (±)-daunomycinone and (±)-carminomycinone. J. Am. Chem. Soc. 98, 1967-1969 (1976)

Knöll, W., Tamm, Ch.: Biosynthese der Verrucarine and Roridine. Teil 5. Synthese von zwei Diastereoisomerenpaaren des [1,8-^{14}C]-α-Bisabolols und Versuche zu deren Einbau in Verrucarol. Helv. Chim. Acta 58, 1162-1171 (1975)

Korzybski, Z., Kowszyk-Gindifer, Z., Kurylowicz, W.: Antibiotics, Origin, Nature and Properties. Oxford-London-Edinburgh-New York-Toronto-Sydney-Paris-Braunschweig: Pergamon Press, Warszawa: Polish Scientific Publishers, 1967, 2 Vols.

Kupchan, S.M., Jarvis, B.B., Dailey, R.G.Jr., Bright, W., Bryan, R.F., Shizuri, Y.: Baccharin, a novel potent antileukemic trichothecene triepoxide from *Baccharis megapotamica*. J. Am. Chem. Soc. 98, 7092-7093 (1976)

Kupchan, S.M., Komoda, Y., Court, W.A., Thomas, G.J., Smith, R.M., Karim, A., Gilmore, C.J., Haltiwanger, R.C., Bryan, R.F.: Maytansine, a novel antileukemic ansa macrolide from *Maytenus ovatus*. J. Am. Chem. Soc. 94, 1354-1356 (1972)

Lancini, G., Sartori, G.: Rifamycin G, a further product of *Nocardia mediterranei* metabolism. J. Antibiotics 29, 466-468 (1976)

Lebet, Cl.-R., Tamm, Ch.: Biosynthese der Cytochalasane. Teil II. Die Grundbausteine von Cytochalasin D. Helv. Chim. Acta 57, 1785-1801 (1974)

Martin, J.R., Egan, R.S., Goldstein, A.W., Collum, P.: Extension of the erythromycin biosynthetic pathway, isolation and structure of erythromycin E. Tetrahedron 31, 1985-1989 (1975)

Masamune, S., Kim, C.U., Wilson, K.E., Spessard, G.O., Georghiou, P.F., Bates, G.S.: Synthesis of macrolide antibiotics. I. Methymycin. J. Am. Chem. Soc. 97, 3512-3513 (1975a)

Masamune, S., Yamamoto, H., Kamata, S., Fukuzawa, A.: Synthesis of macrolide antibiotics. II. Methymycin. J. Am. Chem. Soc. 97, 3513-3515 (1975b)

McGregor, D.N.: Recent developments in the chemistry of penicillins. In: Progress in the Chemistry of Organic Natural Products. Herz, W., Grisebach, H., Kirby, G.W. (eds.). Wien-New York: Springer, 1974, Vol. XXXI, pp. 1-62

Morin, R.B., Jackson, B.G.: Chemistry of cephalosporin antibiotics. In: Progress in the Chemistry of Organic Natural Products. Herz, W., Grisebach, H., Scott, A.I. (eds.). Wien-New York: Springer, 1970, Vol. XXVIII, pp. 343-403

Müller, B., Achini, R., Tamm, Ch.: Biosynthese der Verrucarine und Roridine. Teil 2. Der Einbau von Acetat in die cis,trans-Muconsäure und von Mevalonat in die Roridinsäure. Helv. Chim. Acta 58, 453-470 (1975a)

Müller, B., Achini, R., Tamm, Ch.: Biosynthese der Verrucarine und Roridine. Teil 3. Der Einbau von (3R)-[5-^{14}C]-,[2-^{14}C]- und and C(2) stereospezifisch tritiiertem Mevalonat in Verrucarol. Helv. Chim. Acta 58, 471-482 (1975b)

Müller, B., Tamm, Ch.: Biosynthesis of the verrucarine and roridins. Part 4. The mode of incorporation of (3R)-[(5R)-5-^{1}H]-Mevalonate into verrucarol. Evidence for the identity of the C(11)-hydrogen atom of the trichothecane skeleton with the (5R)-hydrogen atom of (3R)-mevalonic acid. Helv. Chim. Acta 58, 483-488 (1975c)

Nagarajan, R., Boeck, L.D., Gorman, M., Hamill, R.L., Higgens, C.E., Hoelm, M.M., Stark, W.M., Whitney, J.G.: β-Lactam antibiotics from *Streptomyces*. J. Am. Chem. Soc. 93, 2308-2310 (1971)

Nourse, J.G., Roberts, J.R.: Nuclear magnetic resonance spectroscopy. Carbon-13 spectra of some macrolide antibiotics and derivatives. Substituent and conformational effects. J. Am. Chem. Soc. 97, 4584-4594 (1975)

Ovchinnikov, Y.A., Ivanov, V.T.: Conformational states and biological activities of cyclic peptides. Tetrahedron 31, 2177-2209 (1975)

Pachler, K.G.R., Steyn, P.S., Vleggaar, R., Wessels, P.L., Scott, D.B.: Carbon-13 nuclear magnetic assignments and biosynthesis of aflatoxin B_1 and sterigmatocystin. J. Chem. Soc. Perkin I 1976, 1182-1189

Petcher, T.G., Weber, H.P., Rüegger, A.: Crystal and molecular structure of an iodo-derivative of the cyclic undecapeptide cyclosporin A. Helv. Chim. Acta 59, 1480-1489 (1976)

Reiner, R.: Antibiotica und ausgewählte Chemotherapeutica. Stuttgart: Georg Thieme, 1974

Rinehart, K.L.Jr.: Antibiotics with ansa rings. Accounts Chem. Res. 5, 57-64 (1972)

Rinehart, K.L.Jr., Shield, L.S.: Chemistry of the ansamycin antibiotics. In: Progress in the Chemistry of Organic Natural Products. Herz, W., Grisebach, H., Kirby, G.W. (eds). Wien-New York: Springer, 1976, Vol. XXXI, pp. 231-308

Robert, J.-L., Tamm, Ch.: Biosynthesis of cytochalasans. Part 5. The incorporation of deoxaphomin into cytochalasin B (phomin). Helv. Chim. Acta 58, 2501-2504 (1975)

Roberts, J.C.: Aflatoxins and sterigmatocystins. In: Progress in the Chemistry of Organic Natural Products. Herz, W., Grisebach, H., Kirby, G.W. (eds.). Wien-New York: Springer, 1974, Vol. XXXI, pp. 119-151

Rothweiler, W., Tamm, Ch.: Isolation and structure of phomin. Experientia 22, 750-752 (1966)

Rüegger, A., Kuhn, M., Lichti, H., Loosli, H.-R., Huguenin, R., Quiquerez, C., von Wartburg, A.: Cyclosporin A, ein immunosuppressiv wirksamer Peptidmetabolit aus *Trichoderma polysporum (Link ex Pers.) Rifar*. Helv. Chim. Acta 59, 1075-1092 (1976)

Sammes, P.G.: Recent chemistry of the β-lactam antibiotics. Chem. Rev. 76, 113-155 (1976)

Schmidt, P.G., Wang, A.H.J., Paul, I.C.: A structural study on the sodium salt of the ionophore, X-537A (lasalocid), by X-ray and nuclear magnetic resonance analysis. J. Am. Chem. Soc. 96, 6189-6191 (1974)

Schmidt, U., Gombos, J., Haslinger, E., Zak, H.: Hochstereoselektive Totalsynthese des Nonactins. Chem. Ber. 109, 2628-2647 (1976)

Sekita, S., Yoshihara, K., Natori, S., Kuwano, H.: Structures of chaetoglobosin A and B, cytotoxic metabolites of *chaetomium globosum*. Tetrahedron Lett. 1973, 2109-2112

Sekita, S., Yoshihara, K., Natori, S., Kuwano, H.: Structures of chaetoglobosins C, D, E and F, cytotoxic indol-3-yl-[13]cytochalasans from *Chaetomium globosum*. Tetrahedron Lett. 1976, 1351-1354

Sigg, H.P., Weber, H.P.: Isolierung und Strukturaufklärung von Ovalicin. Helv. Chim. Acta 51, 1395-1408 (1968)

Silverton, J.V., Akiyama, T., Kabuto, C., Sekita, S., Yoshihara, K., Natori, S.: X-ray analysis of chaetoglobosin A, an indol-3-yl-[13]cytochalasan from *Chaetomium globosum*. Tetrahedron Lett. 1976, 1349-1350

Smith, T.H., Fujiwara, A.N., Henry, D.W., Lee, W.W.: Synthetic approaches to adriamycin. Degradation of daunorubicin to nonasymmetric tetracyclic ketone and refunctionalization of the A-ring to adriamycin. J. Am. Chem. Soc. 98, 1969-1971 (1976)

Stewart, N.N.: Isolation and proof of structure of wildfire toxin. Nature (London) 229, 174-178 (1971)

Sutherland, J.K.: The nonadrides. In: Progress in the Chemistry of Organic Natural Products. Zechmeister, L. (ed.). Wien-New York: Springer, 1967, Vol. XXV, pp. 131-149

Tamm, Ch.: The antibiotic complex of the verrucarins and roridins. In: Progress in the Chemistry of Organic Natural Products. Herz, W., Grisebach, H., Kirby, G. W. (eds.). Wien-New York: Springer, 1974, Vol. XXXI, pp. 63-117

Turner, W.B.: Fungal Metabolites. London-New York: Academic Press, 1971

Vaněk, Z., Hoštálek, Z.: Biogenesis of Antibiotic Substances. London: Academic Press, 1965

Vederas, J.C., Graf, W., David, L., Tamm, Ch.: Biosynthesis of cytochalasans. Part 4. The mode of incorporation of common naturally-occurring carboxylic acids into cytochalasin D. Helv. Chim. Acta 58, 1886-1898 (1975)

Vederas, J.C., Tamm, Ch.: Biosynthesis of cytochalasans. Part 6. The mode of incorporation of phenylalanine into cytochalasin D. Helv. Chim. Acta 59, 558-566 (1976)

Waksman, S.A.: Microbial Antagonism and Antibiotic Substances. New York: The Commonwealth Fund, 1945

Weber, H.P., Petcher, T.J., Bloch, P., Tamm, Ch.: The crystal and molecular structure of 12,13-dibromopseurotin. Helv. Chim. Acta 59, 137-140 (1976)

Westley, J.W.: A proposed numbering system for polyester antibiotics. J. Antibiotics 29, 584-586 (1976)

Wong, C.M., Schwenk, R., Popien, D., Ho, T.-L.: The total synthesis of daunomycinone. Canad. J. Chem. 51, 466-467 (1973)

Zähner, H.: Biologie der Antibiotica. Berlin-Heidelberg-New York: Springer, 1965

Progress in the Chemistry of Alkaloids with Pharmacological or Biological Activity

H. ACHENBACH

We are all aware of the breath-taking speed of scientific discovery and publication. This report will, therefore, be very fragmentary and certainly incomplete. Some types and classes of alkaloids are intentionally omitted, partly because they are discussed in detail elsewhere in this congress.

The following is an account of recent research, and only occasionally does it refer back as early as 1970.

In accordance with the general theme, most emphasis is placed on the chemistry of the alkaloids. There is an especially useful discussion of the purely pharmacological aspects of new alkaloids by Baumgarth (1).

Before discussing individual alkaloids and classes of alkaloids, it would seem worthwhile to mention the following advances in the methodology of isolation and structural determination:

1. The high pressure liquid chromatography, which is an extremely efficient method for the rapid separation of even very sensitive and thermolabile alkaloids (2).
2. The use of combined gas chromatography-mass spectrometry, which will be referred to later, in connection with the erythrina alkaloids.
3. The ^{13}C-NMR spectroscopy as a new tool in structural elucidation. In the alkaloid field it has contributed to especially by the extensive investigations of Wenkert (3), so that a comprehensive body of data has already been produced. Information from ^{13}C-spectroscopy is an attractive supplement to proton resonance spectroscopy, and it is especially useful in the investigation of structures containing carbons not bound to hydrogen. A fine example of this is provided by vindolinine, where ^{13}C-NMR measurements indicated the necessity for a revision of the structure (4). Vindolinine, which occurs in various species of *Catharanthus*, was orginally thought to have Formula 1. ^{13}C-NMR spectra showed that vindolinine in fact contains one hydrogen-free carbon atom more than shown in Formula 1. The resonance position of the hydrogen-free carbon atom required that it should lie in the neighborhood of a heteroatom, and this led to Formula 2. Encircled in Formula 2 is the C-atom, whose ^{13}C-signal initiated the reconsideration of the structure.

Later, the revised structure was confirmed by extensive proton resonance investigations at 300 MHz (5).

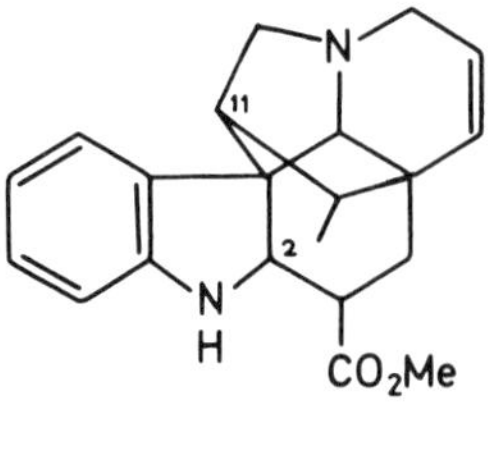

Formula 1

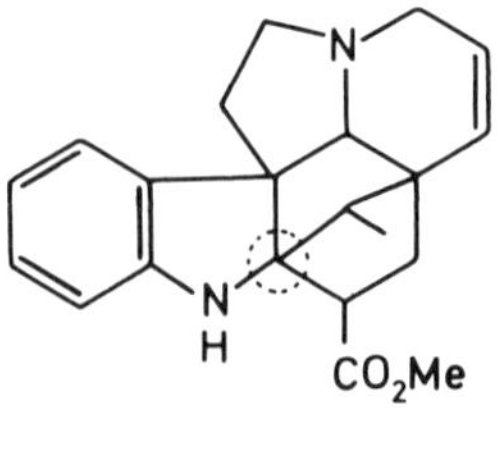

Formula 2: Vindolinine

After these opening remarks, I should like to introduce some simple alkaloids of the pyrrole and pyridine type: The alkaloid codonopsine (Formula 3) from the Campanulaceae *Codonopsis clematidea* possesses hypotensive activity (6). The pyrrolidine ring is tetrasubstituted, and both hydroxyl functions are in the threo-configuration; the configuration of the substituents presented here is the result of recent proton resonance studies (7).

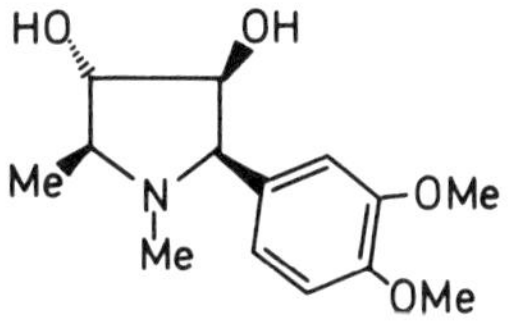

Formula 3: Codonopsine

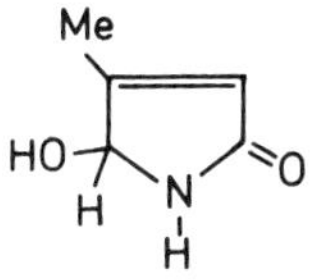

Formula 4: Jatropham

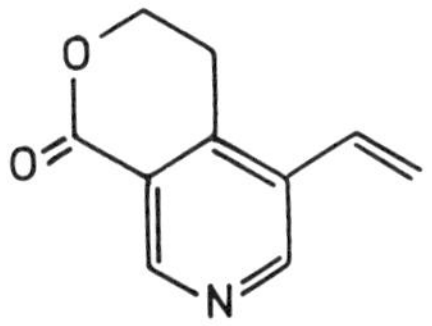

Formula 5: Gentianine

Jatropham (Formula 4) from *Jatropha macrorhiza* (Euphorbiaceae) has antitumor properties (8). Structure Formula 4 is based on its hydrogenation to 4-methyl-pyrrolidine-2-one, and oxidation to α-methyl-maleic acid imide.

Recently, gentianine (Formula 5), which has been known for some considerable time, has attracted keen pharmacological interest . It is a vinyl-pyrido-α-pyrone, which is isolated from various plants, and is also available by synthesis (9). Gentianine is supposed to possess specific antipsychotic activity (10); and its antiinflammatory, sedative, ataractic and analgesic properties have also been studied (11-14).

Investigation of the Australian Leguminosae *Hovea longipes* yielded cytisine and baptifoline, together with the hitherto unknown alkaloid hoveine, which shows marked hypotensive activity in animal tests (15).

The structure (Formula 6) is based essentially on hydrolysis experiments (15): Treatment of hoveine with HCl produces a phenolic acid, which was identified as 4,4'-dimethoxy-α-truxillic acid dimethyl ester (Formula 7) after methylation. The basic moieties of the molecule are two 1,2,3,4-tetrahydroanabasine units with a reactive enamine structure, and these were not stable under the conditions used.

The basic component can, however, be isolated, if hydrolysis is preceded by hydrogenation. It is then obtained as a mixture of two optically active α,β-dipiperidyls, which are epimeric only at C-3 and

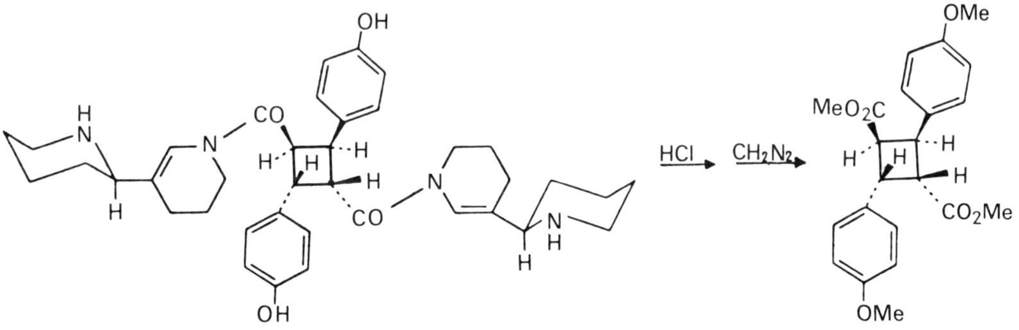

Formula 6: Hoveine

Formula 7

can, therefore, be separated. From the known stereochemistry of the dipiperidyl series, it was possible to derive the absolute configuration as presented in Formula 6.

Carpaine (Formula 8) is the chief alkaloid from *Carica papaya* (Caricaceae). In addition to amoebicidal and antibacterial properties, it also possesses pharmacological activity, which, on the one hand, can be compared with digitalis, and on the other hand with emetine (16).

Chemically, it is characterized by an interesting macrocyclic structure, which is formed by the symmetrical combination of two molecules of carpamic acid (Formula 9) via two lactone groups (17).

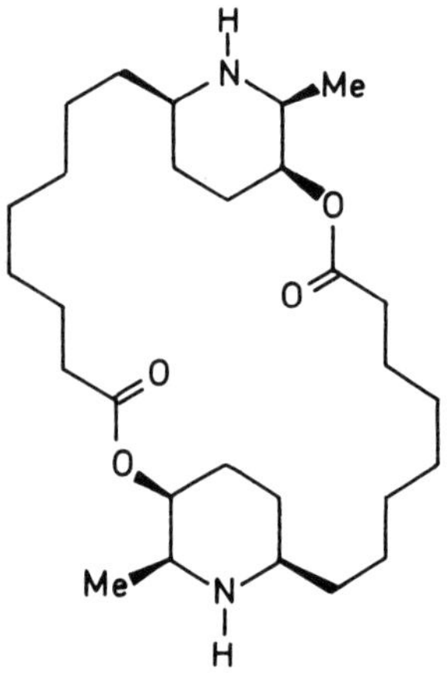

Formula 8: Carpaine

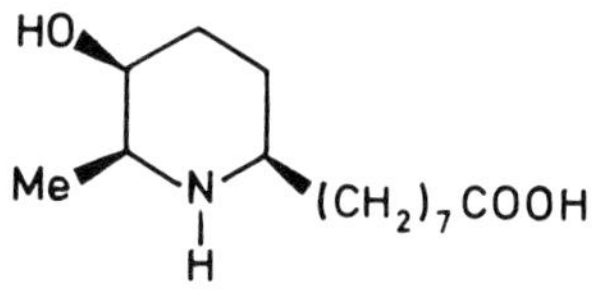

Formula 9: Carpamic acid

Using his method of double activation, Corey has recently devised a pathway (18), for the preparation of carpaine from carpamic acid (19).

This method was originally designed for the intramolecular ring closure of long chain ω-hydroxy fatty acids to form macrocyclic lactones, particularly the type present in the macrolide antibiotics (20) and in the cytochalasans (21).

To achieve the ring closure the carboxyl group is first converted into the 2-pyridinethiol ester (Formula 10). In Formula 10, the nitrogen of the pyridine ring can be protonated by hydroxyl groups. In aprotic solvents at high dilution, this protonation procedes intramolecularly with the production of Formula 11. Macrolactone Formula 13 is formed via intermediate Formula 12 by removal of pyridinethione in a thermic reaction (Fig. 1).

The yields from this efficient and mild procedure are good to excellent for $n > 10$ (18, 22), but in the preparation of intermediate sized rings, dimeric cyclic diesters of Formula 14, like those present in carpaine, are also formed. Thus, a 50 % yield of carpaine is obtained from N-benzyloxycarbonyl carpamic acid (19). A total synthesis of racemic carpamic acid was recently reported (23).

A macrocyclic lactone ring is also present in the Lythraceae alkaloids, which were first isolated and studied by Ferris (24) and Schwarting (25) from species of *Heimia* and *Decodon*. Many of these alkaloids possess a cinnamic or hydrocinnamic acid moiety, whose carboxyl group forms a

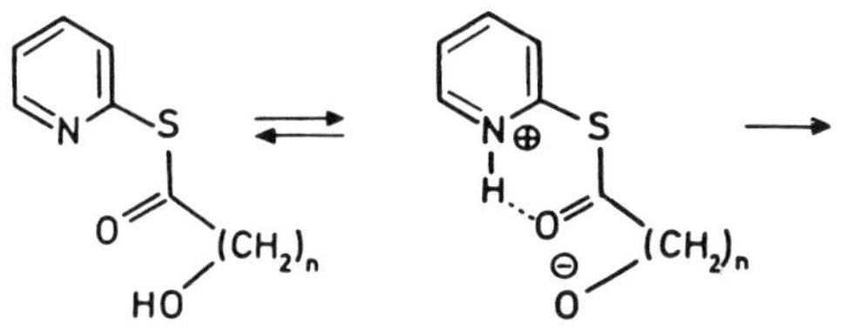

Formula 10 Formula 11

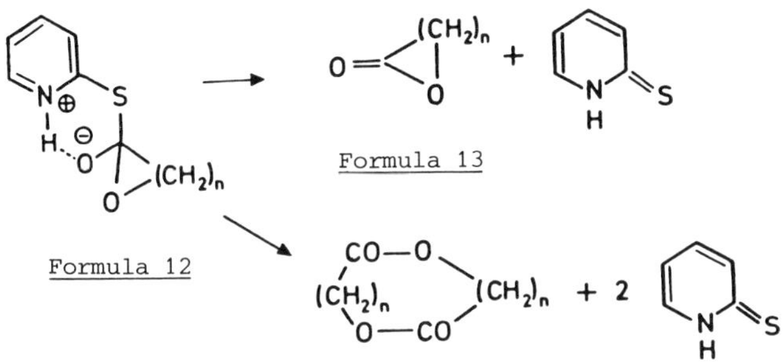

Formula 12 Formula 13 Formula 14

Fig. 1. Formation of macrocyclic lactones by "double activation" according to Corey (18)

lactone linkage with a hydroxyquinolizidine system. This is seen in cryogenine (Formula 15), which is of pharmacological interest, owing to its antiinflammatory activity (26).

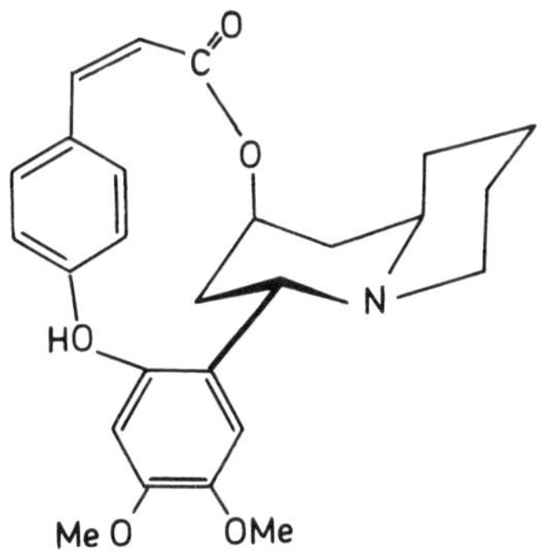

Formula 15: Cryogenine

The Corey method has also been successfully applied to this class of alkaloids: the acid (Formula 16) can be lactonized to the natural alkaloid vertaline (Formula 17) in a yield of about 70 % (19), whereas ring closure of Formula 16 with p-toluenesulfonic acid in benzene yields only 40 % of Formula 17 (27).

Farnsworth has reported the antiviral properties of cryptopleurine (Formula 20), which occurs in *Boehmeria cylindrica* (Urticaceae) and contains a characteristic phenanthroquinolizidine skeleton (28). This report stimulated the interest in synthetic studies and it gives me the opportunity to present an example of the application of electrochemical methods to alkaloid synthesis: the oxidative coupling of the 2,3-diphenyl substituted quinolizidinone (Formula 18), represents a relatively new preparative route to cryptopleurine (29). In a conventional manner phenol coupling is brought about after hydrogenation

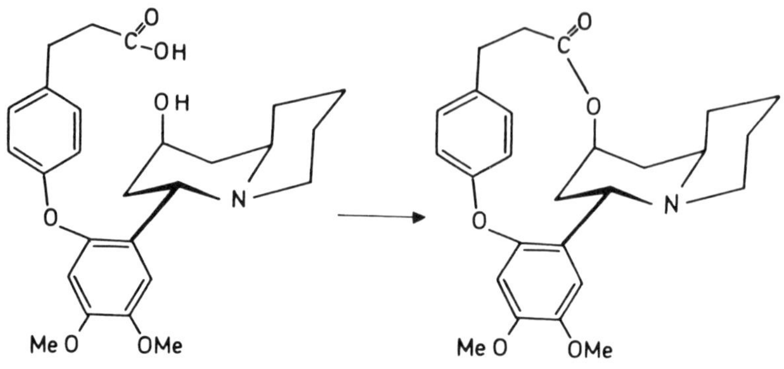

Formula 16

Formula 17: Vertaline

and demethylation with MnO_2 to the spirodienone (Formula 19), a stage which gives only modest yield. (±) Cryptopleurine (Formula 20) can then be easily obtained from the spirodienone in three steps (Fig. 2) (29).

Anodic oxidation in acetonitrile with HBF_4 as the electrolyte brings about the almost quantitative conversion of the precursor (Formula 18) to a mixture of the spirodienone (Formula 21) and the lactam (Formula 22), which can be easily converted into Formula 20 (30, 31).

A new alkaloid, 6,6'-dihydroxythiobinupharidine (Formula 23) has been isolated from *Nuphar luteum* (Nymphaeaceae) (32). It contains two deoxynupharidine units (Formula 24), and it is active against fungi, including human pathogens (33). The encircled methyl groups of the two monomeric units, together with sulphur, form the central thiolane ring of the 6,6'-dihydroxythiobinupharidine. Extensive chemical and spectrochemical studies proved the stereo-configuration shown in Formula 23 (34, 35).

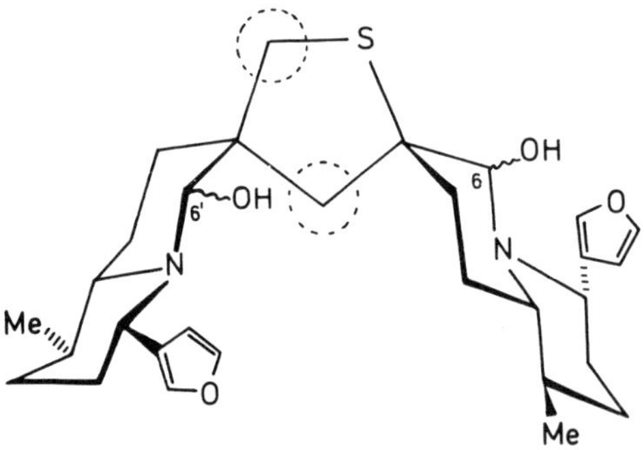

Formula 23: 6,6'-Dihydroxythiobinupharidine

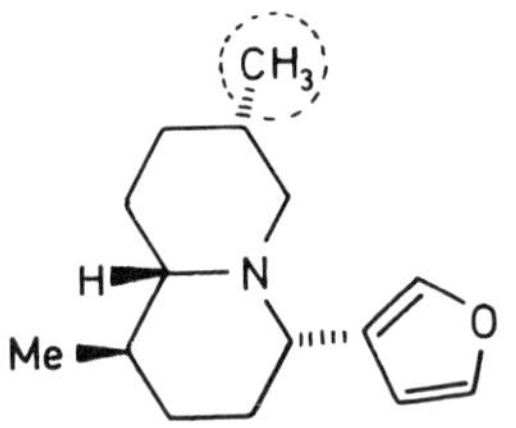

Formula 24: Deoxynupharidine

Chemically and biogenetically closely related to cryptopleurine (Formula 20) are the phenanthroindolizidine alkaloids, which are found in *Tylophora* species (Asclepiadaceae), and which are known for their antitumor activity. The position of the oxygen substituents appears to be crucial for the antitumor activity (36).

Tylophorine (Formula 25) possesses a chiral center at C-13a, whose S-configuration has recently been unequivocally determined by ozonolytic degradation to the S-pyrrolidine-2-acetic acid (37).

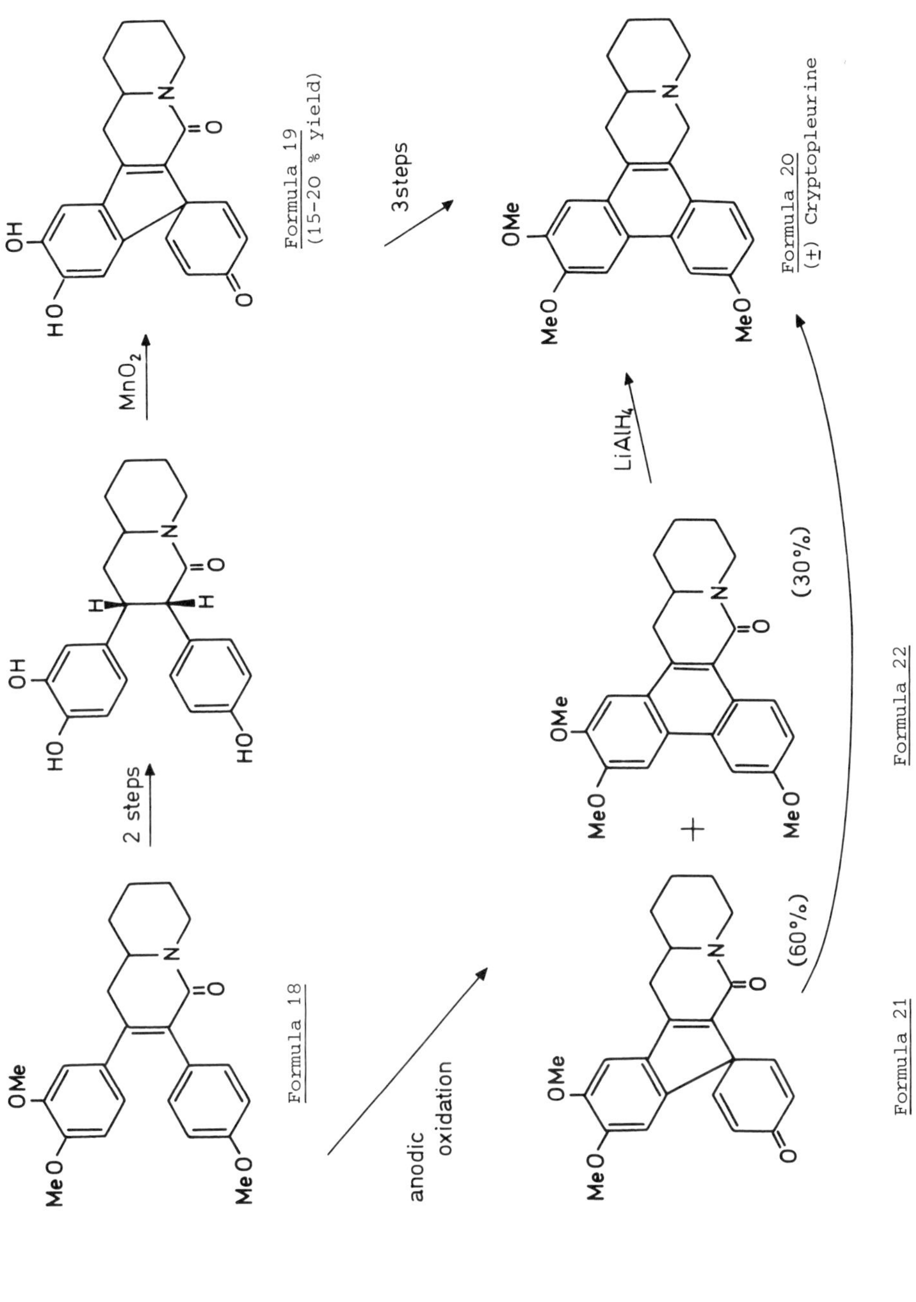

Fig. 2. Preparative route from Formula 18 to the antiviral alkaloid cryptopleurine (Formula 20) by (a) oxidation with MnO_2 and (b) anodic oxidation

More recent studies have led to a revision of the structure of tylophorinidine (Formula 26) (38, 39): contrary to previous assumptions (40), the additional hydroxyl group is in position 14, and it can be removed by hydrogenolysis; it is transdiaxial to the hydrogen at C-13a (39).

A new route for the synthesis of the basic moiety of the tropa alkaloids was reported recently (41, 42). It employs the cycloaddition of pyrroles to substituted acetones, with activation by iron carbonyls. Whereas acetone or 1,3-dibromoacetone do not react, a mixture of the

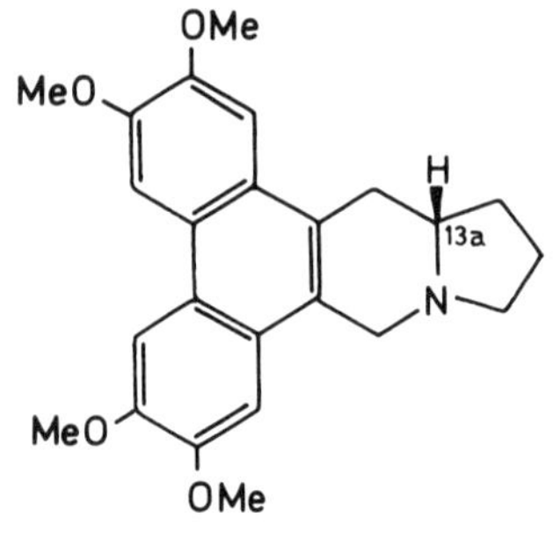

Formula 25: Tylophorine

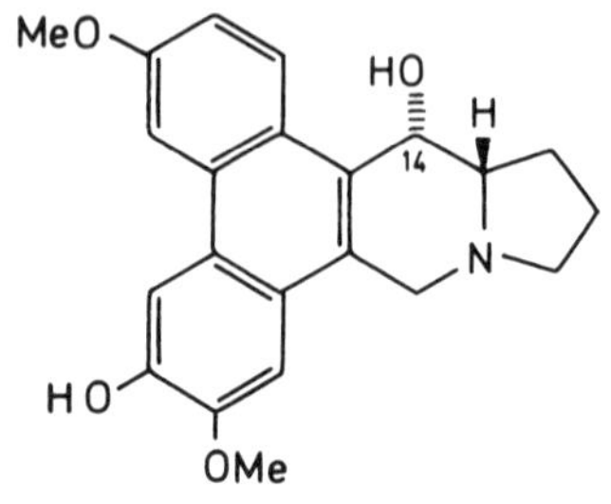

Formula 26: Tylophorinidine

isomeric dibromo products (Formulas 27 and 28) is obtained from the irradiation of tetrabromoacetone and N-methoxycarbonylpyrrole in the presence of di-irone enneacarbonyl (Fig. 3).
Simultaneous catalytic hydrogenation and debromination of these products, followed by treatment with DiBAH (= diisobutylaluminumhydride), produces tropine (Formula 29).

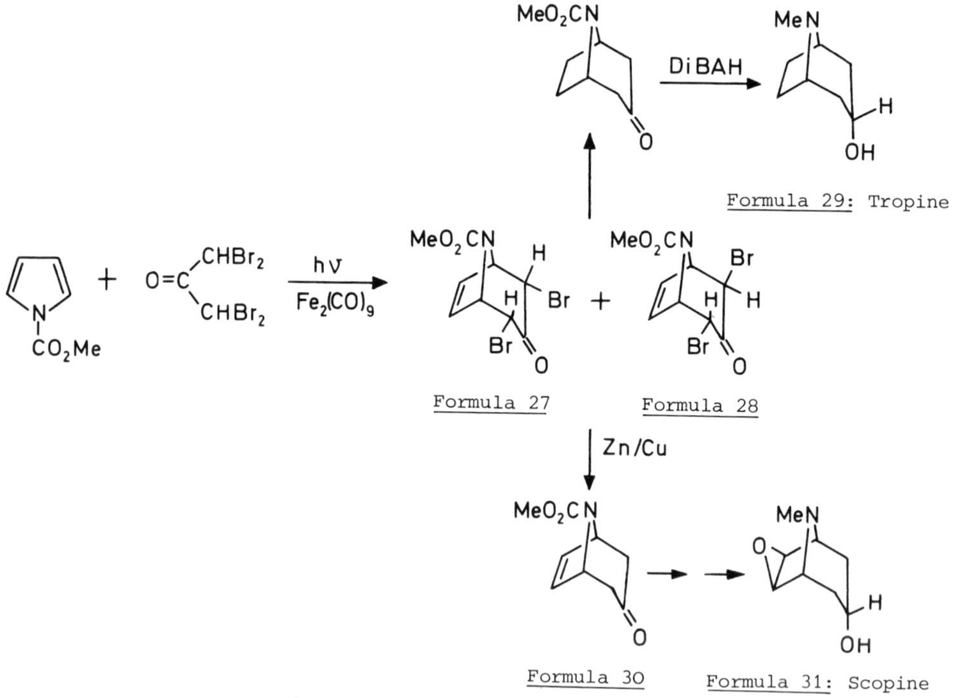

Fig. 3. New synthetic route to tropine (Formula 29) and scopine (Formula 31)

If the bromine is removed with Zn/Cu in methanol, the 6,7-double bond remains intact, and the corresponding unsaturated ketone (Formula 30) is obtained. Reduction and epoxidation of Formula 30 forms scopine (Formula 31), from which scopolamine can be prepared relatively easily.

Erythrina alkaloids are pharmacologically interesting, because they possess curare-like activity (43, 44).

The mass spectra of known erythrina alkaloids have already been the object of earlier studies, in which was found, that essential structural information can be deduced from key fragments (45).

Rinehart recently applied the technique of combined gas chromatography-mass spectrometry to the analysis of silylated crude alkaloid mixtures from two *Erythrina* species, and thereby discovered seven new alkaloids at the first attempt (46). These results motivated two other research groups to use the GC/MS method for the systematic screening of alkaloids in this plant group (44, 47). Thus in a short time, a large number of *Erythrina* species have been investigated, and our knowledge of the erythrina alkaloids has been greatly extended.

I should especially like to refer to cocculine and cocculidine from *Cocculus laurifolius* (Menispermaceae), which, after two structural revisions (48, 49) have Formulas 32 and 33 and thus unequivocally belong to the erythrina alkaloids (50, 51). In animal tests, cocculine (Formula 32) and cocculidine (Formula 33) possess hypotensive activity (52), but no detectable activity on the central nervous system (52).

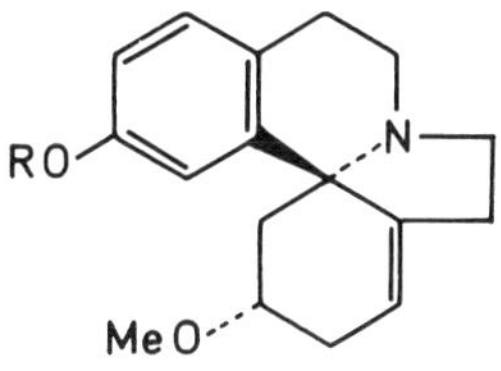

Formula 32: Cocculine : R = H
Formula 33: Cocculidine : R = Me

The proposals for the biogenetic derivation of the erythrina alkaloids from (S)-N-norprotosinomenine (Formula 34) have now received further confirmation (53, 54). Incorporation experiments showed that this in contrast to (+)-N-nororientaline and (±)-N-norreticuline is an efficient precursor of erythraline (Formula 40).

The biosynthesis (Fig. 4) is thought to start with a phenol oxidation of N-norprotosinomenine to Formula 35, followed by rearrangement via the dehydro from (Formula 36) to the dibenzazonine (Formula 37). A transannular attack of the nitrogen in the quinoid structure (Formula 38) then leads to the spiro system (Formula 39), as found in the erythrina alkaloids.

Experimental support for this scheme is as follows:

1. Labeled dibenzazonine (Formula 37) is efficiently incorporated into erythraline.
2. Alkaloids based structurally on the dibenzazonine skeleton have also been found in *Erythrina* species (55).
3. Experiments with correspondingly labeled N-norprotosinomenine require that the biosynthesis should pass through a symmetrical stage, in which the aromatic rings A and C are completely equivalent. This requirement is met in Formulas 37 and 38.

In recent years much attention has been paid to the alkaloids from species of *Cephalotaxus* (*Cephalotaxus harringtonia* var. *drupaceae*, and *Cephalotaxus fortunei* , Taxaceae), owing to their antitumor properties (56). The biologically active compounds are the harringtonines, which are esters of the chief alkaloid cephalotaxine. Cephalotaxine has the

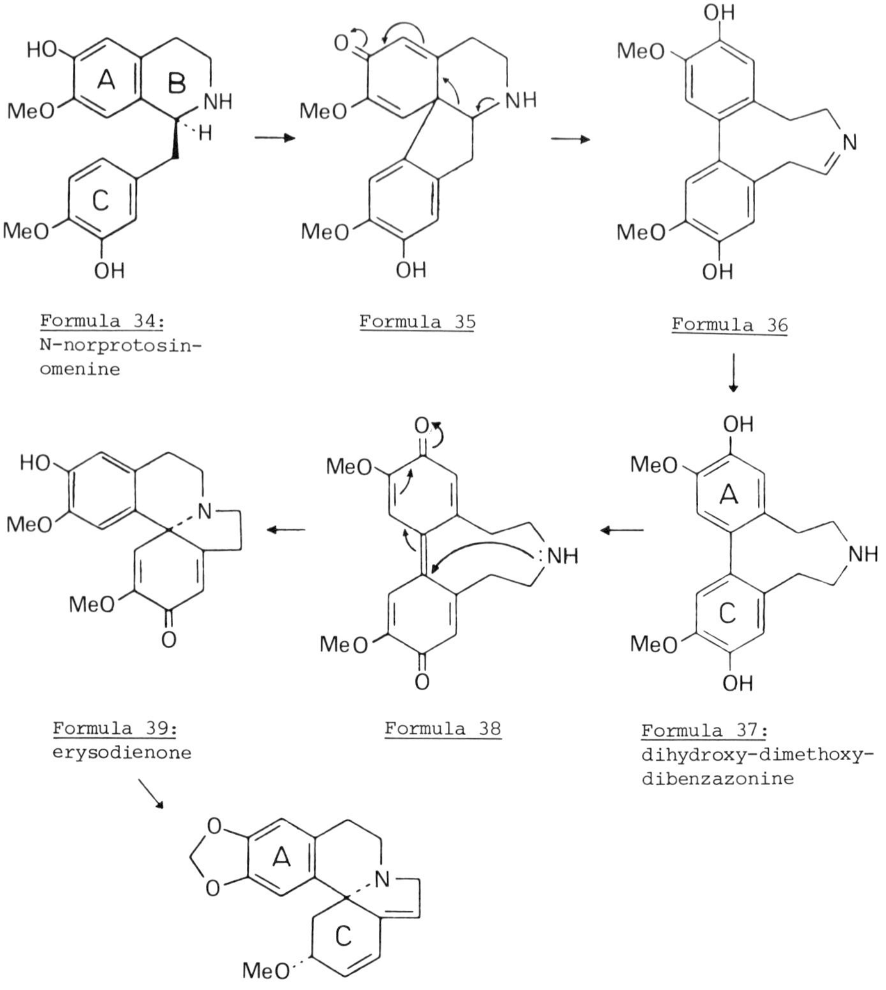

Formula 34: N-norprotosinomenine

Formula 35

Formula 36

Formula 37: dihydroxy-dimethoxy-dibenzazonine

Formula 38

Formula 39: erysodienone

Formula 40: erythraline

Fig. 4. Biosynthesis of the *erythrina* alkaloids according to (53)

unusual tetracyclic spiro-benzazepin structure (Formula 41) and is itself inactive.

Several alkylated and hydroxylated succinic acid monomethyl esters are found as acidic components in the harringtonines (Formulas 42 - 45).

The intensity and type of antitumor activity are apparently strongly dependent on the nature of the acid component, and they are especially marked in the case of homoharringtonine (Formula 44) (57). There is, therefore, an understandable interest in the preparation of harringtonines and possibly even more active analogues (58) with particular attention focused on the total synthesis of cephalotaxine (59 - 61), which can be converted into the harringtonines by acylation.

Since cephalotaxinone (Formula 49), the corresponding ketone can be stereo-selectively reduced to (±)-cephalotaxine with complex hydrides (62), the syntheses procede via this ketone, which has also been shown in plant extracts.

Formula 41 esterified with:

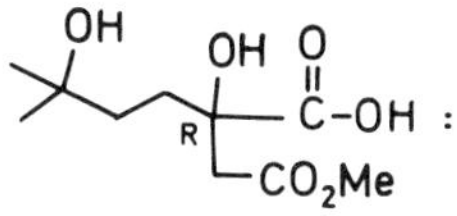

: Formula 42: Harringtonine

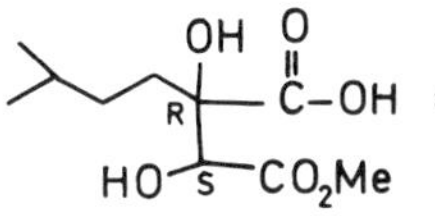

: Formula 43: Isoharringtonine

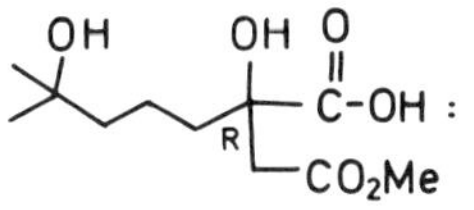

: Formula 44: Homoharringtonine

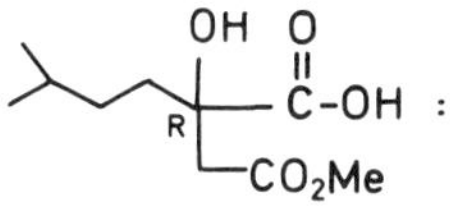

: Formula 45: Deoxyharringtonine

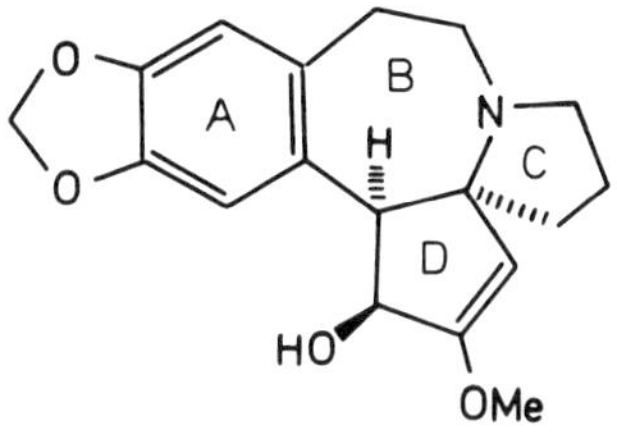

Formula 41: Cephalotaxine

Semmelhack synthesizes cephalotaxinone (Formula 49) via the key compound Formula 48, which he obtains by N-alkylation of the 1-aza-spiro[4.4]-non-en-one (Formula 47) with the tosylate of the o-iodo-phenyl-ethanol (Formula 46) (59). Both substances are relatively easily available.

There have been painstaking investigations of the ring closure of Formula 48 to cephalotaxinone. Systematic investigations under different conditions showed that the photo-SRN1 reaction is better than all other methods, and it gives nearly quantitative yields. The reaction procedes in a basic medium and it activates the aromatic compounds for a nucleophilic attack by photolysis of the iodine.

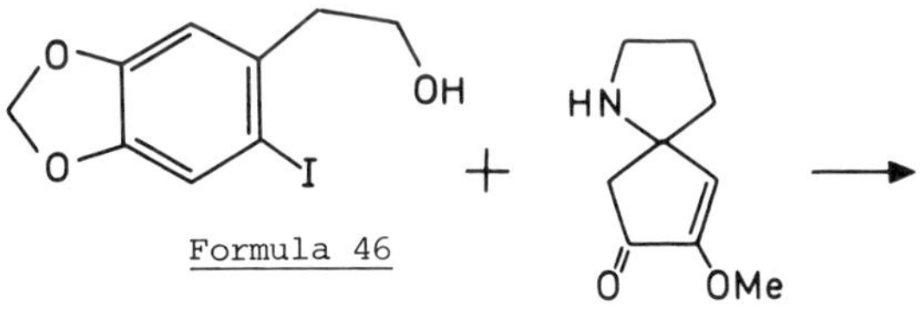

Formula 46

Formula 47

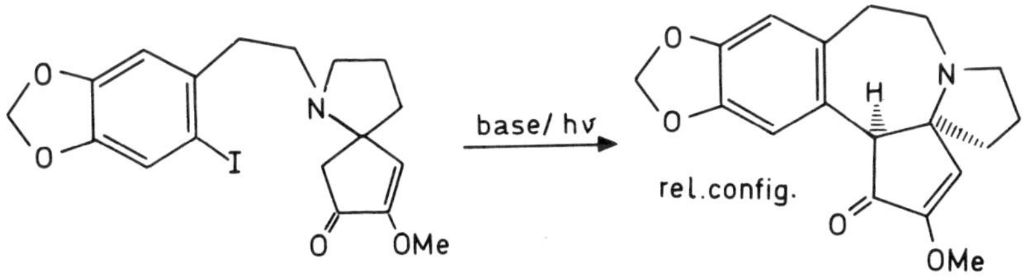

Formula 48

Formula 49: Cephalotaxinone

Camptothecin (Formula 50) from *Camptotheca acuminata* and *Mappia foetida* (Nyssaceae) is characterized by a peculiar indolizidino-quinoline skeleton. Owing to its marked cytostatic properties, it aroused great hopes for cancer therapy, but these have since been disappointed by the high toxicity of the compound (63, 64).

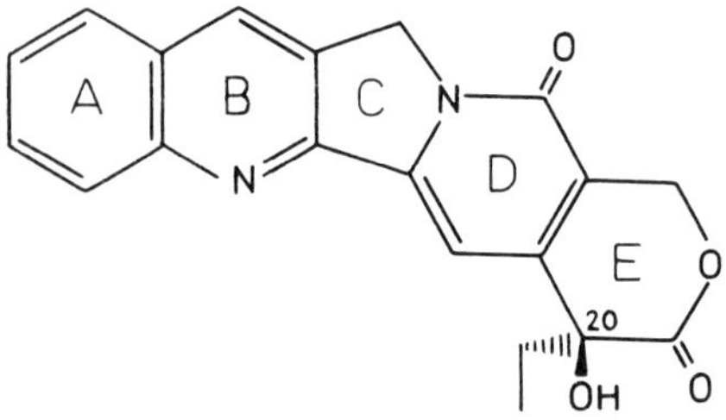

Formula 50: Camptothecin

Nevertheless, camptothecin appears to have some magical attraction as an objective for the synthetic chemist. Since the first total synthesis by Stork and Schultz (65) in 1972, more than 12 other different total syntheses have been reported (66), and the extensive preparative efforts have found special consideration in a monograph (67).

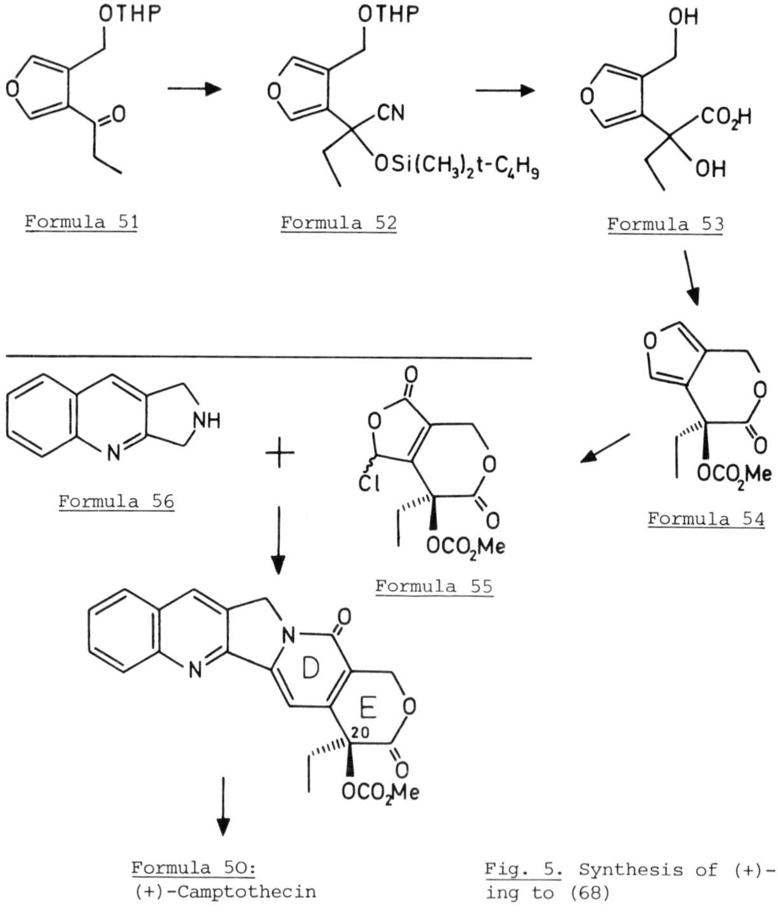

Fig. 5. Synthesis of (+)-camptothecin according to (68)

I should like to describe briefly a new synthetic route, developed by Corey, which leads to natural, optically active camptothecin (Fig. 5) (68).

This is a convergent synthesis, and the pentacyclic ring system of Formula 50 is formed in the penultimate stage from the pyrrolidino-quinoline (Formula 56) and the S-configurated bicyclic compound (Formula 55). The starting point for this component, which has a key position in the synthesis, is 3-hydroxymethyl-4-propionyl-furan (Formula 51), whose OH-group is protected as a tetrahydropyranyl ether. Under specially worked out reaction conditions, treatment with t-butyldimethylsilyl cyanide converts the ketone grouping to the cyanide (Formula 52); the following hydrolysis yields the dihydroxy acid (Formula 53). This chiral acid can be resolved into its antipodes with quinine. The S-configured enantiomer has been lactonized and converted into the furano-α-pyrone (Formula 54), with protection of the OH-group using chloroformic ester. Photo-oxidation, followed by $SOCl_2$ treatment gives Formula 55, which, as already mentioned, is the required key compound for the condensation step.
Removal of the protective group then yields the natural 20(S)-camptothecin.

In view of their biological properties, I feel that the following quinoline alkaloids, found in the *Rutaceae*, are worth mentioning: The quaternary pteleatinium salt (Formula 57) from *Ptelea trifoliata* possesses antibacterial activity (69, 70). The corresponding methyl ether, the O-methyl-balfourodinium cation (Formula 58) is present in *Choisya ternata*, and it is a growth inhibitor (71).

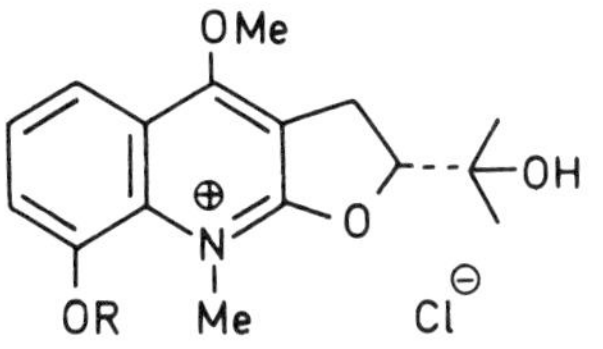

Formula 57: Pteleatinium chlorid : R = H
Formula 58: O-Methyl-balfourodinium chlorid : R = Me

Skimmianine (Formula 59) (from species of *Fagara* and *Zanthoxylum* and others) and dubinidine (Formula 60) from *Haplophylum dubium* have apparently been the subject of extensive pharmacological studies in Russia. They are both supposed to have sedative and hypothermic properties (72, 73) and skimmianine-iron complex also has antimicrobial activity (74). Foliosidine (Formula 61) from *Haplophylum foliosum* is reported to show activity against cardiac arrythmia in animal tests (75).

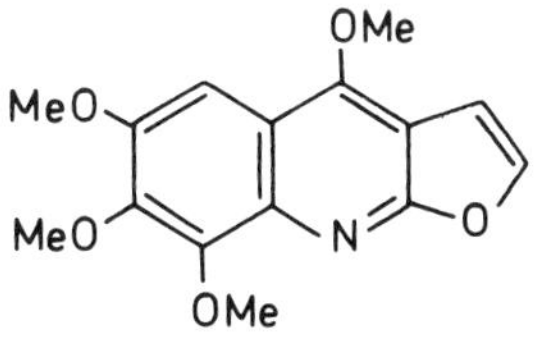

Formula 59:
Skimmianine

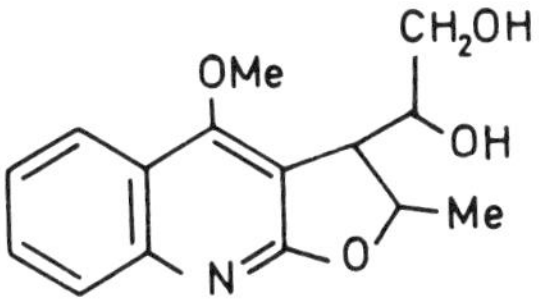

Formula 60:
Dubinidine

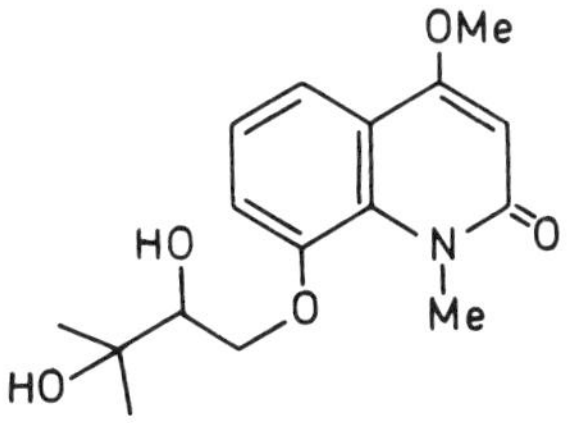

Formula 61:
Foliosidine

Many biologically very active compounds are found amongst the *Amaryllidaceae* alkaloids.

I think some recent results should be mentioned. Thus antimitotic and plant growth inhibitory properties have been reported for narciclasine (Formula 62) (= Lycoricidinol) (76), whose structure and stereochemistry have now been confirmed by X-ray structural analysis (77). Lycorine (Formula 63) and some of its derivatives have hypotensive activity (78), whereas compounds structurally related to mesembrine (Formula 64) are reported to act on the central nervous system (79).

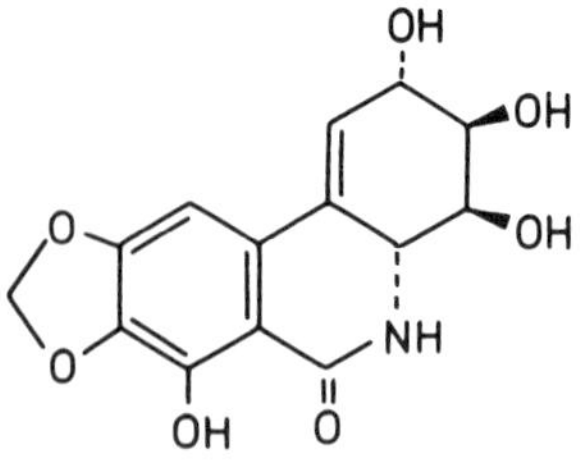

Formula 62:
Narciclasine

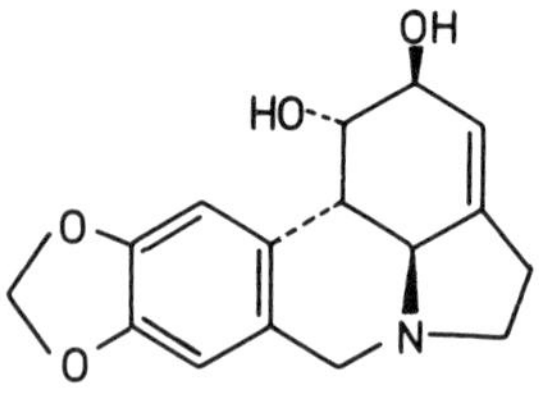

Formula 63:
Lycorine

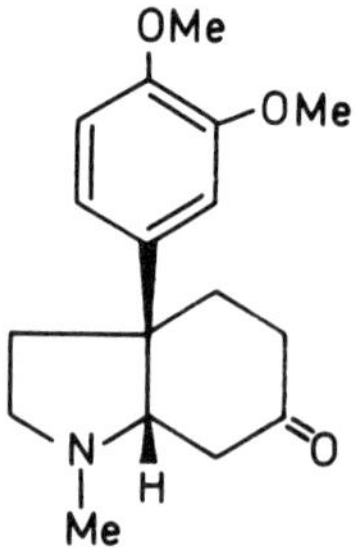

Formula 64:
Mesembrine

Without doubt, it is these reports that have given the essential stimulus for the design of new syntheses (80 - 84).

1-Benzyl-isoquinoline and aporphine alkaloids have again recently been the subject of extensive pharmacological and chemical studies. It would seem that interest in the aporphines was especially engendered by a report that (-)-apomorphine can be used for the treatment of Parkinson's disease (85). A new synthetic route to 1-benzyl-tetrahydroisoquinolines, designed for the total synthesis of thalicarpine, consists of the reaction of the appropriate N-methyl-3,4-dihydroisoquinolinium iodide with an o-nitro toluene under basic conditions (86).

I should also like to mention the new methods for the cyclization of 1-benzyl-isoquinolines to aporphines: the known Pschorr cyclization now has got competition by photochemical methods (87), and by the use of new agents, such as $VOCl_3$, or lead tetraacetate, for the oxidative coupling (88, 89).

Thalicarpine (Formula 68), an alkaloid of the aporphine-benzylisoquinoline dimeric type, is of particular pharmacological interest, owing to its antitumor activity.

The starting point of a new synthesis by Kupchan (Fig. 6), which has been patented (90), is the diphenyl ether (Formula 65), containing rings D and C'.

The aporphine part is first built up via Formula 66 using the o-nitrotoluene grouping of Formula 65, then after ring closure it is selectively formylated and resolved to produce the compound (Formula 67), which occurs naturally in *Hernandia ovigera* (Hernandiaceae) and is called hernandaline (91); finally, the benzyl-isoquinoline component is constructed by Reissert condensation. Thalicarpine also possesses antimicrobial activity (92). It shares this property with some of the macrocyclic bisbenzylisoquinoline compounds that frequently occur in *Thalictrum* species (93).

Structurally, thalicarpine is closely related to the antiinflammatory active (94) fetidine (Formula 69) from *Thalictrum foetidum* (Ranunculaceae), whose structure was recently revised (95). Formally, fetidine is a demethyl-thalicarpine, with the diphenyl ether linkage in ring C' at an alternative position.

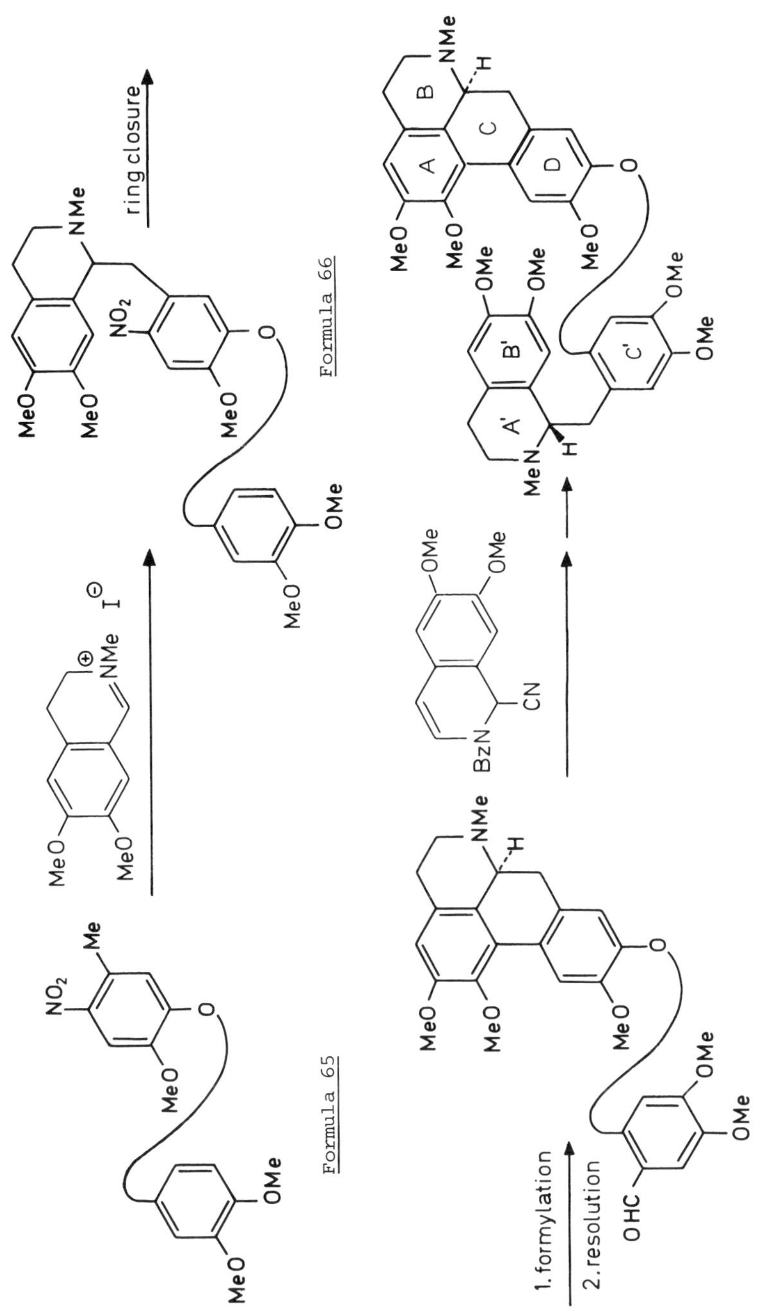

Formula 65

Formula 66

Formula 67

Formula 68: Thalicarpine

Fig. 6. Synthetic route to thalicarpine according to (90)

Proton resonance spectroscopy has made necessary a revision of the structure of tubocurarine chloride. In contrast to earlier assumptions, tubocurarine chloride contains only 3 N-methyl groups and it has only one quaternary nitrogen (96). The new formula has been confirmed and supplemented by crystallographic investigations and conformational studies (97 - 99).

A recently published new variation of the Ullmann diphenyl ether synthesis holds promise of an improved preparative approach to the bis-benzylisoquinoline alkaloids (100).

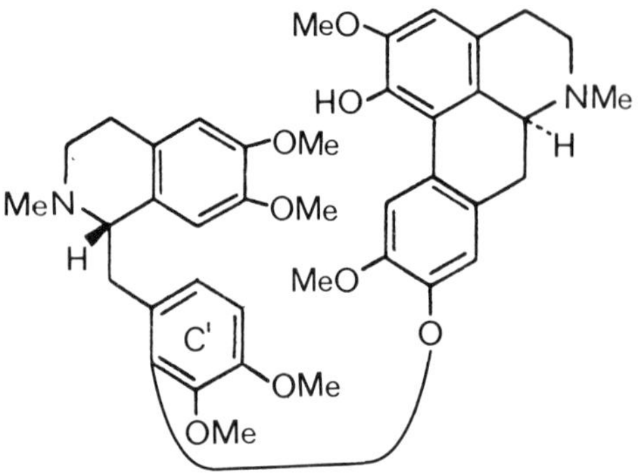

Formula 69: Fetidine

In past years, extensive research work has been carried out on the indole alkaloids. I should like to single out the following points, which are of pharmacological interest: new syntheses in the yohimbine series have been reported by various research groups (101 - 105).

We also have new synthetic routes for the antitumor alkaloid ellipticine (Formula 70) (106 - 108).

9-Hydroxy-ellipticine and other 9-substituted ellipticines have been prepared, which exhibit increased antileukaemic and immuno-suppressive effects, with decreased toxicity (109 - 112).

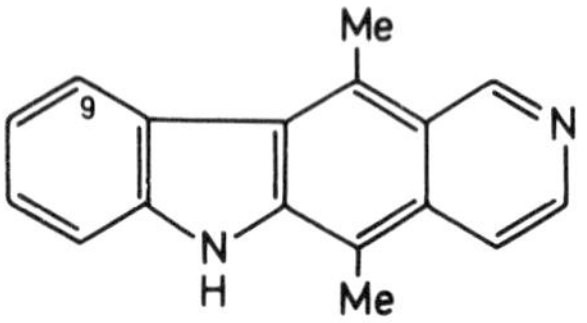

Formula 70: Ellipticine

In particular, further efforts have been made in the synthesis of the vasodilatory vincamine (Formula 71), which is also the subject of much patent literature (113, 114).

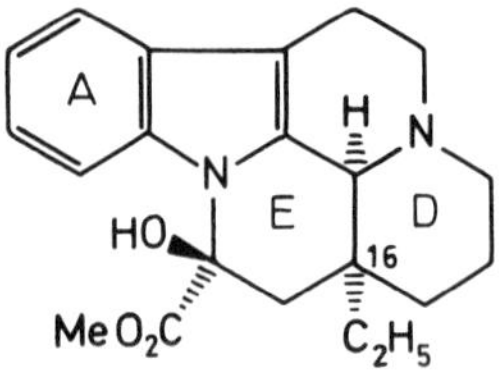

Formula 71: Vincamine

Unlike the earlier methods, these new syntheses are stereoselective with respect to the D/E ring coupling. The crucial stage is an indoloquinolizinium precursor of type Formula 72, whose immonium group can be stereo-selectively reduced according to studies of Wenkert (115).

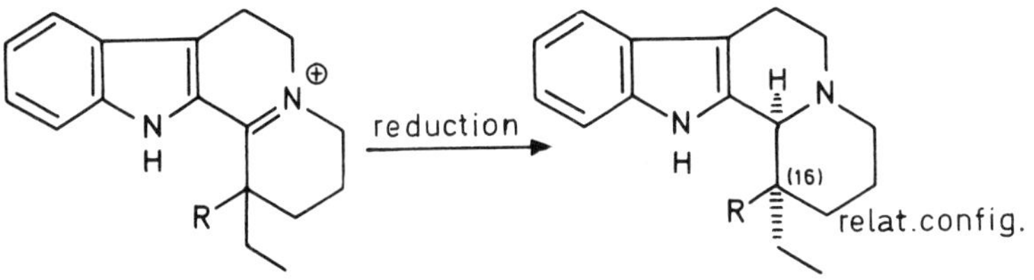

Formula 72

This type of stereo-selective synthesis was also used by Oppolzer to prepare optically active vincamine (116). He introduced the chiral center at C-16 with the correct configuration at a relatively early stage (Fig. 7).

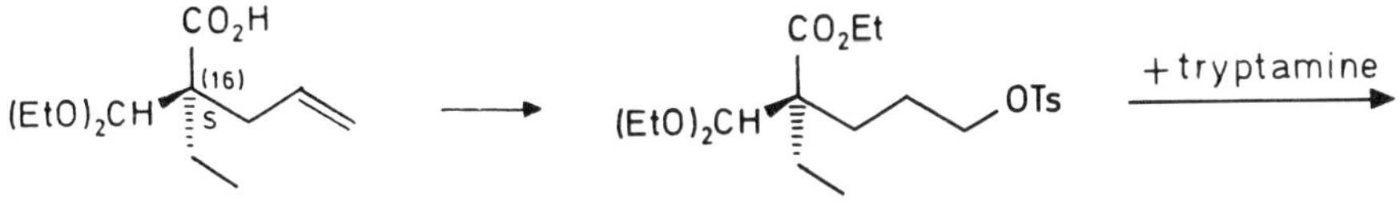

Formula 73 Formula 74

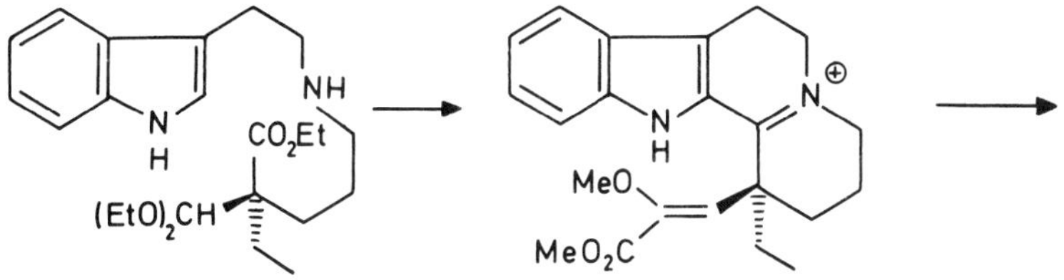

Formula 75 Formula 76

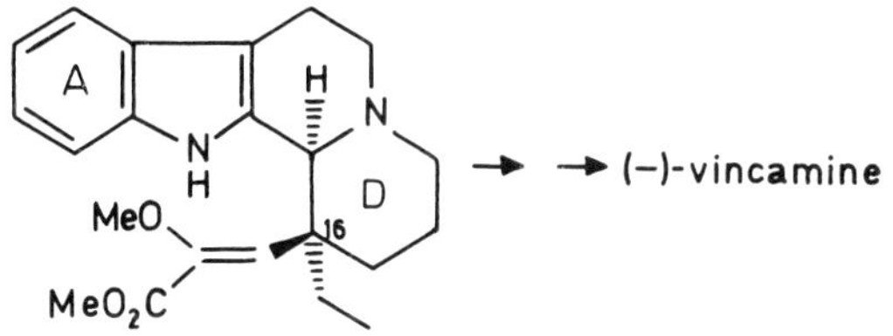

Formula 77

Fig. 7. Synthesis of (-)-vincamine according to (116)

Formula 73 was the optically active compound used, which is readily available by a malonic ester synthesis and subsequent separation into its antipodes via the pseudoephedrine salts. The ethyl ester of Formula 73 was converted in two steps to the tosylate (Formula 74), which was used to alkylate tryptamine. Intramolecular ring closure of the lactam (Formula 75), followed by chain elongation at the freed aldehyde function produces under Bischer-Napieralski conditions Formula 76, which is of the previously mentioned quinolizinium type (Formula 72). Catalytic hydrogenation of the latter preferentially yields the desired cis-compound (Formula 77), which can easily be converted into naturally (-)-vincamine.

The bisindole alkaloids from *Catharanthus roseus* (Apocynaceae) claim special attention; here, efforts, on the one hand, are directed to the isolation and structural elucidation of more new compounds from plant material, with possibly better pharmacological properties; while, on the other hand, there is much interest in the synthesis of these substances.

Of the newly discovered alkaloids in this group, there have to be discussed the antimitotic compounds leurocolombine (Formula 79) (117, 118), vincadioline (Formula 80) (119) and vincathicine (Formula 81) (120); the latter was isolated as early as 1964, but at that time it was wrongly considered to be an oxindole (121). Structural elucidation has depended largely on comprehensive spectroscopic studies, together with ^{13}C-spectroscopic measurements (122), with the following results:

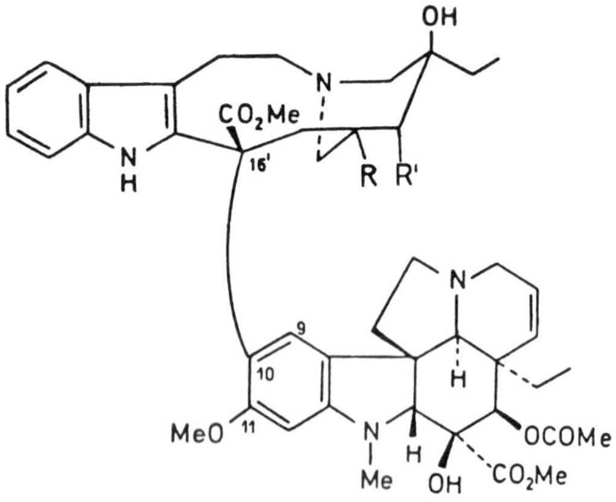

Formula 78: Vinblastine R = H, R' = H
Formula 79: Leurocolombine R =OH, R' = H
Formula 80: Vincadioline R = H, R' =OH*

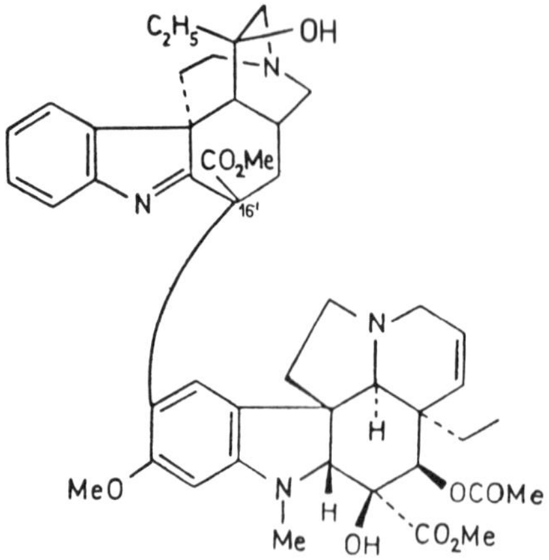

Formula 81: Vincathicine

The three compounds differ from one another and from vinblastine (Formula 78) in the so-called velbanamine (Formula 83) part of the molecule; in all the formulae one can recognize the unchanged vindoline unit, which is bound via C-10. Leurocolombine (Formula 79) and vincadioline (Formula 80) are isomeric hydroxy vinblastines. In leurocolombine the additional OH-group is tertiary and in vincadioline it is secondary. In contrast, vincathicine (Formula 81) possesses a pentacyclic indolenine structure.

Vincathicine can be prepared from the already well known leurosine (Formula 82) (123) by proton catalysis (120):
The proton attacks primarily the oxirane ring. The α,β-double bond of the indole reacts intramolecularly as an enamine, as in the Michael addition, and it attacks at C-15'. This intramolecular nucleophilic reaction, which is sterically favorable, leads to the opening of the oxirane to produce vincathicine (Formula 81).

The absolute configuration at C-16', which hitherto could only be studied with X-ray analysis, has now been investigated with optical rotatory dispersion by Kutney and Scott (124).

It is known that the two clinically important alkaloids vinblastine and vincristine differ only in the substituents on the nitrogen of the vindoline unit (Formula 84). Despite the fact that the structural differences are only slight, these alkaloids have markedly different therapeutic profiles (125) so that a preparative conversion of vin-

*The formula of vincadioline given in (119) has to be revised as Formula 80: pers. comm. September 1976

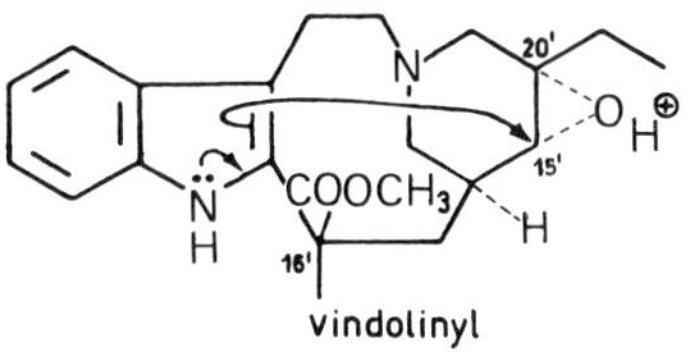

Formula 82: Leurosine

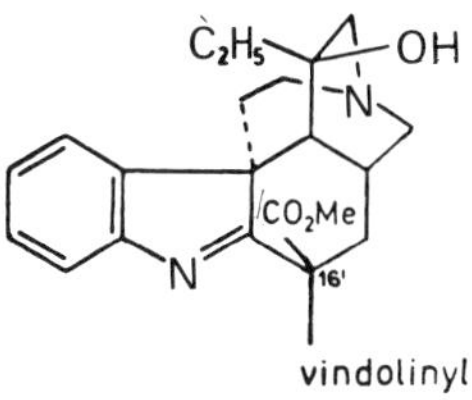

Formula 81: Vincathicine

blastine into vincristine, which is only present in plant material at a level of about 25 ppm, is of interest.

According to a patent, vinblastine can be converted into vincristine by catalytic oxidation with oxygen selectively at the N-methyl group (126). This conversion is also possible with chromium trioxide (127). Finally, one must mention another new method, in which vinblastine is N-demethylated by fermentation with a streptomycete (128).

Synthesis of bisindole alkaloids of the vinblastine type is of considerable practical importance, because their isolation from plant material involves extensive separation procedures. The essential step in the synthesis is the coupling of the two monomeric components. For the synthesis of vinblastine, this means that velbanamine (Formula 83) must be activated at C-1 for an electrophilic attack on vindoline (Formula 84).

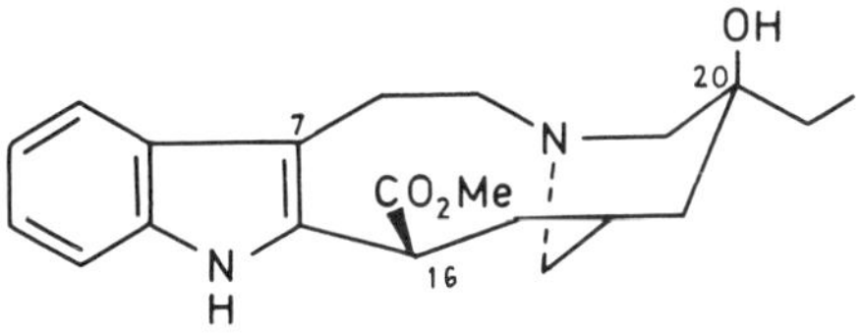

Formula 83: Velbanamine

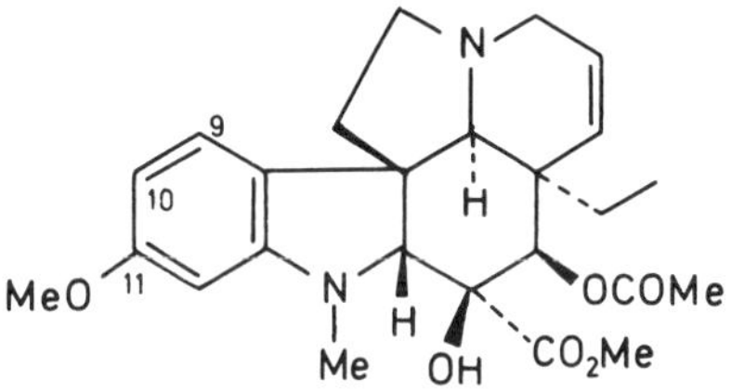

Formula 84: Vindoline

By analogy, and on the basis of reactivities, it is to be expected that the electrophilic reaction will occur very preferentially at C-10 of the vindoline. In model experiments, Kutney reacted vindoline with 7-chloroindolenines of the velbanamine type, which should react in the tautomeric form (Formula 85) (129): the product (Formula 86) was a bisindole with the desired constitution, but with an irregular, "unnatural" epi-configuration at C-16'.

Further investigations showed that the stereochemistry of the coupling can be guided in the required direction, if a suitable pentacyclic compound of the catharanthine type (Formula 87) is used in place of the velbanamine. This coupling partner must be activated by an electron withdrawing substituent on the nitrogen, so that in the nucleophilic attack by the vindoline, the charge, as shown by the arrows in Formula 88, is transferred causing cleavage of the 16/21 bond (130, 131). Finally, the immonium ion (Formula 89) has to be reduced.

Using this modified Polonovski reaction, a series of vinblastine analogues with the correct configuration at C-16' have now been prepared from monomeric precursors (130, 131).

Oxidation of the immonium ion (Formula 89) with osmium tetroxide was recently reported as a means of selectively introducing an hydroxyl

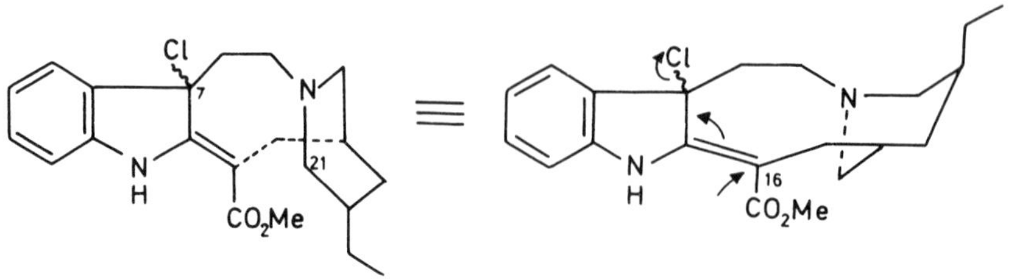

Formula 85

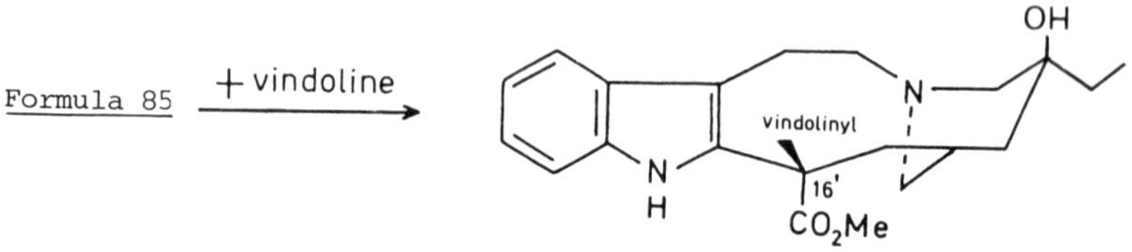

Formula 86

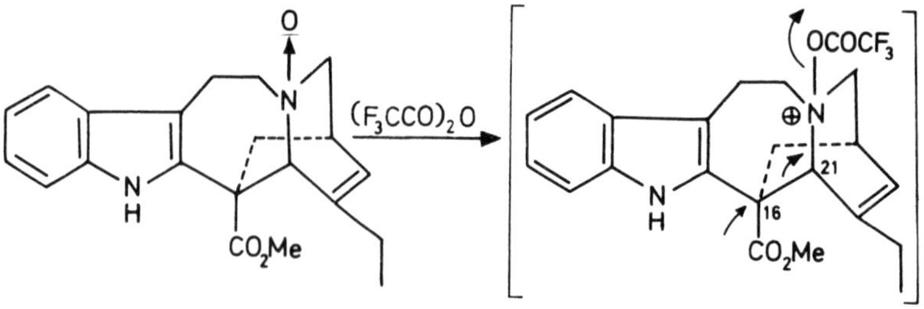

Formula 87: Catharanthine-N-oxide

Formula 88

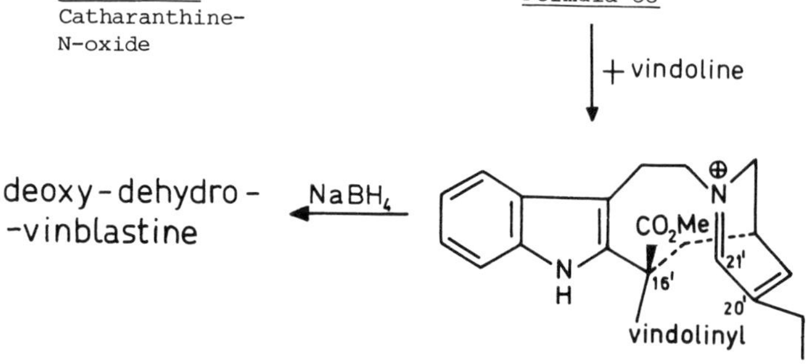

Formula 89

group at C-20', thus producing natural leurosidine (Formula 90) (132). The latter differs from vinblastine only by an epimeric arrangement of the substituents at C-20' (122).

In working with the N-oxides of the catharanthine type, it must be remembered that longer heating causes a [2.3]-sigmatropic rearrangement of the alicyclic ring to an isoxazolidine (133).

Publications and patents concerning the ergoline and lysergic acid alkaloids describe conversion products and derivatives with widely differing properties:
Thus ergoline carbamates of type Formulas 91a or 91b have sympathomimetic, or muscle relaxing properties (134); 8-thiomethylergolines (Formula 92) and their dihydroderivatives inhibit the secretion of prolactine (135); 6-methyl-ergoline-acetonitrile is reported to suppress the production of mammary carcinomas (136) while 1.1-diethyl-

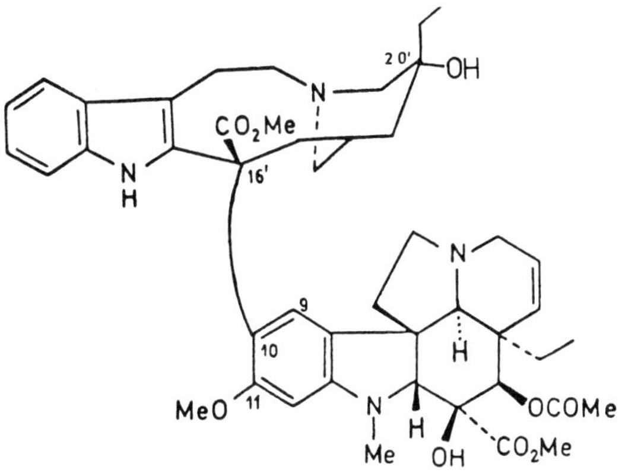

Formula 90: Leurosidine

(6-methylisoergolinyl)- semicarbazide possesses antinidation activity (137). In this connection there seems to be a correlation between the inhibition of prolactin secretion and inhibition of nidation (138).

6-Methyl-8-(nicotinoyl)aminoethylergoline exhibits a pronounced and persistent hypotensive effect (139).

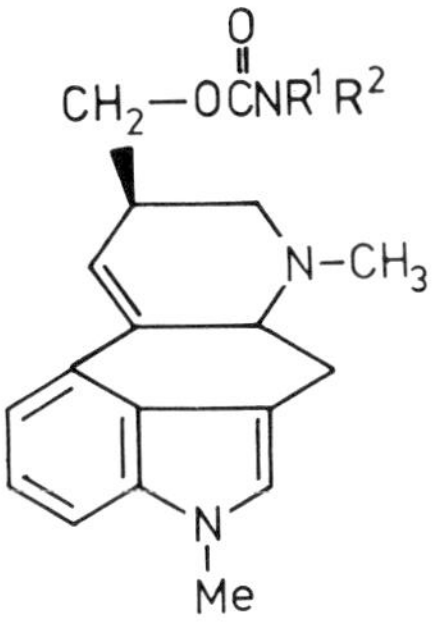

Formula 91a

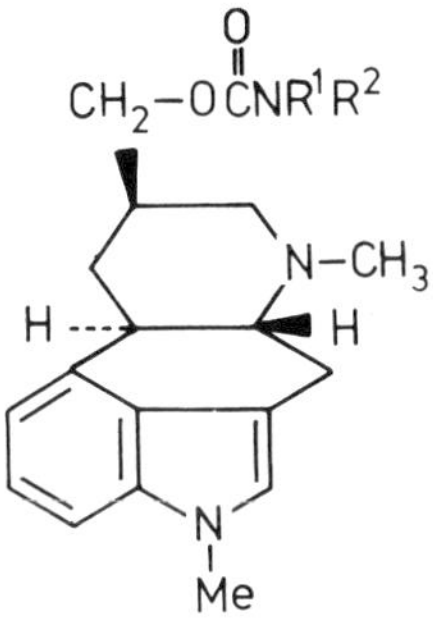

Formula 91b

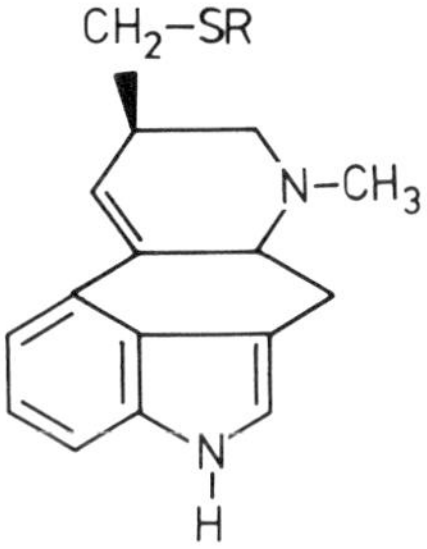

Formula 92

Some attention has also been paid to the separation of natural lysergic acid alkaloid mixtures. In addition to new derivatization techniques (140) and chromatographic methods (141), a procedure has been reported for the separation of ergotamine with the aid of high frequency electromagnetic waves (142).

As a further striking example of the use of microbiological methods in alkaloid chemistry, I must mention mitragynine (Formula 93) from *Mitragyna speciosa* (Rubiaceae). This well-known alkaloid of the corynantheine series possesses analgesic properties (143).
In the microbiological transformation of mitragynine with *Helminthosporum*, a metabolite was isolated with a 10-fold higher analgesic activity. It was identified as mitragyninepseudoindoxyl (Formula 94) and it was also synthesized chemically (144).

The marine alkaloid surugatoxin (Formula 95) belongs also to the indole series. It occurs in *Babylonia japonica*, a carnivorous gastropod, and it causes poisoning if the animal is eaten. Apparently, these snails are poisonous only if they live in the area of Suruga Bay in Japan (145). Environmental influences must, therefore, play an important part in the production of the surugatoxin.

Pharmacologically, surugatoxin shows marked mydriatic properties (145).

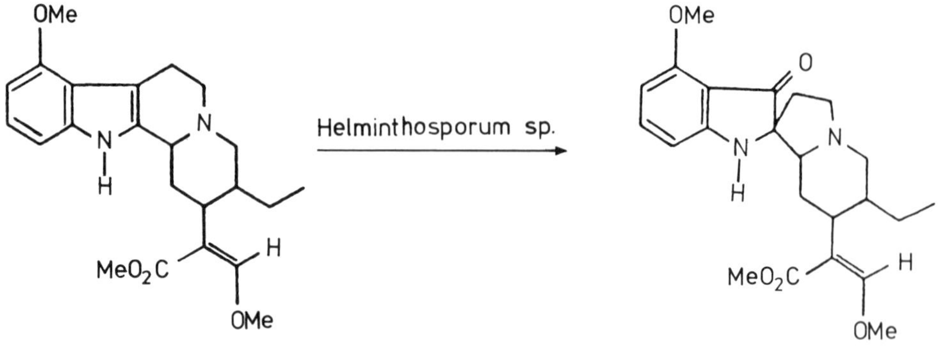

Formula 93: Mitragynine

Formula 94

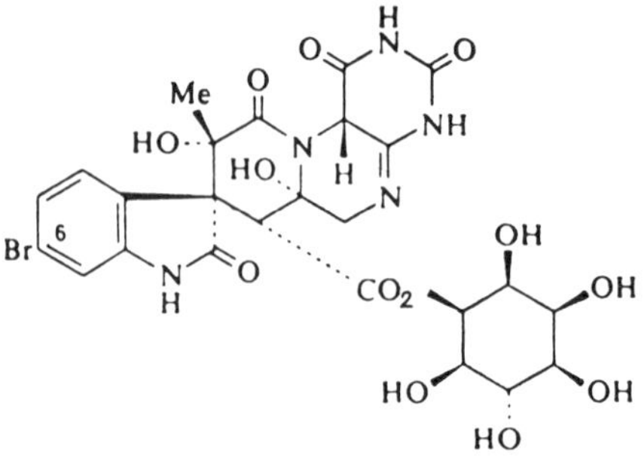

Formula 95: Surugatoxin

X-ray structural analysis (145) led to the completely new type of pentacyclic oxindole structure shown in Formula 95, with a bromine atom at position 6. In the nonindolic part of the molecule, one can recognize the pterine ring system; and finally, on an ester linkage, we see myo-inositol.

Rhazinilam is a new type of alkaloid, which exhibits mild analgesic activity (146) and was discovered during the fractionation of extracts of *Rhazya stricta* (147, 148), *Aspidosperma quebrachoblanco* (149, 150) and *Melodinus australis* (151). Structural elucidation led to the ninemembered lactam ring Formula 96, whose structure contains a phenyl-substituted pyrrolopiperidine (148, 149).

As the stereo Formula 96a shows, the two unsaturated rings stand almost perpendicular to eachother. This explains why the UV-spectrum of rhazinilam does not exhibit the characteristics of a phenyl substituted pyrrole system.

Rhazinilam accumulates in basic extracts of plant material (148). It thus seems probable that rhazinilam is an artefact produced from an alkaloid precursor. It has been proposed that rhazinilam might be derived from or via the hypothetical dihydroxy-aspidospermidine For-

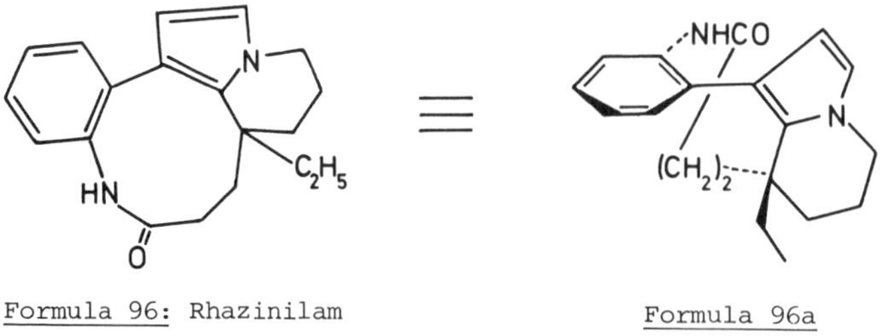

Formula 96: Rhazinilam

Formula 96a

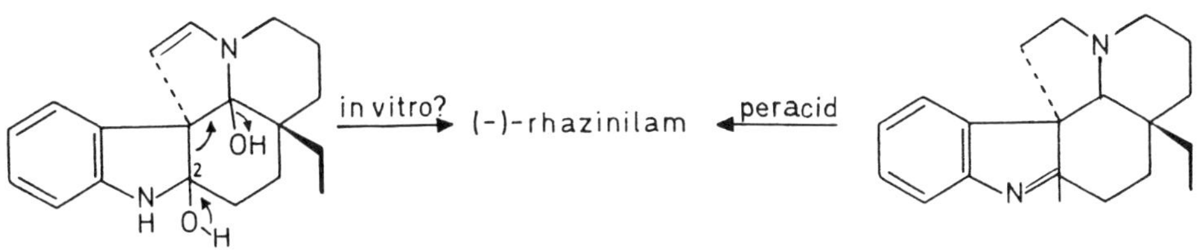

Formula 97 Formula 98

mula 97 (148). Opening of the dihydroindole system is brought about by removal of the proton from the OH-group at C-2 as shown, and this leads directly in a concerted reaction to rhazinilam.

Support for this hypothesis is found in the reaction of (+)-1,2-dehydro-aspidospermidine (Formula 98) with peracid. After additional treatment with Fe^{2+}-sulphate, a 30 % yield of natural (-)-rhazinilam is obtained (152).

A structurally new class of alkaloids is represented by the maytansinoids (153). Owing to their intense antimitotic (154) and antitumor activity (155) they have attracted much attention and already studies on the synthesis of model compounds have been reported (156, 157). Maytansine, the first compound in this class, was isolated from *Maytenus ovatus* (Celastraceae) by Kupchan (153, 158).

Structural studies on maytansine led to the interesting ansa-macrolide structure (Formula 99) (153).

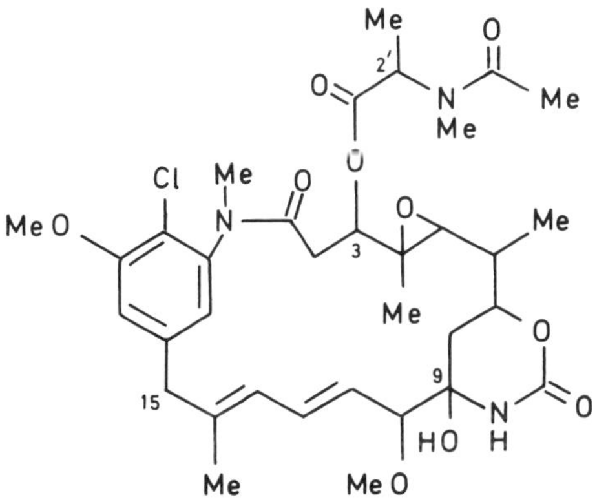

Formula 99: Maytansine

We see a 19 membered amide ring, arranged ansa-like on the chlorine-substituted benzene ring. On the macroring, there is a cyclic carbamate grouping with a carbinolamide arrangement at C-9; and at C-3, we find an N-derivatized glycine bound in an ester linkage.

Isolation of further compounds with the same ansa-macrolide skeleton from specis of *Colubrinus* (159), *Maytenus* (160, 161) and *Putterlickia* has revealed the following structural variations:

1. Alterations of the acyl side chain at C-3, or its nitrogen substituents.
2. Removal of the 3-hydroxy or ester function, leaving on α,β-unsaturated cyclic amide.
3. O-Alkylation of the carbinolamide.
4. Introduction of an OH, or acetoxy group at C-15.

The following structure-activity relationships have been established and supplemented with studies on partial synthesis (162):

The forementioned oxidation or O-alkylation at the ring do not effect the properties substantially, whereas the ester group at C-3 is essential in respect to the biological activity. For maytansinol, the alcohol having a free hydroxyl function at C-3, is inactive. The structure of the acyl side chain seems to be of minor importance, since the acetic acid ester of maytansinol is already active again.

Eritadenine (Formula 100) is an alkaloid from *Lentinus edodes* (Basidiomycetae). Chemically, it is a purine and it is similar to the nucleotides. In animal tests, eritadenine has hypocholesterolaemic activity (163).
The compound can be synthesized easily from adenine and D-erythronolactone (Formula 101) (164). Alkylation of the nitrogen is achieved by reaction of the sodium salt of adenine with the acetonide of D-erythronolactone.

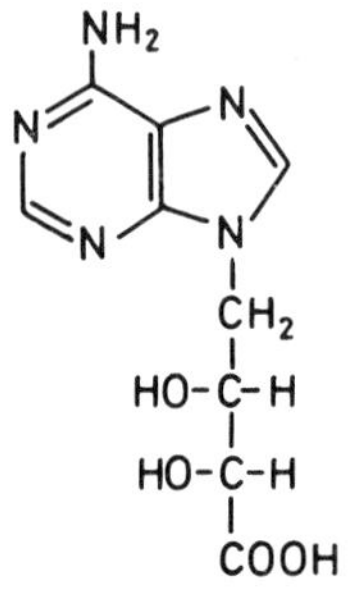

Formula 100:
Eritadenine

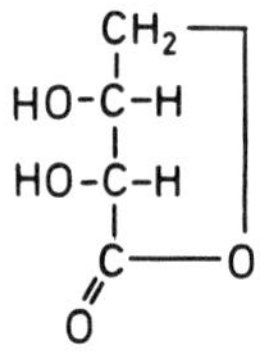

Formula 101:
D-Erythronolactone

Zeatin (Formula 102) is another biologically active purine alkaloid. The trans-form of zeatin occurs in *Zea mays* (Gramineae), and it is one of the most effective natural promotors of plant cell division. Biological activity depends upon the geometry of the molecule, trans-zeatin being about 50 times more active than the cis-isomer (165).

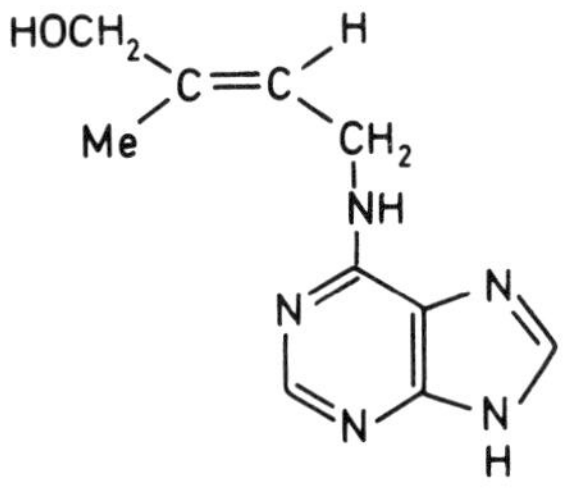

Formula 102: trans-Zeatin

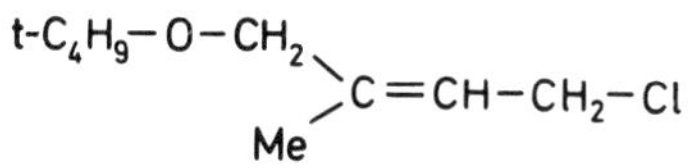

Formula 103

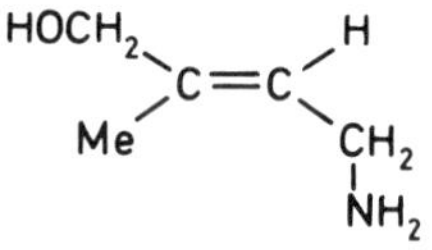

Formula 104

An efficient synthesis was reported recently (166). In order to construct the correct geometrically orientated side chain, the synthesis starts with the 2-methyl-but-2-ene (Formula 103), which is readily available by the addition of t-butyl hypochlorite to isoprene. The chlorine is substituted by reaction with potassium phthalimide and

at the stage of the resulting phthalimide the required transisomer can be easily separated, owing to its rather low solubility. Cleavage of the imide group to the amine (Formula 104), then reaction with 6-chloropurine, leads to trans-zeatin.
Japanese workers have reported a variation of this procedure (167).

As the last compound, we should mention saxitoxin. This is an alkaloid with a hydrogenated purine skeleton, shown in Formula 105 as the hydrated di-cation.

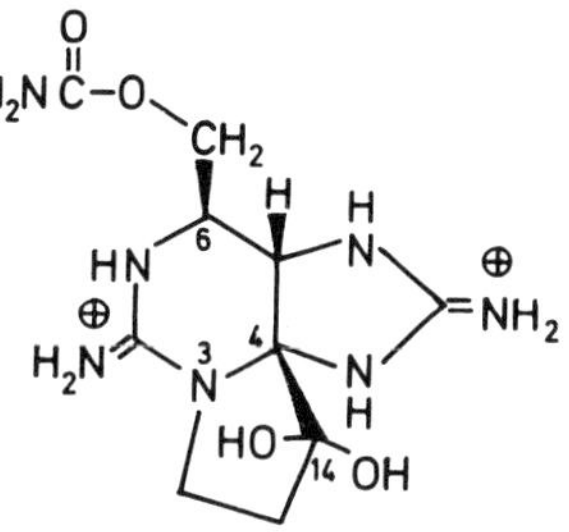

Formula 105: Saxitoxin

Saxitoxin is neurotoxic, and it is one of the most powerful known low molecular weight poisons, with an LD_{50} of 5-10 μg/kg in mice (168). Cases of poisoning arise after eating infected mussels from the West coast of North America. The infective agent is the dinoflagellate *Gonyaulax catanella*.

The structure of saxitoxin has been the subject of intensive chemical and spectroscopic studies, which were very difficult, especially by the high polarity of the molecule and its poor crystallization properties (169).

On the basis of X-ray structural analysis in two different laboratories, the formula is now conclusively established (170, 171). In Formula 105 we see the hydrogenated purine ring system, with a carbamate arrangement at C-6, and two guanidine groups, that are easily protonated and are thereby responsible for the high polarity of the molecule. Positions 3 and 4 are spanned cyclically. At C-14 there is a ketone, which under normal conditions exists as the hydrate, and can only be dehydrated by extreme conditions. The high stability of the hydrate is explained in view of the neighboring powerful electron withdrawing guanidine groups.

The biological effect of saxitoxin, which acts as a sodium ion channel blocker, is ascribed to the molecular properties of the hydrate (171).

That concludes my report on "Progress in the Chemistry of Alkaloids with Pharmacological or Biological Activity." It remains for me to hope and expect that the results of this intense research work will very soon lead to the development of new or improved pharmaceutical or other biologically active substances with practical application.

References

1. Baumgarth, M.: Chemiker-Ztg. 97, 217 (1973)
2. e.g. Verpoorte, R., Baerheim Svendsen, A.: Pharm. Weekbl. 110, 1021 (1975); Verpoorte, R., Baerheim Svendsen, A.: J. Chromatogr. 120, 203 (1976)
3. Wenkert, E., Bindra, J.S., Chang, C.J., Cochran, D.W., Schnell, F.M.: Accounts of Chem. Res. 7, 46 (1974); Cambie, R.C., Burfitt, I.R., Goodwin, T.E., Wenkert, E.: J. Org. Chem. 40, 3789 (1975) and earlier papers in this series; Wenkert, E., Chang, C., Chawla, H.P.S., Cochran, D.W., Hagaman, E.W., King, J.C., Orito, K.: J. Am. Chem. Soc. 98, 3645 (1976)
4. Ahond, A., Janot, M.-M., Langlois, N., Lukacs, G., Potier, P., Rasoanaivo, P., Sangaré, M., Neuss, N., Plat, M., Hagaman, E.W., Wenkert, E.: J. Am. Chem. Soc. 96, 634 (1974)
5. Durham, L.J., Shoolery, J.N., Djerassi, C.: Proc. Natl. Acad. Sci. 71, 3797 (1974)
6. Khanov, M.T., Sultanov, M.B., Egorova, T.A.: Farmakol. Alkaloidov Serdech. Glikozidov 1971, 210 [Chem. Abstr. 77, 135091 (1972)]
7. Yagudaev, M.R., Matkhalikova, S.F., Malikov, V.M., Yunusov, S.Y.: Khim, Prir. Soedin. 1972, 495 [Chem. Abstr. 77, 164902 (1972)]
8. Wiedhopf, R.M., Trumbull, E.R., Cole, J.R.: J. Pharm. Sci. 62, 1206 (1973)
9. Govindachari, T.R., Nagarajan, K., Rajappa, S.: J. Chem. Soc. 1957, 2725; Kametani, T.: Heterocycles 3, 627 (1975)
10. Bhattacharya, S.K., Ghosal, S., Chaudhuri, R.K., Singh, A.K., Sharma, P.V.: J. Pharm. Sci. 63, 1341 (1974)
11. Sadritdinov, F.: Farmakol. Alkaloidov Serdech. Glikozidov 1971, 146 [Chem. Abstr. 78, 79634 (1973)]
12. Tulyaganov, N., Danilevskii, B.L., Sadritdinov, F.S.: Farmakol. Alkaloidov Serdech. Glikozidov 1971, 148 [Chem. Abstr. 78, 66918 (1973)]
13. Danilevskii, B.L., Tulyaganov, N.T., Sadritdinov, F.S.: Dokl. Akad. Nauk Uzb. SSR 1972, 37 [Chem. Abstr. 78, 38001 (1973)]
14. Wan, A.S.C., Macko, E., Douglas, B.: Asian J. Med. 1972, 334 [Chem. Abstr. 78, 11686 (1973)]
15. Fitzgerald, J.S., Johns, S.R., Lamberton, J.A., Redcliffe, A.H., Sioumis, A.A., Suares, H.: Anales de Quimica 68, 737 (1972)
16. Burdick, E.M.: Econ. Botany 25, 363 (1971)
17. Spiteller-Friedmann, M., Spiteller, G.: Monatsh. Chem. 95, 1234 (1964); Coke, J.L., Rice, W.Y.Jr.: J. Org. Chem. 30, 3420 (1965)
18. Corey, E.J., Nicolaou, K.C.: J. Am. Chem. Soc. 96, 5614 (1974)
19. Corey, E.J., Nicolaou, K.C., Melvin, L.S.Jr.: J. Am. Chem. Soc. 97, 654 (1975)
20. Keller-Schierlein, W.: Fortschr. Chem. Org. Naturst. 30, 313 (1973)
21. Binder, M., Tamm, C.: Angew. Chem. 85, 369 (1973); Angew. Chem. Intern. Ed. 12, 370 (1973)
22. Corey, E.J., Nicolaou, K.C., Melvin, L.S.Jr.: J. Am. Chem. Soc. 97, 653 (1975); Corey, E.J., Ulrich, P., Fitzpatrick, J.M.: J. Am. Chem. Soc. 98, 222 (1976)
23. Brown, E., Bourgouin, A.: Chem. Lett. 1974, 109; Brown, E., Bourgouin, A.: Tetrahedron 31, 1047 (1975)
24. Ferris, J.P.: J. Org. Chem. 27, 2985 (1962)
25. Blomster, R.N., Schwarting, A.E., Bobbitt, J.M.: Lloydia 27, 15 (1964)
26. Kaplan, H.R., Wolke, R.E., Malone, M.H.: J. Pharm. Sci. 56, 1385 (1967); Kosersky, D.S., Malone, M.H.: J. Pharm. Sci. 60, 952 (1971)
27. Hanaoka, M., Ogawa, N., Arata, Y.: Chem. Pharm. Bull. 22, 973 (1974)
28. Krmpotic, E., Farnsworth, N.R., Messmer, W.M.: J. Pharm. Sci. 61, 1508 (1972)
29. Paton, J.M., Pauson, P.L., Stevens, T.S.: J. Chem. Soc. C 1969, 1309
30. Kotani, E., Kitazawa, M., Tobinga, S.: Tetrahedron 30, 3027 (1974)
31. Tobinaga, S.: Japan. Kokai 75 59, 398 [Chem. Abstr. 83, 131809 (1975)]
32. LaLonde, R.T., Wong, C.F., Cullen, W.P.: Tetrahedron Lett. 1970, 4477
33. Cullen, W.P., LaLonde, R.T., Wang, C.J., Wong, C.F.: J. Pharm. Sci. 62, 826 (1973)
34. LaLonde, R.T., Wong, C.F., Das, K.C.: J. Am. Chem. Soc. 95, 6342 (1973)
35. Wrobel, J.T., Bobeszko, B., Martin, T.I., MacLean, D.C., Krishnamachari, N., Calvo, C.: Can. J. Chem. 51, 2810 (1973)
36. Schlittler, E.: In: The Alkaloids. A Specialist Periodical Report. London: The Chemical Society 1971, Vol. I, p. 490
37. Govindachari, T.R., Rajagopalan, T.G., Viswanathan, N.: J.C.S. Perkin I, 1974, 1161

38. Wadhawan, V.K., Sikka, S.K., Mulchandani, N.B.: Tetrahedron Lett. 1973, 5091; Wadhawan, V.K., Sikka, S.K., Mulchandani, N.B.: India, A.E.C., Bhabba At. Res. Cent. (Rep.) 1974, BARC-764, 6[Chem. Abstr. 82, 171258 (1975)]
39. Govindachari, T.R., Viswanathan, N., Radhakrishnan, J., Pai, B.R., Natarajan, S., Subramaniam, P.S.: Tetrahedron 29, 891 (1973); Govindachari, T.R.: J. Indian Chem. Soc. 50, 1 (1973)
40. Mulchandani, N.B., Iyer, S.S., Badheka, L.P.: Chem. Ind. 1971, 505
41. Noyori, R., Makino, S., Baba, Y., Hayakawa, Y.: Tetrahedron Lett. 1974, 1049
42. Noyori, R., Baba, Y., Hayakawa, Y.: J. Am. Chem. Soc. 96, 3336 (1974)
43. Ghosal, S., Dutta, S.K., Bhattacharya, S.K.: J. Pharm. Sci. 61, 1274 (1972)
44. Hargreaves, R.T., Johnson, R.D., Millington, D.S., Mondal, M.H., Beavers, W., Becker, L., Young, C., Rinehart, K.L.Jr.: Lloydia 37, 569 (1974)
45. Boar, R.B., Widdowson, D.A.: J. Chem. Soc. B 1970, 1591
46. Millington, D.S., Steinman, D.H., Rinehart, K.L.Jr.: J. Am. Chem. Soc. 96, 1909 (1974)
47. Games, D.E., Jackson, A.H., Khan, N.A., Millington, D.S.: Lloydia 37, 581 (1974)
48. Yunusov, S.Y., Razakov, R.: Khim. Prir. Soedin. 1970, 74[Chem. Abstr. 73, 35585 (1970)]
49. Vul'fson, N.S., Bochkarev, V.N.: Izv. Akad. Nauk SSSR, Ser. Khim. 1972, 500 [Chem. Abstr. 77, 62194 (1972)]
50. Razakov, R., Yunusov, S.Y., Nasirov, S.M., Chekhlov, A.N., Andrianov, V.G., Struchkov, Y.T.: J.C.S. Chem. Commun. 1974, 150
51. Razakov, R., Yunusov, S.Y., Nasirov, S.M., Adrianov, V.G., Struchkov, Y.T.: Izv. Akad. Nauk SSSR, Ser. Khim. 1974, 218[Chem. Abstr. 80, 108727 (1974)]; Nasirov, S.M., Adrianov, V.G., Struchkov, Y.T., Yunusov, S.Y.: Khim. Prir. Soedin. 1975, 395[Chem. Abstr. 84, 59817 (1976)]
52. Zakirov, U.B., Aliev, K.U., Abdumalikova, N.V.: Farmakol. Alkaloidov Serdech. Glikozidov 1971, 197[Chem. Abstr. 77, 135092 (1972)]
53. Barton, D.H.R., Boar, R.B., Widdowson, D.A.: J. Chem. Soc. C 1970, 1213
54. Barton, D.H.R., Potter, C.J., Widdowson, D.A.: J.C.S. Perkin I 1974, 346
55. Ito, K., Furukawa, H., Tanaka, H.: Chem. Pharm. Bull. 19, 1509 (1971)
56. e.g., Arora, S.K., Bates, R.B., Grady, R.A., Powell, R.G.: J. Org. Chem. 39, 1269 (1974); Powell, R.G., Weisleder, D., Smith, C.R.Jr., Rohwedder, W.K.: Tetrahedron Lett. 1970, 815; Mikolajczak, K.L., Powell, R.G., Smith, C.R.Jr.: Tetrahedron 28, 1995 (1972); Powell, R.G., Madrigal, R.V., Smith, C.R.Jr., Mikolajczak, K.L.: J. Org. Chem. 39, 676 (1974); Arora, S.K., Bates, R.B., Grady, R.A., Germain, G., Declercq, J.P., Powell, R.G.: J. Org. Chem. 41, 551 (1976)
57. Powell, R.G., Weisleder, D., Smith, C.R.Jr.: J. Pharm. Sci. 61, 1227 (1972)
58. Mikolajczak, K.L., Smith, C.R.Jr., Powell, R.G.: J. Pharm. Sci. 63, 1280 (1974)
59. Semmelhack, M.F., Chong, B.P., Stauffer, R.D., Rogerson, T.D., Chong, A., Jones, L.D.: J. Am. Chem. Soc. 97, 2507 (1975)
60. Weinreb, S.M., Auerbach, J.: J. Am. Chem. Soc. 97, 2503 (1975)
61. Weinreb, S.M., Semmelhack, M.F.: Accounts Chem. Res. 8, 158 (1975)
62. Powell, R.G., Mikolajczak, K.L.: Phytochemistry 12, 2987 (1973)
63. Schultz, A.G.: Chem. Rev. 73, 385 (1973)
64. Shamma, M., Georgiev, V.S.: J. Pharm. Sci. 63, 163 (1974)
65. Stork, G., Schultz, A.G.: J. Am. Chem. Soc. 93, 4074 (1971)
66. Review: Danieli, B., Palmisano, G.: Fitoterapia 45, 87 (1974); Sugasawa, T., Toyoda, T., Sakasura, K.: Chem. Pharm. Bull. 22, 771 (1974); Sugasawa, T., Toyoda, T., Sakasura, K.: Japan Kogai 74, 117,499 [Chem. Abstr. 82, 125513 (1975)]; Walraven, H.G.M., Pandit, U.K.: Tetrahedron Lett. 1975, 4507; Tang, C.S.F., Morrow, C.J., Rapoport, H.: J. Am. Chem. Soc. 97, 159 (1975); Shanghai, 5th Pharmaceutical Plant, K'o Hsueh T'ung Pao 21, 40 (1976)[Chem. Abstr. 84, 122100 (1976)]; Bradley, J.C., Büchi, G.: J. Org. Chem. 41, 699 (1976)
67. Winterfeldt, E.: In: Recent Developments in the Chemistry of Carbon Compounds. Budapest 1975, Vol.VI, p. 9
68. Corey, A.J., Crouse, D.N., Anderson, J.E.: J. Org. Chem. 40, 2141 (1975)
69. Mitscher, L.A., Bathala, M.S., Beal, J.L.: Chem. Commun. 1971, 1040
70. Mitscher, L.A., Bathala, M.S., Clark, G.W., Beal, J.L.: Lloydia 38, 109 (1975)
71. Garestier, R., Rideau, M.: C.R. Acad. Sci. 274D, 2651 and 3541 (1972)
72. Evdokimova, N.I., Polievtsev, N.P., Sultanov, M.B.: Farmakol. Alkaloidov Serdech. Glikozidov 1971, 167[Chem. Abstr. 78, 119189 (1973)]

73. Polievtsev, N.P., Evdokimova, N.I., Sultanov, M.B.: Farmakol. Alkaloidov Serdech. Glikozidov 1971 [Chem. Abstr. 78, 119191 (1973)]
74. Isamukhamedov, I.: Farmakol. Alkaloidov Serdech. Glikozidov 1971, 224[Chem. Abstr. 78, 92966 (1973)]
75. Polievtsev, N.P., Azimov, M.M.: Farmakol. Alkaloidov Ikh Proizvod. 1972, 58 [Chem. Abstr. 80, 103870 (1974)]
76. Okamoto, T., Torii, Y., Isogai, Y.: Chem. Pharm. Bull. 16, 1860 (1968); Okamoto, T., Torii, Y., Isogai, Y.: In: Plant Growth Substances. Proc. 7th Intern. Conf. 1970. Carr, D.J. (ed.). New York: Springer 1972, p. 311
77. Immirzi, A., Fuganti, C.: J.C.S. Chem. Commun. 1972, 240
78. Zakirov, U.B., Aliev, K.U.: Farmakol. Alkaloidov Serdech. Glikozidov 1971, 111 [Chem. Abstr. 77, 122093 (1972)]; Akzente p. 2 in 'Bild der Wissenschaft' 10 (1973)
79. Oishi, A., Kugita, H.: Japan Pat. 7143,538 and 7143,539 [Chem. Abstr. 76, 59442 and 59443 (1972)]
80. Ohta, S., Kimoto, S.: Tetrahedron Lett. 1975, 2279
81. Tsuda, Y., Sano, T., Taga, J., Isobe, K., Toda, J., Irie, H., Tanaka, H., Takagi, S., Yamaki, M., Murata, M.: J.C.S. Chem. Commun. 1975, 933
82. Lida, H., Aoyagi, S., Kibayashi, C.: J.C.S. Perkin I 1975, 2502
83. Wijnberg, J.B.P.A., Speckamp, W.N.: Tetrehedron Lett. 1975, 3963
84. Stephens, R.V., Lesko, P.M., Lapalme, R.: J. Org. Chem. 40, 3495 (1975)
85. Cotzias, G.C., Papavasiliou, P.S., Fehling, C., Kaufman, B., Mena, E.: New England J. Medicine 282, 31 (1970); Düby, S., Cotzias, G.C., Steck, A., Papavasiliou, P.S.: Federation Proc. 30, 216 (1971)
86. Paull, K.P., Engle, R.R., Twanmoh, L., Wood, H.B.Jr., Driscoll, J.S.: J. Pharm. Sci. 61, 1481 (1972); Kupchan, S.M., Kameswaran, V., Findlay, J.W.A.: J. Org. Chem. 38, 405 (1973)
87. Spangler, R.J., Boop, D.C.: Tetrahedron Lett. 1971, 4851; Kupchan, S.M., Moniot, J.L., Kanojia, R.M., O'Brien, J.B.: J. Org. 36, 2413 (1971); Cava, M.P., Stern, P., Wakisaka, K.: Tetrahedron 29, 2245 (1973); T. Kametani and K. Fukumoto, Accounts Chem. Res. 5, 212 (1972)
88. e.g. Schwartz, M.A.: Synth. Commun. 3, 33 (1973)
89. Hoshino, O., Toshioko, T., Umezawa, B.: Chem. Commun. 1971, 1533
90. Kupchan, S.M., Liepa, A.J., Kameswaran, V., Sempuku, K.: J. Am. Chem. Soc. 95, 2995 (1973); Kupchan, S.M., Liepa, A.J.: U.S. Pat. 3,875,167 [Chem. Abstr. 83, 28433 (1975)]; Kupchan, S.M., Liepa, A.J.: Brit. Pat. 1,373,399 [Chem. Abstr. 83, 59125 (1975)]
91. Cava, M.P., Bessho, K., Douglas, B., Markey, S., Weisbach, J.A.: Tetrahedron Lett. 1966, 4279
92. Gharbo, S.A., Beal, J.L., Doskotch, R.W., Mitscher, L.A.: Lloydia 36, 349 (1973)
93. Mitscher, L.A., Wu, W.-N., Doskotch, R.W., Beal, J.L.: Chem. Commun. 1971, 589; Mitscher, L.A., Wu, W.-N., Beal, J.L.: Experientia 28, 500 (1972); Mitscher, L. A., Wu, W.-N., Doskotch, R.W., Beal, J.L.: Lloydia 35, 167
94. Sadritdinov, F.: Farmakol. Alkaloidov Ikh Proizvod. 1972, 154 [Chem. Abstr. 80, 91211 (1974)]
95. Cava, M.P., Wakisaka, K.: Tetrahedron Lett. 1972, 2309
96. Everett, A.J., Love, L.A., Wilkinson, S.: Chem. Commun. 1970, 1020
97. Gorinsky, C., Palmer, R.A., Reynolds, C.D., Rywater, R.P.: J. Cryst. Mol. Struct. 1, 307 (1971)
98. Codding, P.W., James, M.G.: J.C.S. Chem. Commun. 1972, 1174
99. Egan, R.S., Stanaszek, R.S., Williamson, D.E.W.: J.C.S. Perkin II 1973, 716
100. Cava, M.P., Afzali, A.: J. Org. Chem. 40, 1553 (1975)
101. Review: Töke, L., Szántay, C.: Heterocycles 4, 251 (1976)
102. Töke, L., Honty, K., Szabó, L., Blaskó, G., Szántay, C.: J. Org. Chem. 38, 2496 (1973); Töke, L., Gombos, Z., Blaskó, G., Honty, K., Szabó, L., Tamás, J., Szántay, C.: J. Org. Chem. 38, 2501 (1973); Szántay, C., Honty, K., Töke, L., Szabó, L.: Chem. Ber. 109, 1737 (1976)
103. Stork, G., Guthikonda, R.N.: J. Am. Chem. Soc. 94, 5109 (1972)
104. Mori, K., Takemoto, I., Matsui, M.: Agr. Biol. Chem. 36, 2605 (1972)[Chem. Abstr. 78, 97847 (1973)]
105. Kametani, T., Hirai, Y., Kajiwara, M., Takahashi, T., Fukumoto, K.: Chem. Pharm. Bull. 23, 2634 (1975); Kametani, T., Kajiwara, M., Takahashi, T., Fukumoto, K.: Heterocycles 3, 179 (1975); Kametani, T., Hirai, Y., Fukumoto, K.: Heterocycles 4, 29 (1976)

106. Le Goffic, F., Gouyette, A., Ahond, A.: C.R. Acad. Sci. 274C, 2008 (1972); Le Goffic, F., Gouyette, A., Ahond, A.: Tetrahedron 29, 3357 (1973)
107. Kilmister, K.N., Sainsbury, M.: J.C.S. Perkin I 1972, 2264
108. Besselièvre, R., Thal, C., Husson, H.P., Potier, P.: J.C.S. Chem. Commun. 1975, 90; Langlois, Y., Langlois, N., Potier, P.: Tetrahedron Lett. 1975, 955
109. Hayat, M., Mathé, G., Chenn, E., Janot, M.M., Potier, P., Dat-Xuong, Nguyen, Cave, A., Sevenet, T., Kan-Fan, C., Poisson, J., Miet, J., Le Men, J., Le Goffic, F., Gouyette, A., Ahond, A., Dalton, L.K., Connors, T.A.: Biomedicine 21, 101 (1974)
110. Sainsbury, M., Webb, B.: J.C.S. Perkin I 1974, 1580
111. Le Pecq, J.B., Dat-Xuong, Nguyen, Gosse, C., Paoletti, C.: Proc. Natl. Acad. Sci. 71, 5078 (1974)
112. Dat-Xuong, Nguyen, Adeline, M.T., Lecointe, P., Janot, M.M.: C.R. Acad. Sci. 281C, 623 (1975)
113. Hugel, G., Lêvy, J., Le Men, J.: C.R. Acad. Sci. 274C, 1350 (1972); Thal, C., Sevenet, T., Husson, H.P., Potier, P.: C.R. Acad. Sci. 275C 1295 (1972); Szântay, C., Szabô, L., Kalaus, G.: Tetrahedron Lett. 1973, 191; Herrmann, J. L., Cregge, R.J., Richman, J.E., Semmelhack, C.L., Schlessinger, R.H.: J. Am. Chem. Soc. 96, 3702 (1974)
114. e.g., Centre d'Etudes pour l'Industrie Pharmaceutique, Fr. Demande 2,193,587, [Chem. Abstr. 82, 51782 (1975)]; Giudicelli, D.P.R.L., Najer, H., Iliesco-Branceni, B., Pascal, Y.R.A.: Ger. Offen. 2,421,999 [Chem. Abstr. 82, 57995 (1975)]; Najer, H., Pascal, Y.R.A.: Ger. Offen. 2,362,363 [Chem. Abstr. 82, 4451 (1975)]; Richter, G., Vegyeszeti, G.R.: Brit. Pat. 1,382,609 [Chem. Abstr. 83, 59137 (1975)]; Plat, M.R.M., Plat, M.: Ger. Offen. 2,504,045 [Chem. Abstr. 83, 179358 (1975)]
115. Wenkert, E., Wickberg, B.: J. Am. Chem. Soc. 87, 1580 (1965)
116. Pfäffli, P., Oppolzer, W., Wenger, R., Hauth, H.: Helv. Chim. Acta 58, 1131 (1975)
117. Smith, S.L., Dorman, D.E.: U.S. Pat. 3,890,325[Chem. Abstr. 83, [illegible] (1975)]
118. Tafur, S.S., Jones, W.E., Dorman, D.E., Logsdon, E.E., Svoboda, G.H.: J. Pharm. Sci. 64, 1953 (1975)
119. Jones, W.E., Cullinan, G.J.: U.S. Pat. 3,887,565[Chem. Abstr. 83, 97687 (1975)]
120. Tafur, S.S., Occolowitz, J.L., Elzey, T.K., Paschal, J.W., Dorman, D.E.: J. Org. Chem. 41, 1001 (1976)
121. Svoboda, G.H., Barnes, A.J.Jr.: J. Pharm. Sci. 53, 1227 (1964)
122. Wenkert, E., Hagaman, E.W., Lal, B., Gutowski, G.E., Katner, A.S., Miller, J. C., Neuss, N.: Helv. Chim. Acta 58, 1560 (1975)
123. Neuss, N., Gorman, M., Cone, N.J., Huckstep, L.L.: Tetrahedron Lett. 1968, 783
124. Kutney, J.P., Gregonis, D.E., Imhof, R., Itoh, I., Jahngen, E., Scott, A.I., Chan, W.K.: J. Am. Chem Soc. 97, 5013 (1975)
125. Klener, P.: In: Vinca Alkaloids. Acta Universitatis Carolinae Medica, Monographia LVIII. Prag: Univ. Karlova 1974, p. 119
126. Richter, G., Vegyeszeti, G.R.: Belg. Pat. 823,560 [Chem. Abstr. 84, 59835 (1976)]
127. Jovanovics, K., Szasz, K., Fekete, G., Bittner, E., Dezseri, E., Eles, J.: U.S. Pat. 3,899,493[Chem. Abstr. 83, 179360 (1975)]
128. Brannon, D.R., Neuss, N.: Ger. Offen. 2,440,931[Chem. Abstr. 83, 7184 (1975)]
129. Kutney, J.P., Cook, J., Fuji, K., Treasurywala, A., Clardy, J., Fayos, J., Wright, H.: Heterocycles 3, 205 (1975); Kutney, J., Beck, J., Bylsma, F., Cook, J., Cretney, W.J., Fuji, K., Imhof, R., Treasurywala, A.M.: Helv. Chim. Acta 58, 1690 (1975)
130. Kutney, J.P., Ratcliffe, A.H., Treasurywala, A.M., Wunderly, S.: Heterocycles 3, 639 (1975)
131. Potier, P., Langlois, N., Langlois, Y., Guéritte, F.: J.C.S. Chem. Commun. 1975, 670
132. Langlois, N., Potier, P.: Tetrahedron Lett. 1976, 1099
133. Langlois, Y., Guéritte, F., Andriamialisoa, R.Z., Langlois, N., Potier, P., Chiaroni, Riche, C.: Tetrahedron 32, 945 (1976)
134. Ferrari, G., Krepinski, J.J.: Ger. Offen. 2,424,540[Chem. Abstr. 82, 140365 (1975)]

135. Kornfeld, E.C., Bach, N.J.: U.S. Pat. 3,901,894 [Chem. Abstr. 83, 193578 (1975)]
136. Welsch, C.W., Gribler, C., Clemens, J.A.: Europ. J. Cancer 10, 595 (1974) [Chem. Abstr. 82, 118880 (1975)]
137. Zikán, V., Rezábek, K., Semonský, M.: Collect. Czech. Chem. Commun. 39, 3144 (1974)
138. Rezábek, K., Cassady, J.M., Floss, H.G.: J. Pharm. Sci. 64, 1045 (1975)
139. Cerný, A., Rezábek, K., Seda, M., Trčka, V., Semonský, M.: Collect. Czech. Chem. Commun. 41, 1042 (1976)
140. Wichlinski, L., Trzebinski, J., Skibinski, Z.: Pol. Pat. 77,938 [Chem. Abstr. 84, 105887 (1976)]
141. Heacock, R.A., Langille, K.R., MacNeil, J.D., Frei, R.W.: J. Chromatogr. 77, 425 (1973)
142. Bach, J.: U.S. Pat. 3,880,734 [Chem. Abstr. 83, 183386 (1975)]
143. Macko, E., Weisbach, J.A., Douglas, B.: Arch. Intern. Pharmacodyn. Ther. 198, 145 (1972)
144. Zarembo, J.E., Douglas, B., Valenta, J., Weisbach, J.A.: J. Pharm. Sci. 63, 1407 (1974)
145. Kosuge, T., Zenda, H., Ochiai, A., Masaki, N., Noguchi, M., Kimura, S., Narita, H.: Tetrahedron Lett. 1972, 2545
146. Benoit, P.S., Angry, G., Lyon, R.L., Fong, H.H.S., Farnsworth, N.R.: J. Pharm. Sci. 62, 1889 (1973)
147. Banerji, A., Majumder, P.L., Chatterjee, A.: Phytochemistry 9, 1491 (1970)
148. De Silva, R.T., Ratcliffe, A.H., Smith, G.F., Smith, G.N.: Tetrahedron Lett. 1972, 913
149. Abraham, D.J., Rosenstein, R.D., Lyon, R.L., Fong, H.H.S.: Tetrahedron Lett. 1972, 909
150. Lyon, L., Fong, H.H.S., Farnsworth, N.R., Svoboda, G.H.: J. Pharm. Sci. 62, 218 (1973)
151. Linde, H.H.A.: Helv. Chim. Acta 48, 1822 (1965)
152. Ratcliffe, A.H., Smith, G.F., Smith, G.N.: Tetrahedron Lett. 1973, 5179
153. Kupchan, S.M., Komoda, Y., Court, W.A., Thomas, G.J., Smith, R.M., Karim, A., Gilmore, C.J., Haltiwanger, R.C., Bryan, R.F.: J. Am. Chem. Soc. 94, 1354 (1972)
154. Remillard, S., Rebhuhn, L.I., Howie, G.A., Kupchan, S.M.: Science 189, 1002 (1975)
155. Kupchan, S.M.: Federation Proc. 33, 2288 (1974)
156. Meyers, A.I., Shaw, Chia-Cheng: Tetrahedron Lett. 1974, 717
157. Corey, E.J., Bock, M.G.: Tetrahedron Lett. 1975, 2643
158. Kupchan, S.M., Komoda, Y., Thomas, G.J.: U.S. Pat. 3,896,111 [Chem. Abstr. 83, 209396 (1975)]
159. Wani, M.C., Taylor, H.L., Wall, M.E.: J.C.S. Chem. Commun. 1973, 390
160. Kupchan, S.M., Komoda, Y., Thomas, G.J., Hintz, H.P.J.: J.C.S. Chem. Commun. 1972, 1065
161. Kupchan, S.M., Komoda, Y., Branfman, A.R., Dailey, R.G.Jr., Zimmerly, A.: J. Am. Chem. Soc. 96, 3706 (1974)
162. Kupchan, S.M., Branfman, A.R., Sneden, A.T., Verma, A.K., Dailey, R.G.Jr., Komoda, Y., Nagaó, Y.: J. Am. Chem. Soc. 97, 5294 (1975)
163. Rokujo, T., Kikuchi, H., Tensho, A., Tsukitani, Y., Takenawa, T., Yoshida, K., Kamiya, T.: Life Sci. 9, 379 (1970); Chibata, I., Okamura, K., Takeyama, S., Kotera, K.: Experientia 25, 1237 (1969); Kamiya, T., Saito, Y., Hashimoto, M., Seki, H.: Tetrahedron 28, 899 (1972)
164. Kamiya, T., Saito, Y., Hashimoto, M., Seki, H.: J. Heterocycl. Chem. 9, 359 (1972)
165. Leonard, N.J., Playtis, A.J., Skoog, F., Schmitz, R.Y.: J. Am. Chem. Soc. 93, 3056 (1971)
166. Corse, J., Kuhnle, J.: Synthesis 1972, 618
167. Ohsugi, M., Takahashi, S., Ichimoto, I., Ueda, H.: Nippon Nogei Kagaku Kaishi 47, 807 (1973) [Chem. Abstr. 81, 3280 (1974)]
168. Scheuer, P.J.: Lloydia 38, 1 (1975)
169. Wong, D.L., Oesterlin, R., Rapoport, H.: J. Am. Chem. Soc. 93, 7344 (1971)
170. Schantz, E.J., Ghazarossian, V.E., Schnoes, H.K., Strong, F.M., Springer, J.P., Pezzanite, J.O., Clardy, J.: J. Am. Chem. Soc. 97, 1238 (1975)
171. Bordner, J., Thiessen, W.E., Bates, H.A., Rapoport, H.: J. Am. Chem. Soc. 97, 6008 (1975)

Plant Mono-, Di- and Sesquiterpenoids with Pharmacological or Therapeutical Activity

O. STICHER

A. Introduction

The number of known mono-, di- and sesquiterpenoids has increased explosively in recent years. While the chemistry of certain monoterpenes and isoprene occupied some of the ablest chemists for many years and led to the foundation of modern organic chemistry (Ruzicka, 1959), the chemistry of cyclopentanoid monoterpenes, sesquiterpenes and diterpenes could not be resolved adequately by classical methods and required the development of newer analytical techniques, especially gas chromatography-mass spectrometry (GC-MS), infrared (IR) and nuclear magnetic resonance (NMR) spectroscopy (Loomis and Croteau, 1973).

It is difficult to indicate the exact number of mono-, sesqui- and diterpene-structures known in 1976. According to Devon and Scott (1972), 380 monoterpenes, some 1000 sesquiterpenes and 650 diterpenes were known. The sesquiterpenes therefore are the largest of these terpenoid classes. Herout (1975) wrote: "It is a fact, that up to this time much more than a thousand sesquiterpenoids have been found in natural material. The number of sesquiterpenic lactones alone exceeds six hundred." While the increase of classic structural types in monoterpenes is hardly important, the number and the importance of cyclopentanoid monoterpenes and their derivatives grew in the last years. In this group must be mentioned the β-D-glucosides, known as iridoid- and secoiridoid glucosides. But the use of new methods of isolation and structure elucidation was also very productive for the discovery of new sesqui- and diterpenes. Today we know about 450 monoterpenes, 1200 sesquiterpenes and 1000 diterpenes (mixed-structures, e.g. terpene alkaloids, are not considered). Therefore, this large field of simpler terpenoids cannot be covered exhaustively in this review. The discussion will be confined primarily to a selection of aspects that have some bearing on research into the pharmacological and therapeutical properties of these compounds.

B. Classification

Let us assume that the number of terpenoids produced by plants is larger than of any other group of natural substances. Plants have the ability to produce almost an endless number of chemical variations on a single chemical structure, the simple C_5 isoprenoid unit (Goodwin, 1967; Waller, 1970). This group includes essential oils and resins, steroids, carotenoids, and rubber. A summary of the general classes of terpenoids is shown in Table 1 (see Weissmann, 1966; Waller, 1970).

C. General Biological Properties

During the last ten years several reviews have dealt with broad areas of the occurrence, distribution, chemotaxonomy, chemistry, biochemisty and biosynthesis of monoterpenes (e.g. Weissmann, 1966; Bate-

Table 1. Types of terpenoid compounds

Type	Number of isoprene units	Occurrence/example
Hemiterpenes	1	Combined to some other type of compound, e.g. coumarins, quinones etc.
Monoterpenes	2	Essential oils, iridoids
Sesquiterpenes	3	Essential oils, bitter principles
Diterpenes	4	Resin acids, phytol, vitamin A, gibberellins
Triterpenes	6	Sterols, steroids, saponins
Tetraterpenes	8	Carotenoids
Polyterpenes	n	Rubber, gutta

Smith and Swain, 1966; Loomis, 1967; Sticher, 1969; Bobbitt and Segebarth, 1969; Waller, 1970; Inouye, 1971, 1976; Francis, 1971; Plouvier and Favre-Bonvin, 1971; Devon and Scott, 1972; Banthorpe et al., 1972; Banthorpe and Charlwood, 1972; Nicholas, 1973; Loomis and Croteau, 1973; Thomas, 1974, 1975), sesquiterpenes (e.g. Weissmann, 1966; Parker et al., 1967; Herz, 1968, 1971, 1973; Herout and Šorm, 1969; Waller, 1970; Herout, 1971a,b, 1975; Devon and Scott, 1972; Banthorpe and Charlwood, 1972; Nicholas, 1973; Loomis and Croteau, 1973; Geissman, 1973; Yoshioka et al., 1973; Mills and Money, 1974; Money, 1975) and diterpenes (e.g. Weissmann, 1966; Hanson, 1968, 1971, 1972, 1974, 1975; Hanson and Achilladelis, 1968; Waller, 1970; Devon and Scott, 1972; Banthorpe and Charlwood, 1972; Ourisson, 1973; Nicholas, 1973; Fujita, 1967-1974; Fujita et al., 1974-1975.

In the same period, only a few surveys deal with the biological, pharmacological or therapeutical activity of these compounds or with various specialized aspects of this topic (Orzechowski, 1966, 1974; Goodwin, 1967; Martin-Smith and Sneader, 1969; Herout, 1971b; Rücker, 1973; Wagner and Sprinkmeyer, 1973a; Deininger, 1975; Wheeler, 1976; Wagner, in press). This corresponds to the general fact that the data concerning biological activity are known for only a few hundred natural substances, although in recent years several thousand new natural substances were isolated and characterized. Different reviews in the field of antitumor agents make an exception, but they seldom deal with terpenes only (e.g. Kupchan, 1970a,b, 1972a,b, 1975; Becker, 1971, Rücker, 1972; Artico, 1972; Strauch and Hiller, 1974).

The biological and pharmacological properties of simpler terpenoids described in the literature include a relatively large spectrum of effects. The most important now known biological properties are given in Table 2.

From a medical point of view, the large spectrum of effects of these terpenoids is very limited. Few of the simpler naturally occurring terpenoids are in clinical use today. The most important medicinal applications are quoted in Table 3.

Table 2. Important biological properties of mono-, di- and sesquiterpenoids

Activity	Mono-	Sesqui- terpenoids	Di-
Anesthetic	+		
Analeptic	+	+	
Analgetic		+	
Anthelmintic	+	+	
Antiarrthythmic		+	
Antibiotic (antibacterial, antifungal, antimicrobial, antiseptic, antiviral)	+	+	+
Antiepileptic		+	
Antihistaminic	+		
Antiinflammatory, anti-phlogistic	+	+	
Antirheumatic, antiarthritic	+		
Antitumor (antiblastic, anti-cancer, anticarcinogenic, cytotoxic)	+	+	+
Choleretic, cholagogue		+	
Diuretic	+		
Expectorant	+		+
Hypotensive	+	+	+
Insecticidal	+		+
Irritant	+	+	
Juvenile hormone		+	
Organoleptic (odor, taste)	+	+	+
Pheromone	+	+	
Phytohormone (growth-regu-lating)		+	+
Purgative	+		+
Sedative	+	+	
Spasmolytic	+	+	
Toxic		+	+
Vitamin			+

It would not be correct to place only substances with clinical application in the foreground of our observations. Even if these simpler terpenoids are not of large clinical interest, they nevertheless often have a considerable industrial importance. We also should not forget that even today plants with mono-, di- or sesquiterpenes are often used in the folk medicine of many countries. Especially medicianl plants with essential oils can be found in many pharmacopeias.

Table 3. Important clinical uses of mono-, di- and sesquiterpenoids

Application as	Mono-	Sesqui- terpenoids	Di-
Analeptic agent		+	
Antibiotic		+	
Anthelmintic	+	+	
Disinfectant	+		
Irritant	+		
Sedative	+		
Vitamin			+

D. Monoterpenes

Monoterpenes are predominantly products of the secondary metabolism of plants, although specialized classes occur in some animals and microorganisms. They are most often isolated as the major components of the oils obtained by steam distillation or solvent extraction of plant material. Monoterpenes may also be present in nonsteam distillable forms, for example the cyclopentanoid monoterpenes are normally present in plant tissues as their β-D-glucosides (iridoids and related monoterpenes). Recently, the natural occurrence of monoterpene glucosides with more conventional skeletons has also been discovered. Compounds including the β-D-glucosides of geraniol, nerol, citronellol (Francis and Allcock, 1969), isothujol, neoisothujol (Banthorpe and Mann, 1971), (-)- *cis* -chrysanthenol (Miyakado et al., 1974), thymol and carvacrol (Skopp and Hörster, 1976) were isolated.

Regarding structure, the situation is a wide variation on the theme of a few fundamental carbon skeletons. According to Devon and Scott (1972) there are 15 main skeletons and 15 less common skeletons within monoterpenes. In this survey the monoterpenes are classified into two groups: normal and cyclopentanoid monoterpenes.

I. Normal Monoterpenes

The normal monoterpenes are subdivided into three groups: acyclic, monocyclic, and bicyclic. Among these groups there are hydrocarbons, aldehydes, alcohols, ketones, oxides and others, Figure 1 shows the structure of several representative normal monoterpenes.

The biological, pharmacological, and therapeutical activity of normal monoterpenes (and also of many sesquiterpenes) is very closely connected to that of the essential oils. An exhaustive enumeration of the pharmacological literature known in this field will not be undertaken in this review; on the contrary, aside from general aspects, this review will deal with results of new investigations. A great part of the existing literature is older and was formerly discussed in detail. A good and comprehensive survey is the paper by Hauschild (1956). More recent works were reviewed by Martin-Smith and Khatoon in 1963 and by Wagner and Sprinkmeyer in 1973a. Nearly every textbook of pharmacognosy deals with this matter (e.g. Claus et al., 1970; Steinegger and Hänsel, 1972).

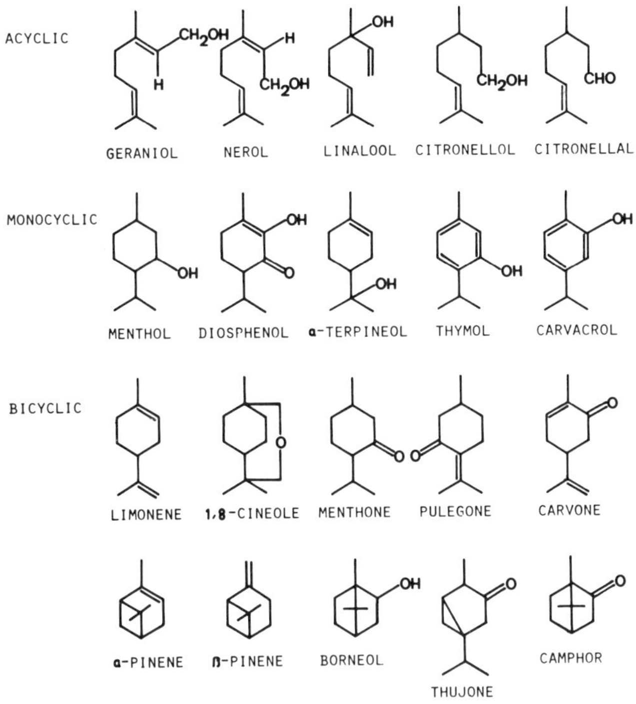

Fig. 1. Some typical normal monoterpenes

Various essential oils and essential oil drugs are used as skin stimulants, antiphlogistic agents, sedatives, expectorants, stomachics, carminatives, diuretics, antiseptics and disinfectants etc. But the most common use of the volatile oil drugs as well as of the separated oils is for flavoring purposes. Therefore, in addition to their proper pharmaceutical uses, the volatile oils are employed as flavors for foods and confections and in the spice, perfume, and cosmetic trades, as well as in pharmacy, where they are often used as flavoring agents to mask the disagreeable taste of certain medicines (Claus et al., 1970; Steinegger and Hänsel, 1972). Many of the pure monoterpenes are also used as ingredients of flavor and fragrance components or as a source of raw materials for chemical modification to provide valuable flavor and perfume materials (Erickson, 1976). The antimicrobial and insecticidal properties of other terpenoids have led to their utilization as pesticides and fungicides in agriculture and horticulture (Martin-Smith and Khatoon, 1963), e.g. the pyrethrins and the cinerins. These technical applications will not be discussed in the present review.

In most cases the activity of volatile oils is produced by the whole terpene-part of an essential oil. Only sporadic certain terpene constituents were detected as the sole carrier of pharmacological action. This circumstance considerably impedes the exact pharmacological and clinical proof of activity. Beside the terpenoids, active principles in essential oils are often other chemical constituents - for example aromatic compounds formed via the shikimic acid - phenylpropanoid pathway.

1. Antiseptic, Disinfectant, Anthelmintic Properties

At one time various essential oils and their constituent terpenoids were applied in combating infections, particularly those of the bronchial and urinary tracts, and in preventing sepsis of burns and wounds. Since the advent of the sulfonamides and the antibiotics, terpenoids have seldom been used for such purposes today (Martin-Smith and Khatoon, 1963). However, it should be noted that some monoterpenoids still find extensive application as disinfectants. Because phenol was often used for the comparison of the efficacy, the carbolic acid coefficient shows how much a compound is more efficacious than phenol.

Table 4. Antiseptic activity of some monoterpenes in comparison with phenol (Rideal et al., 1930)

Monoterpenes	Rideal-Walker carbolic acid coefficient
Phenol	1,0
Carvone	1,5
Citral	5,2
Citronellal	3,8
Geraniol	7,1
Linalool	5,0
Menthol	4,0
Menthone	2,25
Thymol	20,0

As shown in Table 4, the antiseptic activity often exceeds that of phenol. Thymol is about 20 times more efficacious than phenol. Thymol and carvacrol are still used extensively in mouth washes, and various monoterpenoids are incorporated in tooth-pastes, in which their mild antiseptic properties coupled with their rubefacient action on the gums are beneficial (Martin-Smith and Khatoon, 1963).

Besides the determination of the carbolic acid coefficient, series of further methods for proof of antimicrobial properties were used. Not only these methods but also details about further antiseptic active monoterpenes cannot be treated here. For that purpose see the survey of Hauschild (1956), the references by Wagner and Sprinkmeyer (1973a) and Mitschler (1975).

Until now, in spite of numerous experiments, the essential oils, respectively pure monoterpenoids did not gain any importance as real chemotherapeutical agents, i.e. agents that specifically damage pathogenic microorganisms inside the living infected organism. But they are, nevertheless, important in the therapy and prophylaxis of diseases caused by fungi, insects and intestinal worms. For example, thymol inhibits not only bacterial growth but also the growth of yeast and molds. Therefore, it is used in laboratories for the preservation of urine and other easily perishable specimens. Formerly, it was also a component of some helminthicides. Among the monoterpenoids, ascaridole especially has found clinical use as an anthelmintic agent. Ascaridole is the chief constituent of chenopodium oil or American wormseed oil, which until quite recently belonged to the most efficacious anthelmintic. It is efficacious against several types of parasitic intestinal worms in man, especially against roundworms, but also against hookworms. The high toxicity of ascaridole to the host led to considerable opposition to its continued clinical use. Since the discovery of synthetic anthelmintics with larger therapeutic range than chenopodium oil and ascaridole, both remedies are seldom used in human medicine. They are more often applied in veterinary medicine against certain liver flukes (see Hauschild, 1956; Steinegger and Hänsel, 1972).

Several essential oils and their monoterpenoids possess insect-repellent properties. The best known example is citronellal, which enjoyed a reputation as a mosquito-repellent before the introduction of superior synthetic agents. On the other hand, a number of monoterpenoids possesses a pronounced attraction for certain insects, and it is probable that the combination of attractant and repellent properties of essential oils plays a role of considerable importance in the vegetable kingdom, just as their mild antibacterial and antifungal properties serve to protect the plant against noxious bacteria and fungi (Martin-Smith and Khatoon, 1963; Martin-Smith and Sneader, 1969).

2. *Irritant, Skin Stimulant, Expectorant, Diuretic Properties*

Many of the simpler terpenoids are characterized by the possession of irritant properties. Certain essential oils may still be used externally as counter-irritants and as rubefacients in the form of embrocations and liniments. They produce an initial feeling of warmth and smarting, which is often followed by a mild local anesthesia, making them valuable in antipruritic preparations. Similar preparations are used to relieve rheumatic pain and neuralgia and in the treatment of the common cold and bronchitis (Martin-Smith and Khatoon, 1963).

Monoterpenoids containing essential oils are also used as inhalants with expectorant and cough stimulant properties due to their mild irritation of the bronchial glands. Certain essential oils, such as oil of juniper, are used as diuretics because they produce irritation in the kidneys (Table 5).

Table 5. Irritant, expectorant and diuretic properties of essential oils and their constituent monoterpenoids

Essential oil	Main constituent	Main use
Turpentine oil	α-Pinen, β-pinen, Δ^3-Carene	Irritant
Camphor oil	Camphor	Irritant
Eucalyptus oil	Cineol	Expectorant
Pine needle oil	Bornyl acetate, phellandrene, limonene	Expectorant
Buchu oil	Diosphenol	Diuretic
Juniper oil	Terpinen-4-Ol	Diuretic

3. Sedative, Carminative, Spasmolytic Properties

Another group of essential oils with monoterpenoids that may be mentioned is the group acting on the central nervous system. It can be a question of central stimulating, central sedative or narcotic effects.

Noteworthy in this connection is camphor, which was supposed to have a stimulating effect even on the circulation. The pharmacological investigations show, however, that the central camphor effect or the action on the respiratory is small and results from reflex actions caused by the painful local irritations following its injection (see Martin-Smith and Khatoon, 1963; Deininger, 1975).

The best known essential oil with sedative activity is the valerian oil. Calamus oil, melissa oil and lavender oil also have a sedative effect. The most important papers on this topic were recently summarized by Wagner and Sprinkmeyer (1973a). These authors also made a survey about the pharmacological works that deal with carminative activity. The carminative activity of volatile oils depends on the spasmolytic effect (Gordonoff and Rodel, 1960). For further details see the review of Wagner and Sprinkmeyer (1973a) and the references cited therein.

First it was mentioned that the general part of pharmacological literature about essential oils is of older date. The national board of control of the European Community and of other countries, e.g. Intercantonal Office for the Control of Medicaments in Switzerland (IKS), today require proof of efficacy and harmlessness even for medicaments which already have been marketed for several decades (Orzechowski, 1974). These requirements not only have the suspected negative aspects but also positive ones. Investigations are now made that would have seemed to be unnecessary in former times. Also, many old medicaments which have to conform to present requirements of efficacy will probably profit from this regulation. As a result, in the years 1973 and 1974 some new papers about pharmacological properties of lower terpenoids were published.

Wagner and Sprinkmeyer (1973b) investigated "Melissengeist" (spirit of Carmelite), an aqueous alcoholic distillate from drug mixture containing essential oil, for its volatile constituents using a combination of chromatographic (TLC and GLC) and spectroscopic (IR and MS) techniques. By this means it was possible to identify the main terpene constituents, thereby affording a reliable method for clinical and pharmacological studies. Use of capillary gas chromatography enabled the detection of the presence of some 100 individual terpenoids, 20 of which could be unambiguously identified by comparison with test substances and through infrared and mass-spectrometry. In another work, Wagner and Sprinkmeyer (1973a) investigated the sedative, spasmolytic and bacteriostatic activity of Melissengeist, melissa oil and pure terpenoids. The acute toxicity of Melissengeist was also determined. For the employed methods see the corresponding literature.

Using the sedative test Wagner and Sprinkmeyer found that terpenoids like citral, limonene, linalool etc. were very efficacious in a dose range of 1 to 31.6 mg/kg. The examination of sedative action of melissa oil and its identified main terpene alcohols and aldehydes citronellol, geraniol, citronellal and citral, showed that the greatest sedative activity was produced by citronellal. Melissengeist possesses a sedative effect in all doses tested. The effect is evidently better than that of the alcohol contained in Melissengeist.

The authors conclude that not only certain terpenoids, but all indicated principal terpenoids and phenylpropan-derivatives of the distillate are responsible for the evident sedative and spasmolytic activity of Melissengeist. It is remarkable that the sedative effect has already been observed with small dosages. In the spasmolytic activity, some terpenoids of the distillate attain values that can be compared with papaverine.

The bacteriostatic activity of volatile oil included in Melissengeist was indicated on a great number of test bacteria. In part, inhibitions exceeding the spectrum of broad-range antibiotics could be determined.

It was shown that with the present total content of essential oils in the investigated Melissengeist, additional pharmacological effects are obtained that qualitatively and quantitatively surpass the effect of particular terpenoids. The shown range of action of the combination of drugs, respectively of their total distillates appeared to have a therapeutic significance.

Holm et al. (1974) electrophysiologically analyzed the influence of terpenoids on the brain of the cat. The question was whether terpenoids modify electric brain activities, as is the case with some psychotropic, respectively neurotropic substances. The most remarkable result of these investigations was an activating effect on the hippocamp. A tranquilizing effect of investigated terpenoids mixtures can be deduced from these results. Certainly, other mechanisms than by the tranquilization with benzodiazepines seem to be responsible for it.

Clinical investigations about therapeutical effects of Melissengeist on psycho-vegetative syndroms were made by Lingen (1974), Hammer (1974) and Büchner et al. (1974). In a randomized double blind study the latter treated 102 subjects, aged 20 to 55, with Melissengeist and placebo. The analysis of the data lead to the following results: significant improvement of the clinical state could be found at the 5 p.c. level ($p < 0{,}05$). The discriminating analysis showed that primarily the symptoms characteristic of vegetative disturbances had improved, i.e. inner restlessness, unaccountable-excitability, blushing, palpitation, and headache. These results, together with psychological tests, point to a positive therapeutic efficacy of Melissengeist in vegetative dystonia.

II. Cyclopentanoid Monoterpenes and Derivatives

In recent years the class of the naturally occurring compounds known as the cyclopentanoid or methylcyclopentanoid monoterpenes or iridoids gained increased recognition because of their varied types of biological activity and because they provide a structural link between terpenes and alkaloids (Waller, 1970).

The iridoids are characterized by a cyclopentanpyran ring system. The term "iridoids," as suggested by Briggs et al. (1963), shows a relationship with the name of the simplest compound of this class of substances, iridodial (Fig. 2), which was first reported (Cavill et al., 1956) as an extractive of the common Australian meat ant, *Iridomyrmex detectus*.

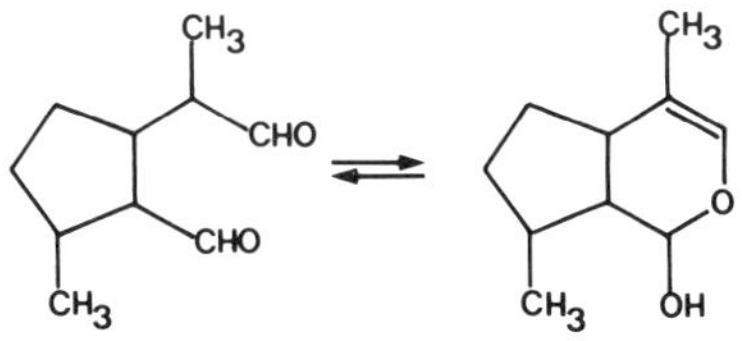

Fig. 2. Iridodial

However, usually not all natural substances which can be derived from iridodial are today characterized as iridoids (Sticher and Junod-Busch, 1975). Figure 3 shows the main groups of the iridoid plant compounds as suggested by Sticher and Junod-Busch (1975) on the basis of a proposal by Hegnauer (1966).

Fig. 3. The main groups of the iridoid plant compounds (Sticher and Junod-Busch, 1975)

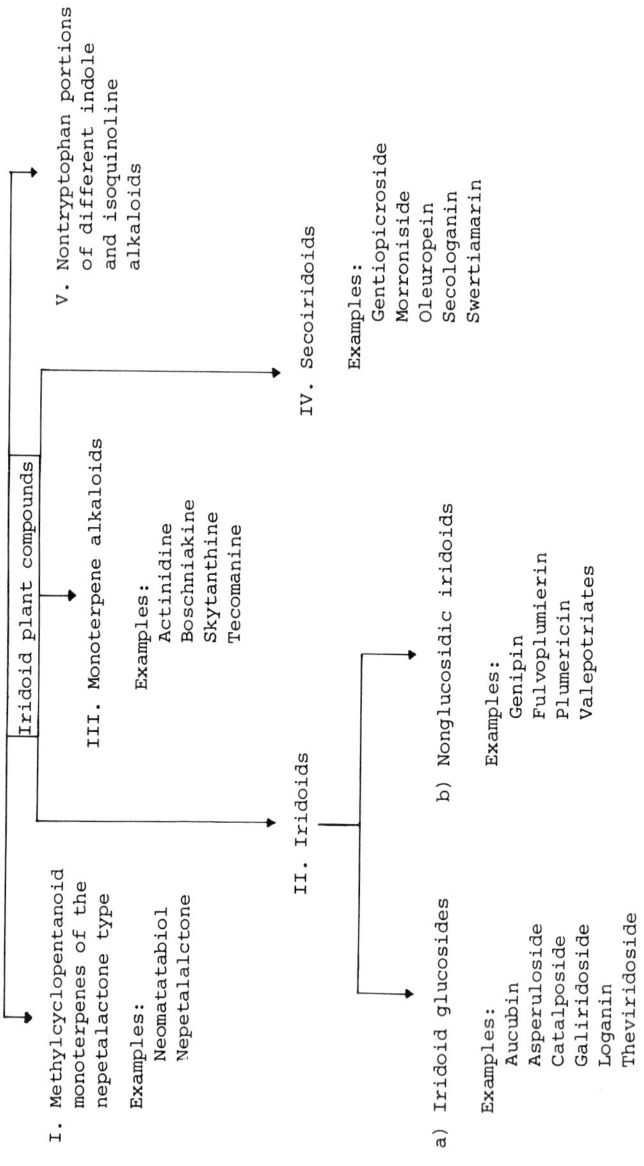

From the five groups, only the β-D-glucosides and the nonglucosidic compounds of the group II are today classified as real iridoids, whereas substances arising from loganin by cleavage of the cyclopentane ring (group IV) are called secoiridoids. The other groups are not classified as real iridoids. The methylcyclopentanoid monoterpenes (group I) of the nepetalactone type are normally volatile and occur in essential oils. Furthermore, many of the known defensive secretions of insects, for example iridomyrmecin, iridodial, dolichodial, etc. also belong in this category. Plouvier and Favre-Bonvin (1971) referred to this group as "simple iridoids." Group III includes the monoterpene alkaloids and group V the indole and isoquinoline alkaloids, of which the nontryptophan portions have been shown to be biosynthesized from the iridoid loganin. Figure 4 to 6 show the structures of several iridoid compounds of the discussed groups.

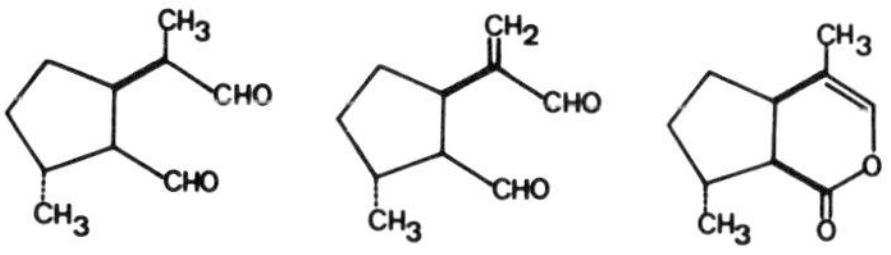

Iridodial Dolichodial Nepetalactone

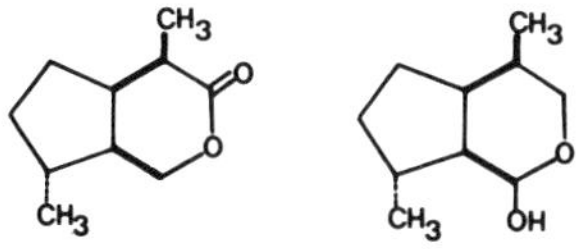

Iridomyrmecin Neomatatabiol

Fig. 4. Metylcyclopentanoid monoterpenes of the nepetalactone type (simple iridoids)

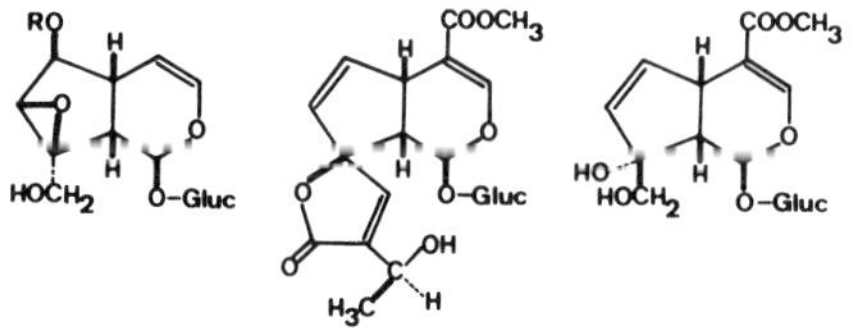

Catalpol R=H Plumieride Monotropein

Catalposide R=p-Hydroxybenzoyl

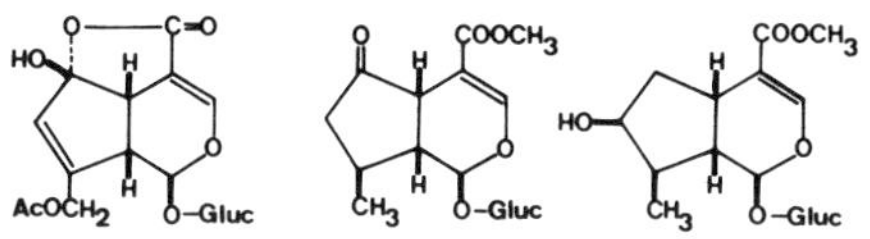

Asperuloside Verbenalin Loganin

Fig. 5. Iridoid glucosides

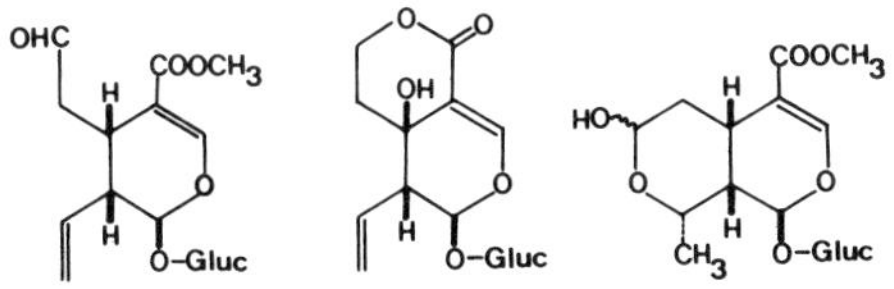

Secologanin Swertiamarin Morroniside

Fig. 6. Secoiridoid glucosides

1. Biological Activity of the Methylcyclopentanoid Monoterpenes of the Nepetalactone Type

Many of the methylcyclopentanoid monoterpenes of the nepetalactone type have a powerful biological activity. The most remarkable property of some of these substances is to act as insect repellent and attractant. Similar biological activity, including feline attractant, canine attractant and arthropod defense, also belong to this category. However, because normally they have no pharmacological activity on mammals and are not clinically used, consideration of these biological aspects is not within the scope of this review.

Accounts about occurrence and chemistry of this group of monoterpenes are reviewed by Cavill (1969) and by Plouvier and Favre-Bonvin (1971). Accounts about more biological aspects can be found in papers of Martin-Smith and Khatoon (1963), Hegnauer (1966), Martin-Smith and Sneader (1969) and as literature references by Cavill (1969) and Waller (1970).

2. Pharmacological Activity of the Iridoids and Secoiridoids

The iridoids and secoiridoids are not an especially important class of compounds as physiologically active substances. Their bitterness is an exception. However, they are the active ingredients of a number of folk medicines and have been used for centuries, e.g. as bitter tonic, sedative, febrifuge, cough medicine, remedy for wounds, against skin diseases and because of their insecticidal or hypotensive effects. Any discussion of this topic is somewhat complicated because the properties attributed to a plant or drug are not necessarily due to its iridoid constituents (Bobbitt and Segebarth, 1969). For more details about the use of iridoid- and secoiridoid-containing drugs in folk medicine, see the papers of Hänsel (1966), Hegnauer (1966), Bobbitt and Segebarth (1969), Buchbauer (1974) and Swiatek (1975).

The properties of specific pure iridoids have been investigated only in a few cases:

Antimicrobial Activity. Many biological and pharmacological papers deal with the remarkable antimicrobial activity of some iridoids. But this activity is not analogous to the known bacteriostatic and fungicidal activities of certain essential oils, i.e. the normal monoterpenes. For example, the effect of iridoid glucosides occurs only under exclusively external conditions. Besides, the antimicrobial activity is, especially with regard to the structure dependence and the antibiotic spectrum, much more specific than that of essential oils (Hänsel, 1966).

Concerning iridoid glucosides, aucubin, agnuside and asperuloside were investigated for an antibiotic activity (Rombouts and Links, 1956; Elich, 1962; Hänsel, 1966). Thereby, the genuine glucosides were proved to be inefficacious, while aucubin was efficacious under the influence of β-glucosidase (e.g. emulsin). Against a culture of *Staphylococcus aureus* , 1 ml of 2 % aqueous solution of aucubin had in the presence of β-glucosidase the same effect as 600 I.U. penicillin (Elich, 1962). The constitution of the real active structure is today still unknown.

Under the influence of β-glucosidase or an acid hydrolysis, the aglucone, aucubigenin (Fig. 7), is set free. This aglucone is extremely unstable and, therefore, it has never been isolated (Karrer and Schmid, 1946). After hydrolysis poorly soluble dark colored polymerization products result. Most of the other known iridoid glucosides sustain a similar decomposition on acid treatment. Therefore, formerly

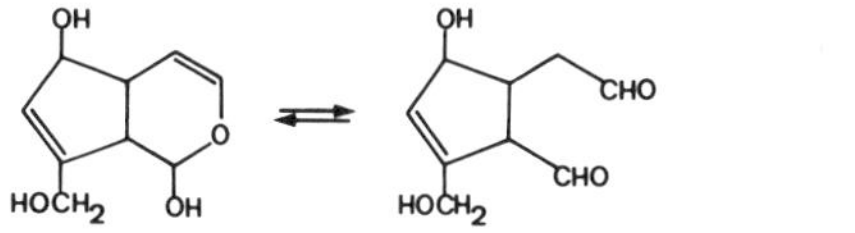

Aucubigenin   Dialdehyde structure of aucubigenin

Fig. 7. Theoretical structure of aucubigenin

these plant constituents were also called "acid-labile glucosides" or "glucosides with acid-labile aglucone" (see Sticher, 1969, and references cited therein). These final products, formed by the influence of β-glucosidase on aucubin, are inefficacious just as the glucoside itself (Hänsel, 1966). For this reason, it was impossible to decide whether the aglucone itself possesses the antibiotic properties or whether this is due to the formation of a di- or polymere (Rombouts and Links, 1956). It was also suggested that the theoretical possible dialdehyde structure (Fig. 7) of the aglucone could be active (Hänsel, 1966). But his supposition may be improbable because of the extreme instability of the aglucone.

Beside aucubin, only the iridoid glucoside plumieride showed a weak activity against fungi (Jewers et al., 1975). The main antimicrobial potency of iridoids is caused by nonglucosidic compounds (Fig. 8) such as plumericin (Little and Johnstone, 1951; Jewers et al., 1975), isoplumericin (Jewers et al., 1975), fulvoplumierin (Grumbach et al., 1952; Bencze, 1954; Jewers et al., 1975), genipic acid and genipinic acid (Tallent, 1964), the valepotriates (Thies, 1971), and by the aglucone of the secoiridoid glucoside oleuropein and its hydrolysis product elenolic acid (Fleming et al., 1973).

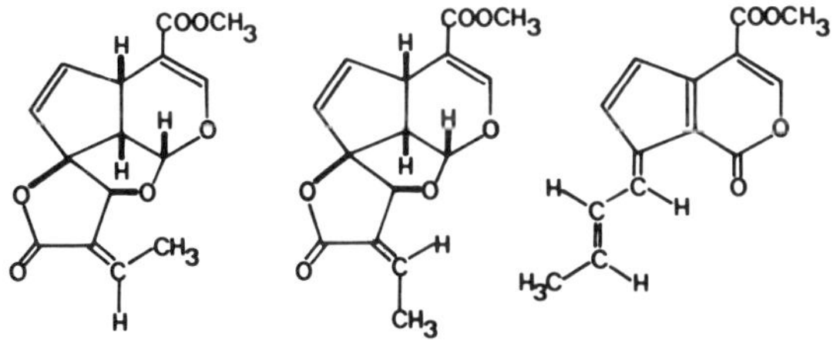

Plumericin   Isoplumericin   Fulvoplumierin

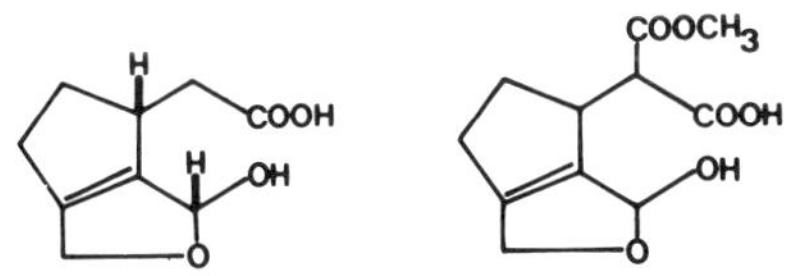

Genipic acid   Genipinic acid

Fig. 8. Nonglucosidic iridoids with antibiotic activity

Plumericin, isoplumericin and fulvoplumierin inhibited the growth of a number of Gram-positive and Gram-negative bacteria and fungi. Among the Gram-positive bacterial the growth of various strains of *Mycobacterium tuberculosis* is also inhibited.

Fleming et al. (1969) isolated a compound from green olives that appeared to have the antimicrobial properties noted earlier during the fermentation of brined olives (Etchells et al., 1966; Fleming and Etchells, 1967). The compound, a bitter phenolic material was considered to be an enzymatic degredation product of oleuropein. Walter et al. (1973) undertook to develop a procedure to produce sufficient amounts of oleuropein and its hydrolysis products (Fig. 9) so that the chemical and antimicrobial properties could be determined.

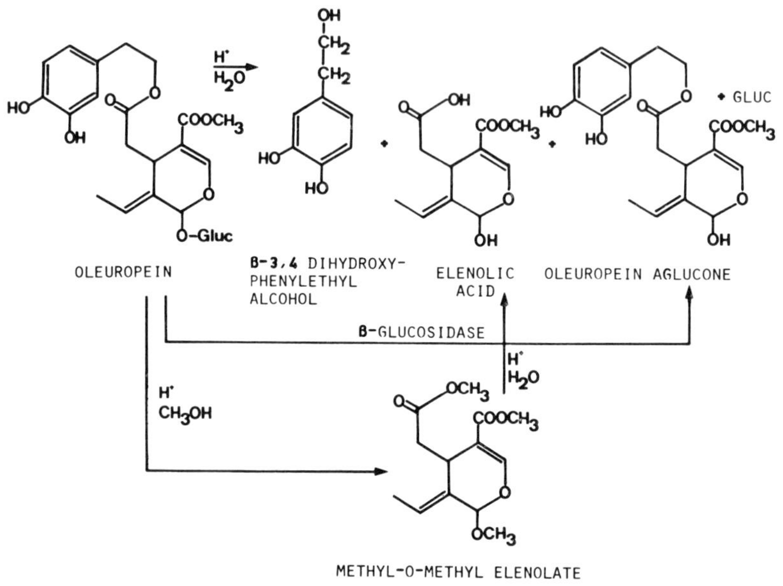

Fig. 9. Structure of oleuropein and its hydrolysis products (Walter et al., 1973)

Effects of these compounds on selected species of bacteria and yeasts are reported by Fleming et al. (1973). They found that oleuropein was not inhibitory, but two of its hydrolysis products, the aglucone and elenolic acid, inhibited growth of four species of lactic acid bacteria tested. Another hydrolysis product, β-3,4-dihydroxyphenylethyl alcohol was not inhibitory. Neither oleuropein nor products of its hydrolysis were inhibitory to the yeast species tested.

Hypotensive Effect. The secoiridoid oleuropein is of interest because of its hypotensive effect. Empirical clinical data about a healing effect of the olive leaves in the case of hypertensive diseases have been known since 1950. The degredation product of oleuropein, elenolic acid, which was prepared by hydrolysis of olive extracts with phosphoric aicd, has for a long time been known as a hypotensive agent (Walter, 1973). According to a recent study by Petkov and Manolov (1972), oleuropein is the hypotensive principle of the leaves of the olive tree. In different pharmacological investigations including acute toxicity, effect on blood pressure, coronary action, antiarrhythmic action, effect on the intestinal smooth muscles, it was possible to demonstrate that oleuropein has a hypotensive action as well as coronary dilating, antiarrhythmic and spasmolytic actions.

Analgetic and Antiphlogistic Properties. Harpagoside was investigated some years ago. Harpagoside (Fig. 10) was first isolated from the root of *Harpagophytum procumbens*, a South African drug. New surveys about the plant, the crude drug and their constituents as well as the pharmaco-

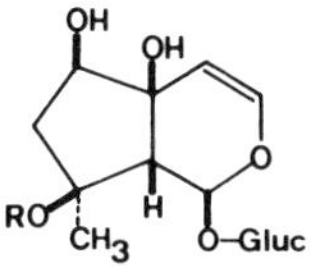

Harpagide
R=H
Harpagoside
R=trans-Cinnamoyl

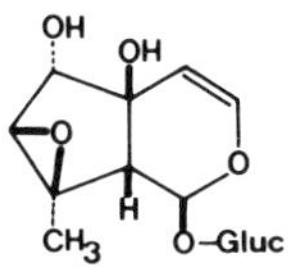

Procumbide

Fig. 10. Iridoid glucosides from *Harpagophytum procumbens*

logical, clinical and analytical investigations have just been published (Kämpf, 1976; Sticher, 1977). Whereas different authors report about acute toxicity, clinical and pharmacological tests for preparations of crude drug, (references cited by Sticher, 1977) there exists only one pharmacological work about the main iridoid glucoside, harpagoside - Eichler and Koch (1970). They tested the whole plant extract of the root of *H. procumbens*, the isolated glucoside and also the glucoside split by emulsin, for the antiphlogistic, analgetic and spasmolytic effects. The results of these tests were compared with those of phenylbutazone.

Table 6. Pharmacological investigation of harpagoside (Eichler and Koch, 1972)

Test	Harpagoside	Harpagoside split by emulsin	Water extract
Edema of the rat	O	O	O
Granuloma pouch produced by croton oil	+	+	not investigated
Formalin-induced arthritis	O	+	+
Rabbit ear test (analgetic effect)	+	O	O
Contractions on the isolated guinea pig ileum	O	not investigated	not investigated

In the formalin-induced arthritis test in the rat, an effect comparable with that of phenylbutazone was shown both with the whole extract and with the emulsin-split glucoside. No effect was obtained with the glucoside harpagoside.

The granuloma pouch test was positive for harpagoside and for the split glucoside, similar to phenylbutazone. An analgetic effect comparable to phenylbutazone was obtained only with harpagoside.

In this case, the same phenomenon already described for aucubin, namely the difficulty in deciding what the real active structure is - the intact glucoside, the aglucone or a polymerization product - seems to be present.

Bitter Tonic. Crude drugs containing loganin and related iridoid glucosides, such as the herb of the buckbean (*Menyanthes trifoliata*), and containing gentiopicroside and the related secoiridoid glucosides amarogentin, amaroswerin and amaropanin, such as gentian root (*Gentiana* species) and the indian gentian (*Swertia chirata*), are used as bitter tonic due to the mentioned glucosides. Amarogentin and amaroswerin are among the most bitter substances we know (Fig. 11; Table 7).

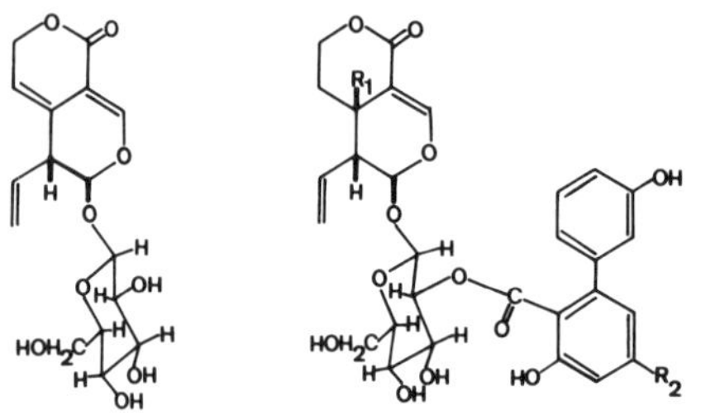

Gentiopicroside Amaropanin R_1=H, R_2=H
Amarogentin R_1=H, R_2=OH
Amaroswerin R_1=OH, R_2=OH

Fig. 11. Bitter principles of gentian

Table 7. Bitter value of gentian constituents (Wagner and Vasirian, 1974)

Bitter principle	Bitter value	Average amount in the roots
Amarogentin	58 000 000	0.05 - 0.3 %
Amaroswerin	58 000 000	0.03 - 0.1 %
Amaropanin	20 000 000	0.05 - 0.2 %
Gentiopicroside	12 000	2 - 4 %
Gentiobiose	120	5 - 8 %

The bitter values of these glucosides are normally determined with organoleptic methods. Recently, Wagner et al. (Wagner and Vasirian, 1974; Münzing-Vasirian, 1974; Wagner and Münzing-Vasirian, 1975) proposed a chemical determination of the bitter principles in gentian. They separated the main bitter principles with thin-layer chromatography. After elution and reaction with a color reagent the developed color is measured in a spectrophotometer. The total bitter values of the crude drug can be calculated from the content of amaroids.

In our opinion, the best future method for proof and determination of iridoid and secoiridoid glucosides is the high pressure liquid chromatography (HPLC). Over the past two years, we have occupied ourselves with this method and gained the rudiments for the separation of pure glucosides. Now we are able to employ these examples of separation to the standardization of particular glucosides in medicinal drugs (Meier and Sticher, 1976; Meier, in prep.; Sticher, in press). In a short lecture, Meier has reported to this Congress about the standardization of iridoid and secoiridoid glucosides in various crude drugs.

Sedative Agents. Whereas the bitter principles are not therapeutically used as pure substances but only as extractives of crude drugs, there exist among the iridoids a group of nonglucosidic compounds, known under the collective name "valepotriates" (Fig. 12), which are used as therapeutic agents. These compounds were isolated from the roots of *Valeriana wallichii* and other plants of the Valerianaceae family (see Thies, 1966-1976; Thies et al., 1966, 1973; Inouye et al., 1974a). In Germany the valepotriates exist as a prescription speciality with the name Valmane®. Valmane® is produced by Kali-Chemie and is used as a weak sedative.

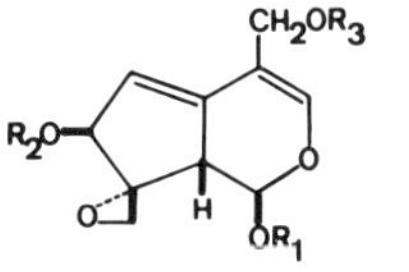

Valtratum $R_1=R_2=COCH_2CH(CH_3)_2$
$R_3=Ac$

Ace-valtratum R_1 or $R_2=COCH_2CH(CH_3)_2$
R_1 or $R_2=COCH_2C(CH_3)_2OAc$
$R_3=Ac$

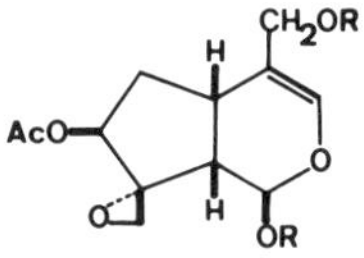

Didrovaltratum
$R=COCH_2CH(CH_3)_2$

Fig. 12. Examples of valepotriates

In pharmacological experiments a tranquilizing effect and an improved coordination capacity of the genuine mixture of valepotriates could be proved (Eickstedt and Rahman, 1969). Further they acted antagonistically against the hypotensive effect of ethanol (Eickstedt, 1969). Till now, these effects on the central nervous system could be determined only in men in clinics and psychological institutes. They were verified by long-term tests and double blind studies (Buchthala, 1968; Dziuba, 1968; Standl, 1968; Straube, 1968;, Krueger, 1969; Broeren, 1969; Boeters, 1969; Hübler, 1969; Jauch, 1969;, Wittig, 1969).

Laxative Properties. Recently another drug, the fruit of *Gardenia jasminoides*, which has long been used as an important component of several preparations in Chinese traditional medicine, was pharmacologically investigated by Yamauchi et al. (1974). The crude drug has a fecal softening activity which is mainly due to geniposide. But also the other iridoid glucosides occurring in *Gardenia* ssp. and further iridoid glucosides have purgative activities (Inouye et al., 1974b). Inouye et al. (1974b) investigated the relative purgative activities of 13 naturally occurring iridoid glucosides and of 3 chemical derivatives (Table 8).

Table 8 indicates that all the iridoid compounds tested in mice were found to be more or less active though they differ considerably in the onset time of production of diarrhea. Among others, although the purgative activities of verbenalin and plumieride are approximately 1/7 as potent as that of sennosides, the main active principles of senna or rhubarb, these iridoid glucosides characteristically reveal their activity after a very short time compared to those of sennosides.

These data also suggest that the purgative activity was significantly reduced by the presence of the free carboxylic group at the 11 position in the molecule (Fig. 13). Thus, for example geniposidic acid, deacetylasperulosidic acid and monotropein are weaker purgatives compared with geniposide and deacetylasperulosidic acid methylester. On the other hand, the hydroxy group at the 6 position generally exerted

Table 8. Purgative activity of iridoid glucosides (Inouye et al., 1974)

Iridoid compound	50 % Cathartic dose (ED_{50} g/kg)	Onset of diarrhea after dose h
Geniposide	0.30	3
Geniposidic acid	> 0.8	5
Deacetylasperulosidic acid methylester	0.53	> 6
Deacetylasperulosidic acid	≫ 0.6	-
Asperuloside	0.24	> 6
Paederoside	0.30	> 6
Gardenoside	1.20	3
Monotropein	> 0.5	> 6
Plumieride	0.12	1
Aucubin	0.39	> 6
Catapol	0.34	> 6
Catalposide	> 0.3	> 6
Verbenalin	0.11	1
Loganin	0.54	4
Deoxyloganin	0.80	3
Deoxygeniposide	> 1.2	4

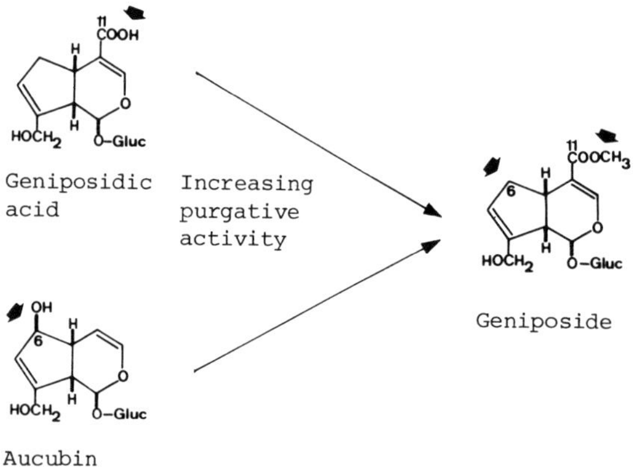

Fig. 13. Structural dependency of purgative activity

delayed actions as suggested by the slower onset of diarrhea for asperuloside, aucubin, catalpol and deacetylasperulosidic acid methylester.

The most recent paper by Yamauchi et al. (1976) deals with the mechanism of purgative action of geniposide. It was found that geniposide cause diarrhea in mice after oral administration, although not after parenteral injection. It was then found that this glucoside caused a propulsive action in the large intestine by examining the movement and the evacuation of a charcoal meal in the intestins. After an oral dose of geniposide, the aglucone genipin was detected in all of the gastrointestinal segments, especially in the cecum and the colon. Direct injection of genipin into the cecum remarkably reduced the time required for the onset of diarrhea compared with the case of the injection of geniposide. Accordingly, it has been concluded, that the aglucone genipin is effective and acts as a propulsive agent in the large intestine.

Antileukemic Activity. Recently Kupchan et al. (1974) reported the isolation and structural elucidation of a new antileukemic lactone, allamandin (Fig. 14), with iridoid structure. Usually, tumor-inhibitory natural products are especially known among the sesquiterpenes

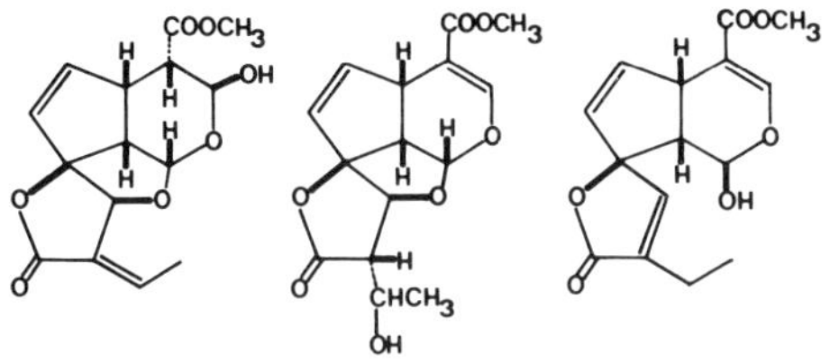

Allamandin   Allamandicin   Allamdin

Fig. 14. New nonglucosidic iridoids from *Allamanda catharthica* (Kupchan et al., 1974)

and the diterpenes (see Sect. E. III). Allamandin belongs to the nonglucosidic iridoids and was isolated together with the new companion iridoids, allamandicin and allamdin and the known plumericin and isoplumericin from an ethanolic axtract of *Allamanda cathartica*. Allamandin was found to show significant activity in vivo against the P-388 leukemia in the mouse and in vitro against cells derived from human carcinoma of the nasopharynx (KB).

Various Other Effects. The potency of iridoid glucosides is not yet exhausted. Various minor effects have been reported. Verbenalin has a low toxicity (Cheymol, 1938a), it possesses activity on the uterus similar to ergot (Cheymol, 1938b, and references cited therein) and is a weak parasympathomimetic (Cheymol, 1938c). Catalpol and catalposide are the active diuretic principles of the fruit of *Catalpa ovata* (Kimura et al., 1963; Suzuki, 1964). The effect of asperuloside on the blood pressure was investigated, but not definitely established (Knott and McCutcheon, 1961). Aucubin stimulates the uric acid excretion of the kidneys (Kato, 1946). Its excretion through the kidney was ascertained (Ogata and Nishioji, 1924).

First it was mentioned that the iridoids are not an especially important class of compounds as pharmacologically active substances. That is quite true, although to date various effects have been proved. In the future, the iridoids perhaps will turn out to be interesting elements in the search for new or better synthetic compounds (Sticher, 1974). The beginning in this direction has already been made (Thies, 1971, 1976). For the understanding of this prophecy, the mentioned group V (Fig. 3) must be additioned to the spectrum of iridoids, namely iridoids which occur as nontryptophan portions of different indole and isoquinoline alkaloids. The question is whether these compounds are reckoned to the alkaloid- or terpenoid-group. Martin-Smith and Sneader (1969) class them with terpenoid derivatives. Because the nitrogen certainly plays an important role, semisynthetic iridoids with a molecule containing nitrogen may perhaps turn out to be more active substances than iridoids as such.

3. Cantharidin

Cantharidin is a well-known compound with pronounced irritant properties. At one time it was used medicinally to produce prolonged counter-irritation, but at considerable risk, due to the toxic effects of the drug (Martin-Smith and Khatoon, 1963).

In this review the long-known pharmacological and clinical data will not be discussed (see e.g. Martin-Smith and Khatoon, 1963, and references cited therein).

Today cantharidin is of interest because new biogenetic investigations showed that the assumed theoretical relationship to the monoterpenoids is wrong. The very obvious hypothesis consists of a tail to tail linkage of two isoprene units (see Schlatter et al., 1968; Steinegger and Hänsel, 1972; Teuscher, 1975) (Fig. 15).

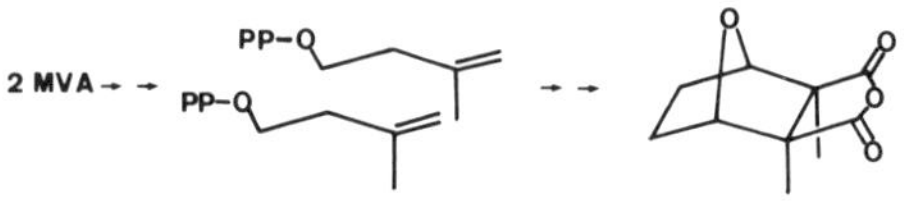

Tail to tail linkage of 2 isoprene units

Cantharidin

Fig. 15. Theoretical biogenesis of cantharidin (Schlatter et al., 1968)

It is owing to a team of Schmid from the University of Zürich that we know much more today about the biosynthesis of cantharidin. Schlatter et al. (1968) showed in feeding experiments that cantharidin is not formed by a tail to tail linkage of two isoprene units. They suggested that 3 isoprene units participate in cantharidin (Fig. 16). It was clearly proved that farnesol is the biogenetic precursor of cantharidin. The C atoms 1, 5, 6, 7 and 7' of farnesol are eliminated during the biosynthesis of cantharidin, whilst the C atoms 2, 4, 11' and 12 are incorporated. The favored precursor for cantharidin is all-transfarnesol (Schlatter and Dürsteler-Meier, 1970; Woggon, 1974).

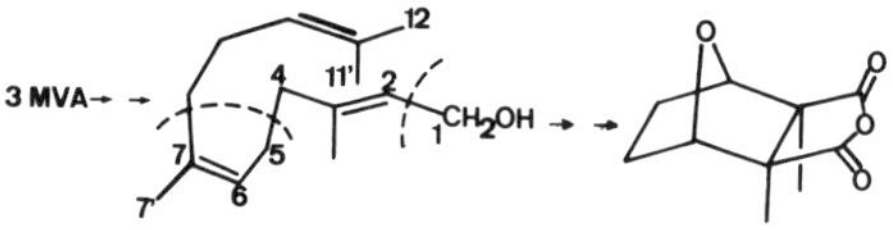

Farnesol

Cantharidin

Fig. 16. Biosynthesis of cantharidin (Schlatter et al., 1968; Schlatter and Dürsteler-Meier, 1970; Woggon, 1974)

It has, therefore, been proven that cantharidin is a sesquiterpene derivative and not a monoterpene.

E. Sesquiterpenes and Diterpenes

As was previously mentioned, up to this time about 1200 sesquiterpenes and 1000 diterpenes have been found in natural materials, originally mainly in the plant kingdom, but more recently also among the fungi and quite recently in the animal kingdom as well (sea organisms, insects etc.) (Herout, 1971b, 1975; Scheuer, 1973). Parallel to the broad occurrence of sesquiterpenes and diterpenes, there is also a rich variety of structures of these compounds. Devon and Scott's Index (1972) listed 30 main structural types of sesquiterpenes (total 1000) which represent over 700 of the compounds, the remainder being described by 70 less common skeletons. The diterpenes (total 650) are placed into 20 main classes accounting for 560 of the compounds. The remaining diterpenes with less common skeletons have been divided into four subclasses. Today these numbers are rather incomplete. In the scope of this lecture, the different carbon skeletons cannot be discussed. There are sufficient excellent accounts which describe the chemistry and biochemistry of sesquiterpenoids and diterpenoids (see Sect. C).

Originally the carbon skeletons of the sesquiterpenic and diterpenic compounds were grouped according to chemical principles, mainly according to the number of the rings in the molecule. Today it is possible to classify these terpenic substances by using clear biogenetic principles (Hanson and Achilladelis, 1968; Herout, 1971b).

Beside the general surveys about sesquiterpenes and diterpenes, there also exist some excellent reviews about the biological and pharmaceutical properties of these naturally occurring compounds. Sesquiterpenes were treated manifoldly (see Sect. C). Diterpenoids have become more important during the past years because of the wide range of biological activity that these substances show. The biological activity of diterpenoids ranges from bitter principles through antibiotics, insecticidal compounds and tumor inhibitors to the gibberellin plant growth hormones. They represent the major constituents of a number of plant resins, some of which are of commercial importance and which may function in the plant as inhibitors of dehydration and microbial attach (Hanson, 1971, 1974).

Since an extensive treatment of this field is not possible now, only the pharmacological properties of some compounds of certain pharmaceutical importance will be discussed; for the general biological properties or economic uses see the cited literature.

I. Antiphlogistic and Spasmolytic Agents

For a long time, antiinflammatory sesquiterpenes, such as guaiazulene and chamazulene (Fig. 17), have been known. Azulenes practically do not exist naturally. They are formed as artifacts from sesquiterpenic precursors such as matricin, achillin or artabsin during steam distillation, via the equally unstable chamazulene-carboxylic acid (see Isaac, 1974, and references cited therein).

A number of clinical and pharmacological tests were made on the antiphlogistic activity of azulene, but not in all investigations was it possible to demonstrate any antiinflammatory activity (Martin-Smith and Khatoon, 1963). Today this fact is absolutely certain (Isaac and Schimpke, 1965; Jakovlev and Schlichtegroll, 1969).

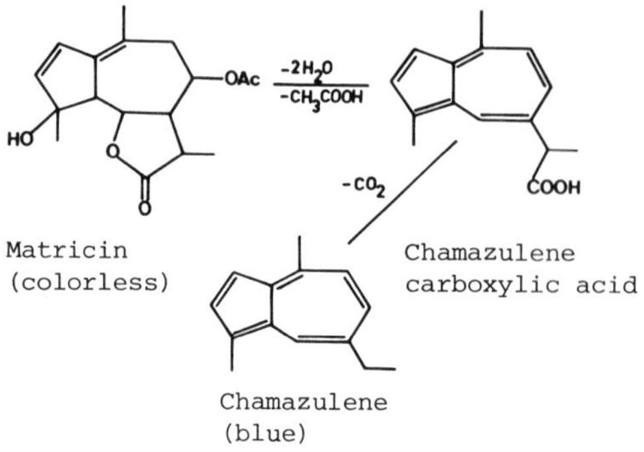

Fig. 17. Formation of chamazulene from matricin

Furthermore, (-)-α-bisabolol (Fig. 18) showed a clear antiinflammatory action against the carrageenine edema of the rat food and against the cotton pellet granuloma of the rat. The antiphlogistic effect is quantitatively comparable to that of guaiazulene but bisabolol is clearly less toxic (Jakovlev and Schlichtegroll, 1969; Isaac, 1969).

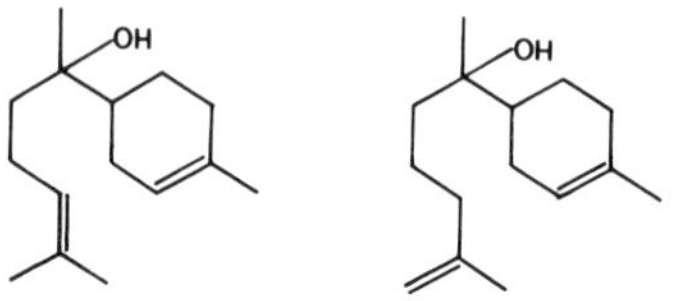

Fig. 18. α-Bisabolol

The usual naturally occurring levorotatory form of bisabolol (e.g. in camomile oil) has more powerful antiphlogistic and spasmolytic activity than the dextrorotatory form or the racemate (see Isaac, 1974). Latest biochemical studies showed that (-)-α-bisabolol has a primary antipeptic action depending on dosage, which is not caused by an alteration of the pH-value. The proteolytic activity of pepsin is reduced by 50 % through addition of bisabolol in the ratio 1/0.5 (Isaac and Thiemer, 1975).

Although spasmolytic activity is found rather widely among the sesquiterpenes, now only the petasins shall be mentioned. Petasin and isopetasin are beside S-petasin and S-isopetasin (Fig. 19) the spasmolytic agents of the leaves and roots of *Petasites hybridus* (Bucher, 1951;

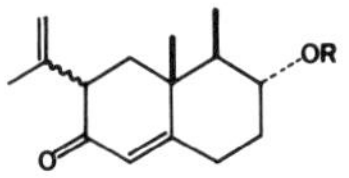

Petasin R = Angelic acid
S-Petasin R = β-Methylthioacrylic acid

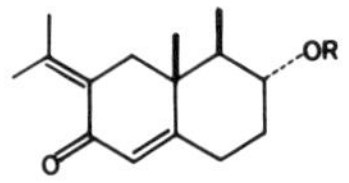

Iso-Petasin R = Angelic acid
Iso-S-Petasin R = β-Methylthioacrylic acid

Fig. 19. The petasins and isopetasins

Aebi et al., 1955, 1958; Stoll et al., 1956). The petasins belong to the group of eremophilane sesquiterpenes. They are esters of the C_{15}-alcohol petasol or isopetasol, with angelic or β-methylthioacrylic acid, respectively. Petasin is 14 times more active than papaverine. The esters of isopetasol are less active (Aebi et al., 1958).

Two months ago Wagner et al. (1976) reported about a thin-layer and gas chromatographic determination of the crude drug and extracts of *Petasites* species. They suggest a quantitative gas chromatographic standardization for petasin and isopetasin.

II. Bitter Substances

Bitterness is typical for a great number of sesquiterpenoids, being particularly marked in the majority of lactones present in the family of Compositae (Herout, 1971b). But only *Artemisia absinthium* and *Cnicus benedictus* are important in pharmacy and in the food industry. The bitter taste of *Artemisia* is due to the guaianolide lactone absinthin (Vokáč et al., 1968; Herout, 1971b) and related compounds (Fig. 20). Cnicin, the bitter principle of *C. benedictus*, is an ester of 3,4-dihydroxy-1-butene-2 carboxylic acid with a sesquiterpene lactone of the germacrane type (Samek et al., 1969; Yoshioka et al., 1970).

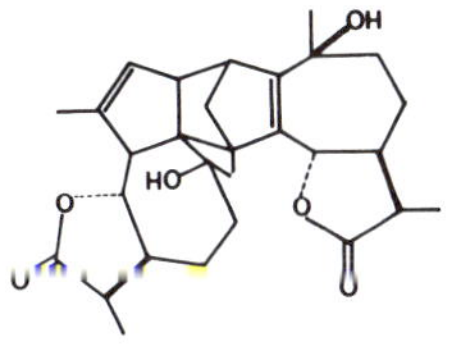

Absinthin
(Vokáč et al., 1968; Herout, 1971)

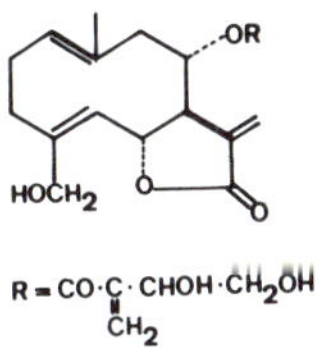

Cnicin
(Samek et al., 1969; Yoshioka et al., 1970)

Fig. 20. Important sesquiterpene lactones with bitter taste

Bitterness is a phenomenon of certain diterpenoids, especially of lactones like marrubiin and columbin too (Fig. 21).

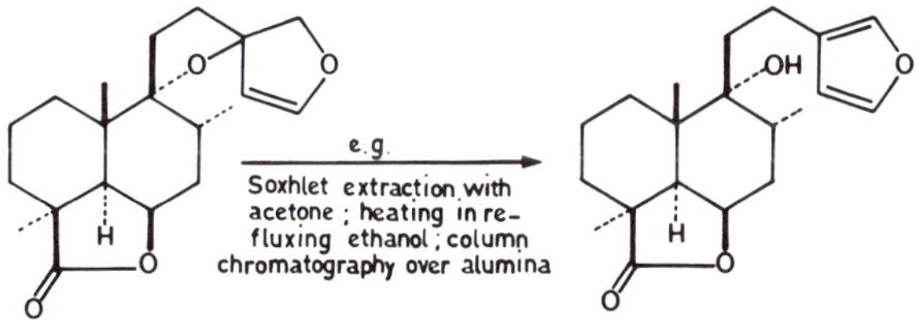

Premarrubiin (genuine)

Marrubiin (artifact)

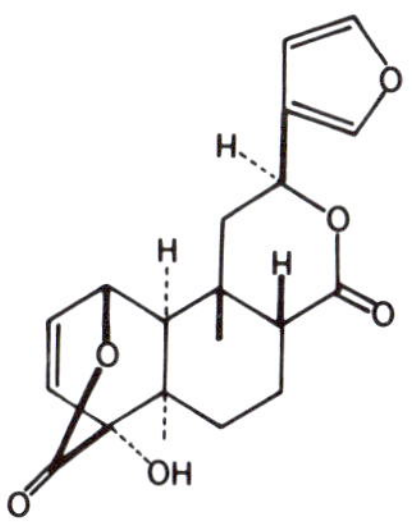

Columbin

Fig. 21. Examples of diterpene lactones with bitter taste

Marrubiin was isolated from *Marrubium vulgare*, a plant whose herb is used in folk medicine as expectorant. Marrubiin itself is now regarded as an artifact of isolation, while premarrubiin occurs as genuine diterpene in the plant (Henderson and McCrindle, 1969). Earlier published procedures for isolation of marrubiin have all involved use of conditions which generate marrubiin from premarrubiin, e.g. Soxhlet extraction of the plant with acetone, dissolution of an extract in refluxing ethanol, and column chromatography of an extract over alumina. Pure premarrubiin can be transformed into marrubiin by distillation in vacuo, heating in refluxing ethanol or dissolution in chloroform (Henderson and McCrindle, 1969).

Columbin is a bitter principle of the root of *Jatrorrhiza palmata*, which formerly was used for the preparation of bitter tonics. A review about some aspects of the chemistry of diterpene bitter principles have been published by Cocker (1966).

Like the iridoid bitter principles, the sesquiterpenic and diterpenic bitter agents are not used as such, but only in crude drug preparations. The pharmaceutical usefulness of the bitter drugs is primarily due to their stimulation of stomach secretion (Schmid, 1966; Glatzel, 1966a,b; Blumberger and Glatzel, 1966).

III. Antitumor Activity

The sesquiterpene lactone cnicin and its hydrolysis products also show, according to new papers (Vanhaelen-Fastré, 1972; Vanhaelen-Fastré and Vanhaelen, 1976), antibiotic and cytotoxic activity. In the following the antitumor activity of sesquiterpenoids and diterpenoids will be discussed; for the antibiotic and antifungal activity we refer to the cited literature (see Sect. C; Herout, 1971b).

The availability of modern, refined methods for testing anticarcinogenic agents has encouraged the systematic search for cancerostatic agents among natural products (Wagner, in press). Many of the sesquiterpenes in the Compositae family, chiefly lactones from the germacranolide, guaianolide, pseudoguaianolide and elemanolide class are especially active. Table 9 shows the sesquiterpene lactones that have so far been isolated and shown to have antitumor activity.

Table 9. Sesquiterpenes with antitumor activity[a,b,c]

Germacranolides		
Substance	Plant	References
Elephantin	*Elephantopus elatus*	Kupchan et al., 1966
Elephantopin		Kupchan et al., 1969c
Molephantin	*Elephantopus mollis*	Lee et al., 1973
Phantomolin		McPhail et al., 1974a
Molephantinin		Lee et al., 1975a
Deoxyelephantopin	*Elephantopus carolinianus*	Lee et al., 1975b
Onopordopicrin	*Onopordon acanthium*	Drozdz et al., 1968 Hladon et al., 1975
Vernomygdin	*Vernonia amygdalina*	Kupchan et al., 1969b
Eupatoriopicrin	*Eupatorium cannabinum*	Drozdz et al., 1972 Hladon et al., 1975 Hladon and Chodera, 1975

Table 9 (Continued)

Eupacunin Eupacunoxin Eupatocunin Eupatocunoxin Eupacunolin	*Eupatorium cuneifolium*	Kupchan et al., 1971b Kupchan et al., 1973b
Eupatolide	*Eupatorium formosanum*	Lee et al., 1972b Hladon et al., 1975
Eupaformonin		McPhail et al., 1974b
Eupahyssopin	*Eupatorium hyssopifolium*	Lee et al., 1976c
Eupaserrin	*Eupatorium semiserratum*	Kupchan et al., 1973a
Deacetyleupaserrin		
Liatrin	*Liatris chapmannii*	Kupchan et al., 1971a
Provincialin	*Liatris provincialis*	Herz and Wahlberg, 1973
Eleganin	*Liatris elegans*	Herz and Sharma, 1975
Ovatifolin Erioflorin acetate Erioflorin methacrylate	*Podanthus ovatifolius*	Gnecco et al., 1973
Alatolide	*Jurinea alata*	Drozdz et al., 1973 Hladon et al., 1975 Hladon and Chodera, 1975
Ursiniolide A + B	*Ursinia anthemoides*	Grabarczyk, 1973 Hladon et al., 1975 Hladon and Chodera, 1975
Cnicin	*Cnicus benedictus*	Vanhaelen-Fastré, 1972 Vanhaelen-Fastré and Vanhaelen, 1976
Tagitinin F	*Tithonia tagitiflora*	Pal et al., 1976
Lipiferolide Epitulipinolide diepoxide	*Liriodendron tulipifera* (Magnoliaceae)	Doskotch et al., 1972 Doskotch et al., 1975
Costunolide		Doskotch and El-Feraly, 1969
Tulipinolide		Doskotch and El-Feraly, 1970
Epitulipinolide		
	Guaianolides and Pseudoguaianolides	
Gaillardin	*Gaillardia pulchella*	Kupchan et al., 1965
Euparotin Euparotin acetate Eupachlorin Eupachlorin acetate Eupatoroxin	*Eupatorium rotundifolium*	Kupchan et al., 1967 Kupchan et al., 1968a Kupchan et al., 1969d

Table 9. (Continued)

Eupatundin 10-Epieupatoroxin Eupachloroxin		
Damsin Damsinic acid	*Ambrosia ambrosioides*	Doskotch and Hufford, 1969 Doskotch and Hufford, 1970
Cynaropicrin	*Cynara scolymus*	Samek et al., 1971 Corbella et al., 1972 Hladon et al., 1975
Zaluzanin C	*Zaluzania robinsonii*	Jolad et al., 1974
Angustibalin Helenalin	*Balduina angustifolia*	Lee et al., 1972a
Helenalin Autumnolide	*Helenium autumnale* var. *montanum*	Pettit et al., 1973 Pettit et al., 1974
Microlenin Microhelenin-A	*Helenium microcephalum*	Lee et al., 1976a Lee et al., 1976b
Grosheimin	*Cynara scolymus* *Grossheimia macrocephala*	Samek et al., 1972 and references Hladon et al., 1975
Multiradiatin Pleniradin Radiatin Fastigilin C Fastigilin A Baileyin	*Baileya multiradiata*	Pettit et al., 1975
Trilobolide	*Laser trilobium* (Umbelliferae)	Holub et al., 1973 Hladon et al., 1975)
	Elemanolides	
Vernolepin Vernomenin	*Vernonia hymenolepis*	Kupchan et al., 1968b Kupchan et al., 1969a
Vernodalin	*Vernonia amygdalina*	Kupchan et al., 1969b
	Related compounds	
Arnicolide A	*Arnica montana*	Poplawski et al., 1971 Hladon et al., 1975
Eremantholide A	*Eremanthus eleagnus*	Rauffauf et al., 1975

[a]With exception of *Liridodendron tulipifera* (Magnoliaceae) and *Laser trilobium* (Umbelliferae) all plant species mentioned, belong to the Compositae family. [b]Sesquiterpenes belonging to the antibiotics, e.g. illudin M and S, fumagillin, vertisporin, are not enumerated. [c]For further sesquiterpene lactones, not enumerated in the table, e.g. tamaulipin A and B, chammissonin diacetate, coronophilin, 3-hydroxydamsin, desacetylconfertiflorin, parthenin, ambrosin, aromaticin and mexicanin I see Kupchan et al. (1971c)

The tested sesquiterpene lactones were active against different tumors, e.g. in vitro against human carcinoma of the nasopharynx (KB cells), HeLa cells (carcinoma cervicis uteri), normal rabbit kidney cells RK 13, Ehrlich ascites carcinoma cells and in vivo against Walker carcinosarcoma-256 in the rat, P-388 lymphocytic leukemia in the mouse or sarcoma Sa-180, Ehrlich ascites carcinoma and exudative leukemia L-1210 in the mouse (see e.g. Kupchan, 1975; Hladon et al., 1975; Hladon and Chodera, 1975).

The structures of some representatives of the germacranolide-, guaianolide-, pseudoguaianolide- and elemanolide class are shown in Figure 22.

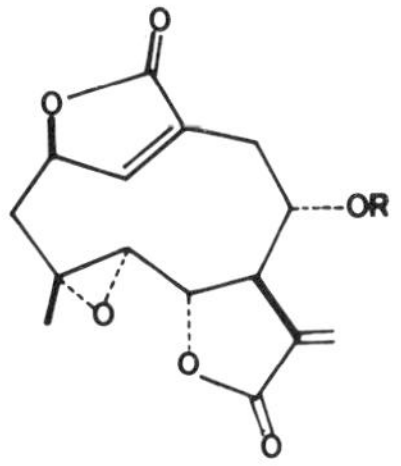

Elephantin R=$(CH_3)_2C$=CHCO-
Elephantopin R=CH_2=C(CH_3)CO-
(Germacranolides)

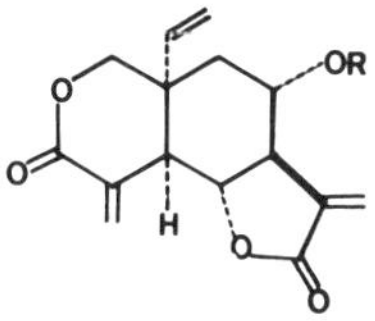

Vernolepin R=H
Vernodalin R=CH_2=C(CH_2OH)CO-
(Elemanolides)

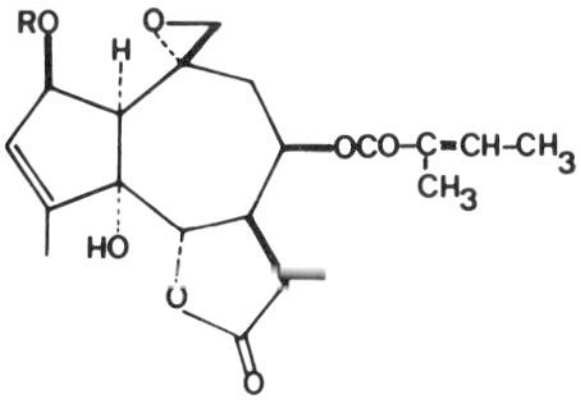

Euparotin R=H
Euparotin acetate R=CH_3CO-
(Guaianolides)

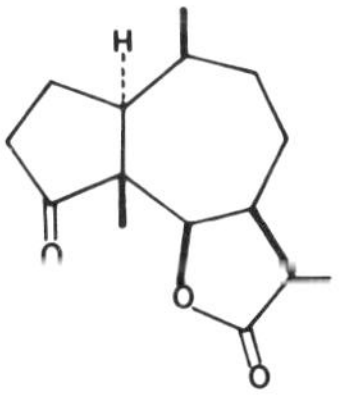

Damsin
(Pseudoguaianolide)

Fig. 22. Examples of tumor-inhibitory sesquiterpene lactones

The structure of the cytotoxic sesquiterpene lactones show considerable variation in carbon skeletons, and contain a variety of combinations of functional groups. However, it has been possible to demonstrate that the cytotoxicity is primarily dependent upon the presence of a free conjugated α-methylene-γ-lactone grouping (see e.g. Kupchan et al., 1971c; Kupchan, 1975). Modification of the α-methylene-γ-lactone results in a diminution in cytotoxicity or leads to derivatives which are essentially inactive (Kupchan, 1975). According to Kupchan et al. (1971c), a second unsaturated carbonyl function is necessary for in vivo tumor-inhibitory activity. Since the double bond of the lactone ring reacts extremely easily with the sulfhydryl-group of cysteine at pH 7,4 (Jones and Young, 1968; Kupchan, 1970a; Kupchan et al., 1970a; Hanson et al., 1970), the mechanisms by which these compounds exert their biological activities appear to depend on an interaction of α-methylene-γ-lactones and other conjugated systems with biologically important sulfhydryl groups of enzymes.

More recent studies of several cytotoxic sesquiterpene lactones and related compounds confirmed the requirement for an unsaturated lactone ring for cytotoxicity. As a rule, activity of germacranolides was higher than that of guaianolides (Hladon et al., 1975).

Not only sesquiterpenic tumor-inhibitoring substances are known but also diterpenic. In contrary to the sesquiterpene lactones, they have been isolated from various plant families. Table 10 shows the diterpenoids that have so far been isolated and shown to have antitumor activity.

Table 10. Diterpenes with antitumor activity[a]

Substance	Plant (family)	References
Taxodione Taxodone	*Taxodium distichum* (Taxodiaceae)	Kupchan et al., 1968c Kupchan et al., 1969e
Taxol	*Taxus brevifolia* (Taxaceae)	Wani et al., 1971
Nagilactones B - E	*Podocarpus* sp. (Taxaceae)	Hayashi et al., 1975
Podolide	*Podocarpus gracilior* (Taxaceae)	Kupchan et al., 1975a
Triptolide Tripdiolide	*Tripterygium wilfordii* (Celastraceae)	Kupchan et al., 1972c Kupchan and Schubert, 1974
Crassin acetate	*Pseudoplexaura* sp. (marine invertebrates)	Weinheimer et al., 1975
Gnididin Gniditrin Gnidicin	*Gnidia lamprantha* (Thymelaeaceae)	Kupchan et al., 1975b
Mezerein	*Daphne mezereum* (Thymelaeaceae)	Kupchan and Baxter, 1975
Jatrophone	*Jatropha gossypiifolia* (Euphorbiaceae)	Kupchan et al., 1970b Kupchan et al., 1976b
Jatrophatrione	*Jatropha macrorhiza* (Euphorbiaceae)	Torrance et al., 1976
Ingenol 3,20-dibenzoate	*Euphorbia esula* (Euphorbiaceae)	Kupchan et al., 1976a
Phorbol 12-tiglate 13-decanoate	*Croton tiglium* (Euphorbiaceae)	

[a]The simaroubaceae bitter principles with antitumor activity, e.g. bruceantin, burceantarin, bruceine B are not enumerated because of their biogenetical relationship with the triterpenes (see Polonsky, 1973; Connolly, 1974)

The quinone methide derivatives taxodione and taxodone (Fig. 23) might exert their biological effect by interaction with a biological nucleophile at C(7) (Kupchan, 1975). It is suggested that they may act via alkylation of biologically important sulfhydryl groups (Hanson et al., 1970). The quite recently described reaction of jatrophone with thiols

Fig. 23. Examples of tumor-inhibitory diterpenoids

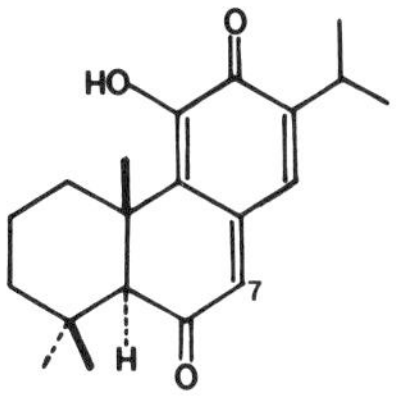

Taxodione

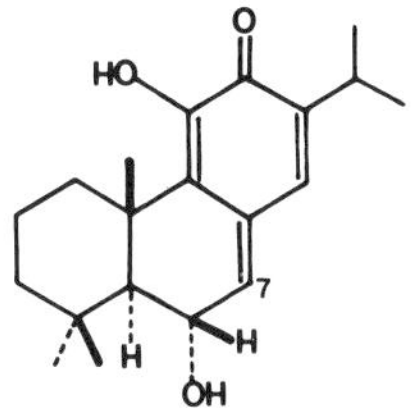

Taxodone

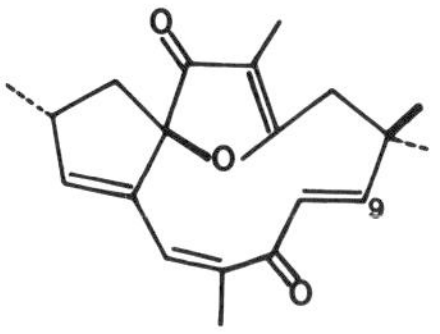

Jatrophone

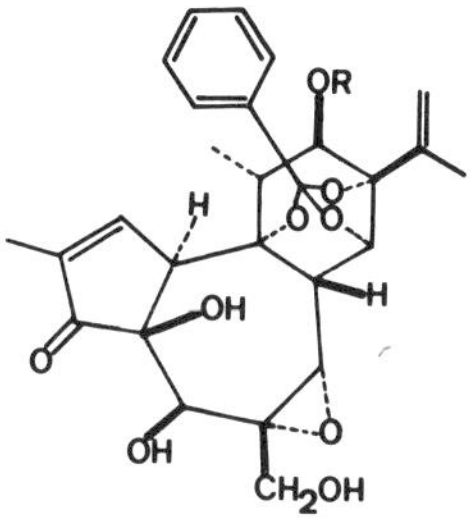

Gnididin

R= $COCH\underset{t}{=}CHCH\underset{t}{=}CH(CH_2)_4CH_3$

at C(9) support further the hypothesis that jatrophone and other electrophilic tumor inhibitors may act by selective alkylation of growth-regulatory biological macromolecules (Kupchan et al., 1976b).

The therapeutic use of the cytotoxic sesquiterpenoids and diterpenoids has hitherto been prevented by their relatively high toxicity. Attempts to increase the activity of the molecule by chemical modification have so far been unsuccessful (Pettit et al., 1974).

Beside the cytotoxic diterpenoids, other diterpenic substances are of interest because of their irritant, toxic or cocarcinogenic activity. Examples are the phorbol esters (Hecker, 1971; Fürstenberger and Hecker, 1972) from *Croton* and *Euphorbia* species, mezerein and daphnetoxin (Ronlan and Wickberg, 1970) from *Daphne* species and the grayanotoxins (see Martin-Smith and Khatoon, 1963) from various species of the Ericaceae family.

For further sesquiterpenoids and diterpenoids with pharmacological activities see the contributions of G.A. Cordell and T.R. Govindachari.

F. Conclusion

Many biological active lower terpenoids and diterpenoids were not treated in this survey. Especially di- and sesquiterpenic agents such as the plant growth-regulating hormones (e.g. Goodwin, 1967; Cross, 1968; MacMillan, 1974; Milborrow, 1974), vitamin A, antibiotic compounds (e.g. Herout, 1971b), toxic sesquiterpenes (e.g. Rücker, 1973), picrotoxin (Coscia, 1969), the sweet substance stevioside and related diterpene glycosides (Khoda et al., 1976; Wagner, in press) as well as substances which are of economic importance have not been mentioned. For all these active terpenic principles and for the terpene alkaloids (e.g. Wildman et al., 1969; Edwards, 1969; Pelletier and Page, 1973, 1974) we refer to the existing literature.

Acknowledgments. Financial support by the Swiss National Science Foundation is gratefully acknowledged.

References

Aebi, A., Büchi, J., Waaler, T., Eichenberger, E., Schmutz, J.: Inhaltsstoffe von *Petasites hybridus* (L.) Fl. Wett. Pharm. Acta Helv. 29, 277-279 (1955)

Aebi, A., Waaler, T., Büchi, J.: Petasin und S-Petasin, die spasmolytisch wirksamen Inhaltsstoffe von *Petasites officinalis* (L.) F. Wett. Pharm. Weekbl. 93, 397-406 (1958)

Artico, M.: Chemioterapia dei tumori. Il Farmaco, Ed. Sci. 27, 683-712 (1972)

Banthorpe, D.V., Charlwood, B.V.: Biogenesis of terpenes. In: Chemistry of Terpenes and Terpenoids. Newman, A.A. (ed.). London-New York: Academic Press, 1972, pp. 337-411

Banthorpe, D.V., Charlwood, B.V., Francis, M.J.O.: The biosynthesis of monoterpenes. Chem. Rev. 72, 115-155 (1972)

Banthorpe, D.V., Mann, J.: Monoterpene glucosides from petals of *Tanacetum vulgare*. Phytochemistry 11, 2589-2591 (1971)

Bate-Smith, E.C., Swain, T.: The asperulosides and the aucubins. In: Comparative Phytochemistry. Swain, T. (ed.). London-New York: Academic Press, 1966, pp. 159-174

Becker, H.: Cancerostatisch wirksame Inhaltsstoffe höherer Pflanzen. Mitt. Deut. Pharm. Ges. 41, 309-321 (1971)

Bencze, V.L.: Konstitution des Fulvoplumierins. Diss. Univ. Zürich, 1954

Blumberger, W., Glatzel, H.: Über die Speichelwirksamkeit von Bitterstoffen. In: Pflanzliche Bitterstoffe. Planta Med. Suppl. Schratz, E. (ed.). Stuttgart: Hippokrates, 1966, pp. 52-60

Bobbitt, J.M., Segebarth, K.-P.: The iridoid glycosides and similar substances. In: Cyclopentanoid Terpene Derivatives. Battersby, A.R., Taylor, W.I. (eds.). New York: Dekker, 1969, pp. 1-145

Boeters, M.: Behandlung vegetativer Regulationsstörungen mit Valepotriaten (Valmane®). Münch. Med. Wochenschrift 111, 1873-1876 (1969)

Briggs, L.H., Cain, B.F., Le Quesne, P.W., Shoolery, J.N.: The structure of asperuloside. Tetrahedron Lett. 1963, 69

Broeren, W.: Zur post-experimentellen Erfassung variierender Reaktionen auf psychotrope Substanzen. Pharmakopsychiatrie, Neuropsychopharmakologie 2, 34-50 (1969)

Buchbauer, G.: Iridoide und ihre pharmazeutische Bedeutung. Oesterr. Apoth. Z. 28, 173-178 (1974)

Bucher, K.: Über ein antispastisches Prinzip in *Petasites officinalis* Moench. Arch. Exp. Pathol. Pharmakol. 213, 69-71 (1951)

Buchthala, M.: Klinische Beobachtungen bei der Anwendung eines neuen Aequilans. Hippokrates 39, 466-468 (1968)

Büchner, K.H., Hellings, H., Huber, M., Peukert, E., Späth, L., Deininger, R.: Doppelblindstudie zum Nachweis der therapeutischen Wirkung von Melissengeist bei psychovegetativen Syndromen. Med. Klin. 69, 1032-1036 (1974)

Cavill, G.W.K.: Insect terpenoids and nepetalactone. In: Cyclopentanoid Terpene Derivatives. Battersby, A.R., Tylor, W.I. (eds.). New York: Dekker, 1969, pp. 203-238

Cavill, G.W.K., Ford, D.L., Locksley, H.D.: The chemistry of ants. I. Terpenoid constituents of some Australian *Iridomyrmex* species. Australian J. Chem. 9, 288-293 (1956)

Cheymol, J.: Le verbênaloside: toxicité, élimination. Absence d'action sur l'hêmolyse et de temps du coagulation du sang. J. Pharm. Chim. 27 (8), 325-339 (1938a)

Cheymol, J.: Action du verbênaloside sur deux organes isolés (intestin du Lapin et utêrus du Cobaye). J. Pharm. Chim. 27 (8), 386-397 (1938b)

Cheymol, J.: Le verbênaloside est un parasympathomimêtique faible. J. Pharm. Chim. 27 (8), 374-386 (1938c)

Claus, E.P., Tyler, V.E., Brady, L.R.: Pharmacognosy, 6th ed. Philadelphia: Lea and Febiger, 1970
Cocker, W.: Some aspects of the chemistry of diterpene bitter principles. Planta Medica 14, 78-85 (1966)
Connolly, J.D.: Triterpenoids. In: Terpenoids and Steroids. Overton, K.H. (ed.). London: The Chemical Society, 1974, pp. 183-220
Corbella, A., Gariboldi, P., Jommi, G., Samek, Z., Holub, M., Drozdz, B., Bloszyk, E.: Absolute stereochemistry of cynaropicrin and related guaianolides. J.C.S. Chem. Commun. 1972, 386-387
Coscia, C.J.: Picrotoxin. In: Cyclopentanoid Terpene Derivatives. Taylor, W.I., Battersby, A.R. (eds.). New York: Dekker, 1969, pp. 147-201
Cross, B.E.: Biosynthesis of the gibberellins. In: Progress in Phytochemistry. Reinhold, L., Liwschitz, Y. (eds.). London-New York-Sydney: Interscience, 1968, Vol. I, pp. 195-222
Deininger, R.: Zentrale Wirkung der Terpene. Erfahrungsheilkunde 24, 261-264 (1975)
Devon, T.K., Scott, A.I.: Handbook of Naturally Occurring Compounds. Terpenes. New York-London: Academic Press, 1972, Vol. II
Doskotch, R.W., El-Feraly, F.S.: Tulipinolide, a new germacranolide sesquiterpene, and costunolide. Two cytotoxic substances from *Liriodendron tulipifera* L. J. Pharm. Sci. 58, 877-880 (1969)
Doskotch, R.W., El-Feraly, F.S.: The structure of tulipinolide and epitulipinolide. Cytotoxic sesquiterpenes from *Liriodendron tulipifera* L. J. Org. Chem. 35, 1928-1936 (1970)
Doskotch, R.W., Hufford, C.D.: Damsin, the cytotoxic principle of *Ambrosia ambrosioides* (Cav.) Payne. J. Pharm. Sci. 58, 186-188 (1969)
Doskotch, R.W., Hufford, C.D.: The structure of damsinic acid, a new sesquiterpene from *Ambrosia ambrosioides* (Cav.) Payne. J. Org. Chem. 35, 486-490 (1970)
Doskotch, R.W., Keely, S.L.Jr., Hufford, C.D.: Lipiferolide, a cytotoxic germacranolide, and γ-liriodenolide, two new sesquiterpene lactones from *Liriodendron tulipifera*. J.C.S. Chem. Commun. 1972, 1137-1138
Doskotch, R.W., Keely, S.L.Jr., Hufford, C.D., El-Feraly, F.S.: Nes sesquiterpene lactones from *Liriodendron tulipifera*. Phytochemistry 14, 769-773 (1975)
Drozdz, B., Grabarczyk, H., Samek, Z., Holub, M., Herout, V., Šorm, F.: Sesquiterpenic lactones from *Eupatorium cannabinum* L. Revision of the structure of Eupatoriopicrin. Coll. Czechosl. Chem. Commun. 37, 1546-1554 (1972)
Drozdz, B., Holub, M., Samek, Z., Herout, V., Šorm, F.: The constitution and absolute configuration of onopordopicrine - a sesquiterpenic lactone from *Onopordon acanthium* L. Coll. Czechosl. Chem. Commun. 33, 1730-1737 (1968)
Drozdz, B., Samek, Z., Holub, M., Herout, V.: The structure of alatolide, a sesquiterpenic lactone from *Jurinea alata* CASS. Coll. Czechosl. Chem. Commun. 38, 727-730 (1973)
Dziuba, K.: Erfahrungen mit dem Aequilans Valmane in ambulanter Praxis. Med. Welt 19 (N.F.), 1866-1868 (1968)
Edwards, O.E.: Sesquiterpene alkaloids. In: Cyclopentanoid Terpene Derivatives. Taylor, W.I., Battersby, A.R. (eds.). New York: Dekker, 1969, pp. 357-408
Eichler, O., Koch, C.: Über die antiphlogistische, analgetische und spasmolytische Wirksamkeit von Harpagosid, einem Glykosid aus der Wurzel von *Harpagophytum procumbens* DC. Arzneim.-Forsch. (Drug Res.) 20, 107-109 (1970)
Eickstedt, K.-W.: Die Beeinflussung der Alkohol-Wirkung durch Valepotriate. Arzneim.-Forsch. (Drug Res.) 19, 995-997 (1969)
Eickstedt, K.-W., Rahman, S.: Psychopharmakologische Wirkungen von Valepotriaten. Arzneim.-Forsch. (Drug Res.) 19, 316-319 (1969)
Elich, J.: Die antibakterielle Aktivität einiger einheimischer *Plantago*-Arten. Diss. Freie Univ. Berlin, 1962
Erickson, R.E.: The industrial importance of monoterpenes and essential oils. Lloydia 39, 8-19 (1976)
Etchells, J.L., Borg, A.F., Kittel, I.D., Bell, T.A., Fleming, H.P.: Pure culture fermentation of green olives. Appl. Microbiol. 14, 1027-1041 (1966)
Fleming, H.P., Etchells, J.L.: Occurrence of an inhibitor of lactic acid bacteria in green olives. Appl. Microbiol. 15, 1178-1184 (1967)

Fleming, H.P., Walter, W.M.Jr., Etchells, J.L.: Isolation of a bacterial inhibitor from green olives. Appl. Microbiol. 18, 856-860 (1969)

Fleming, H.P., Walter, W.M.Jr., Etchells, J.L.: Antimicrobial properties of oleuropein and products of its hydrolysis from green olives. Appl. Microbiol. 26, 777-782 (1973)

Francis, M.J.O.: Monoterpene biosynthesis. In: Aspects of Terpenoid Chemistry and Biochemistry. Goodwin, T.W. (ed.). London-New York: Academic Press, 1971, pp. 29-51

Francis, M.J.O., Allcock, C.: Geraniol β-D-glucoside; occurrence and synthesis in rose flowers. Phytochemistry 8, 1339-1347 (1969)

Fujita, E.: The chemistry on diterpenoids in 1966. Bull. Inst. Chem. Res., Kyoto Univ. 45, 229-265 (1967)

Fujita, E.: The chemistry on diterpenoids in 1968. Bull. Inst. Chem. Res., Kyoto Univ. 48, 111-145 (1970a)

Fujita, E.: The chemistry on diterpenoids in 1969. Bull. Inst. Chem. Res., Kyoto Univ. 48, 294-345 (1970b)

Fujita, E.: The chemistry on diterpenoids in 1970. Bull. Inst. Chem. Res., Kyoto Univ. 49, 423-466 (1971)

Fujita, E.: The chemistry on diterpenoids in 1971. Bull. Inst. Chem. Res., Kyoto Univ. 52, 519-560 (1974)

Fujita, E., Fuji, K., Nagao, Y., Node, M.: The chemistry on diterpenoids in 1972. Bull. Inst. Chem. Res., Kyoto Univ. 52, 690-739 (1974)

Fujita, E., Fuji, K., Nagao, Y., Node, M.: The chemistry on diterpenoids in 1973. Bull. Inst. Chem. Res., Kyoto Univ. 53, 319-366 (1975a)

Fujita, E., Fuji, K., Nagao, Y., Node, M., Ochiai, M.: The chemistry on diterpenoids in 1974. Bull. Inst. Chem. Res., Kyoto Univ. 53, 494-545 (1975b)

Fujita, E., Fujita, T.: The chemistry on diterpenoids in 1967. Bull. Inst. Chem. Res., Kyoto Univ. 47, 522-551 (1969)

Fürstenberger, G., Hecker, F.: Zum Wirkungsmechanismus cocarcinogener Pflanzeninhaltsstoffe. Planta Medica 22, 241-266 (1972)

Geissman, T.A.: The biogenesis of sesquiterpene lactones of the Compositae. In: Terpenoids: Structure, Biogenesis and Distribution. Runeckles, V.C., Mabry, T.J. (eds.). New York-London: Academic Press, 1973, pp. 65-95

Glatzel, H.: Bemerkungen zur Physiologie der Geschmacksstoffe, insbesondere der Bitterstoffe. In: Pflanzliche Bitterstoffe. Planta Med. Suppl. Schratz, E. (ed.). Stuttgart: Hippokrates, 1966a, pp. 46-50

Glatzel, H.: Bemerkungen zur Physiologie der Geschmacksstoffe, insbesondere der Bitterstoffe. Deut. Apoth. Z. 106, 817-819 (1966b)

Gnecco, S., Poyser, J.P., Silva, M., Sammes, P.G., Tyler, T.W.: Sesquiterpene lactones from *Podanthus ovatifolius*. Phytochemistry 12, 2469-2477 (1973)

Goodwin, T.W.: The biological significance of terpenes in plants. In: Terpenoids in Plants. Pridham, J.B. (ed.). London-New York: Academic Press, 1967, pp. 1-23

Gordonoff, T., Rodel, S.: Über die Pharmakologie der Karminativa. Hippokrates 31, 335-338 (1960)

Grabarczyk, H.: Search for sesquiterpene lactones in the species of genera *Ursinia*, *Venidium* and *Arctotis*. Pol. J. Pharmacol. Pharm. 25, 469-475 (1973)

Grumbach, A., Schmid, H., Bencze, W.: Über ein pflanzliches Antibiotikum. Experientia 8, 224-225 (1952)

Hänsel, R.: Glykosidische Bitterstoffe der Monoterpenreihe. In: Pflanzliche Bitterstoffe. Planta Med. Suppl. Schratz, E. (ed.). Stuttgart: Hippokrates, 1966, pp. 61-77; Deut. Apoth. Z. 106, 1761-1767 (1966)

Hammer, O.: Zur therapeutischen Anwendung von Terpenen. Folia Phytotherapeutica 4, 6 (1974)

Hanson, J.R.: Recent advances in the chemistry of the tetracyclic diterpenes. In: Progress in Phytochemistry. Reinhold, L., Liwschitz, Y. (eds.). London-New York-Sydney: Interscience, 1968, Vol. I, pp. 161-193

Hanson, J.R.: The biosynthesis of the diterpenes. In: Progress in the Chemistry of Organic Natural Products. Herz, W., Grisebach, H., Kirby, G.W. (eds.). Vienna-New York: Springer, 1971, pp. 395-416

Hanson, J.R.: The bicyclic diterpenes. In: Progress in Phytochemistry. Reinhold, L., Liwschitz, Y. (eds.). London-New York-Sydney-Toronto: Interscience, 1972, Vol. III, pp. 231-285
Hanson, J.R.: Diterpenoids. In: Terpenoids and Steroids. Overton, K.H. (ed.). London: The Chemistral Society, 1974, pp. 145-170
Hanson, J.R.: Diterpenoids. In: Terpenoids and Steroids. Overton, K.H. (ed.). London: The Chemical Society, 1975, pp. 93-121
Hanson, J.R., Achilladelis, B.: The biosynthesis of diterpenes. Perfum. Essent. Oil Record 59, 802-807 (1968)
Hanson, R.L., Lardy, H.A., Kupchan, S.M.: Inhibition of phosphofructokinase by quinone methide and α-methylene lactone tumor inhibitors. Science 168, 378-380 (1970)
Hauschild, F.: Pharmakologie der ätherischen Öle. In: Die ätherischen Öle. Gildemeister, E., Hoffmann, Fr., Treibs, W. (eds.). Berlin: Akademie, 1956, Vol. I, 4th ed., pp. 110-229
Hayashi, Y., Sakan, T., Sakurai, Y., Tashiro, T.: Antitumor activity of nagilactones. Gann 66, 587-588 (1975)
Hecker, E.: Cocarcinogens from Euphorbiaceae and Thymeleaceae. In: Pharmacognosy and Phytochemistry. Wagner, H., Hörhammer, L. (eds.). Berlin-Heidelberg-New York: Springer, 1971, pp. 147-165
Hegnauer, R.: Aucubinartige Glucoside. Über ihre Verbreitung und Bedeutung als systematisches Merkmal. Pharm. Acta Helv. 41, 577-587 (1966)
Henderson, M.S., McCrindle, R.: Premarrubiin. A diterpenoid from *Marrubium vulgare* L. J. Chem. Soc. (C) 1969, 2014-2015
Herout, V.: Chemotaxonomy of the family Compositae (Asteraceae). In: Pharmacognosy and Phytochemistry. Wagner, H., Hörhammer, L. (eds.). Berlin-Heidelberg-New York: Springer, 1971a, pp. 93-110
Herout, V.: Biochemistry of sesquiterpenoids. In: Aspects of Terpenoid Chemistry and Biochemistry. Goodwin, T.W. (ed.). London-New York: Academic Press, 1971b, pp. 53-94
Herout, V.: Recent results in the study of the chemistry of terpenoids. Herba Hungarica 14, 109-122 (1975)
Herout, V., Šorm, F.: Chemotaxonomy of the sesquiterpenoids of the Compositae. In: Perspectives in Phytochemistry. Harborne, J.B., Swain, T. (eds.). London-New York: Academic Press, 1969, pp. 139-165
Herz, W.: Pseudoguaianolides in Compositae. In: Recent Advances in Phytochemistry. Mabry, T.J. (ed.). Amsterdam: North-Holland, 1968, Vol. I, pp. 229-269
Herz, W.: Sesquiterpene lactones in Compositae. In: Pharmacognosy and Phytochemistry. Wagner, H., Hörhammer, L. (eds.). Berlin-Heidelberg-New York: Springer, 1971, pp. 64-92
Herz, W.: Pseudoguaianolides in Compositae: In: Chemistry in Botanical Classification. Nobel Symposium 25. Bendz, G., Santesson, J. (eds.). Stockholm: Nobel Foundation. New York-London: Academic Press, 1973, pp. 153-172
Herz, W., Sharma, R.P.: New germacraloides from *Liatris* species. Phytochemistry 14, 1561-1567 (1975)
Herz, W., Wahlberg, I.: Provincialin, a cytotoxic germacranolide from *Liatris provincialis* Godfrey with an unusual ester side chain. J. Org. Chem. 38, 2485-2489 (1973)
Hladon, B., Chodera, A.: Sesquiterpene lactones. Cytostatic and pharmacological activity. Arch. Immunol. Ther. Exp. 23, 857-865 (1975)
Hladon, B., Drozdz, B., Holub, M., Bobkiewicz, T.: In vitro studies on cytotoxic properties of sesquiterpene lactones in tissue cultures of human and animal malignant cells. Arch. Immunol. Ther. Exp. 23, 845-855 (1975)
Holm, E., Haselberger, J., Reith, H.-J., Fischer, B., Fiene, R.: Elektrophysiologische Analyse der Einflüsse von Terpenen auf das Gehirn der Katze. Die Heilkunst 87, 70-75 (1974)
Holub, M., Samek, Z., De Groote, R., Herout, V., Šorm, F.: The structure of the sesquiterpenic triester lactone trilobolide. Coll. Czechoslov. Chem. Commun. 38, 1551-1562 (1973)
Hübler, B.: Erfahrungen mit dem Aequilans Valmane als Zusatztherapeutikum bei vertebragenen Erkrankungen. Z. für Allgemeinmedizin 45, 1591-1594 (1969)

Inouye, H.: Biosynthesis of iridoid- and secoiridoid glucosides. In: Pharmacognosy and Phytochemistry. Wagner, H., Hörhammer, L. (eds.). Berlin-Heidelberg-New York: Springer, 1971, pp. 290-313

Inouye, H., Takeda, Y., Uobe, K., Yamauchi, K., Nabuuchi, N., Kuwano, S.: Purgative activities of iridoid glucosides. Planta Medica 25, 285-288 (1974b)

Inouye, H., Ueda, S., Takeda, Y.: Biosynthesis of secoiridoid glucosides. Heterocycles 4, 527-565 (1976)

Inouye, H., Ueda, S., Uesato, S., Shingu, T., Thies, P.W.: Die absolute Konfiguration von Valerosidatum und von Didrovaltratum. Tetrahedron 30, 2317-2325 (1974a)

Isaac, O.: Fortschritte in der Kamillenforschung. Struktur und Wirkung des (-)-α-Bisabolols. Präparative Pharmazie 5, 189-199 (1969)

Isaac, O.: Fortschritte in der Kamillenforschung. Deut. Apoth. Z. 114, 255-260 (1974)

Isaac, O., Schimpke, H.: Alte und neue Erkenntnisse in der Kamillenforschung. Arch. Pharm. Mitt. Deut. Pharm. Ges. 35, 133-147, 157-170 (1965)

Isaac, O., Thiemer, K.: Biochemische Untersuchungen von Kamilleninhaltsstoffen. III. In-vitro-Versuche über die antipeptische Wirkung des (-)-α-Bisabolols. Arzneim.-Forsch. (Drug Res.) 25, 1352-1354 (1975)

Jakovlev, V., von Schlichtegroll, A.: Zur entzündungshemmenden Wirkung von (-)-α-Bisabolol, einem wesentlichen Bestandteil des Kamillenöls. Arzneim.-Forsch. (Drug Res.) 19, 615-616 (1969)

Jauch, H.: Valmane® in der Geriatrie. Med. Klinik 64, 437-439 (1969)

Jewers, K., Coppen, J.J.W., Manchanda, A.H., Paisley, H.M., Castillo, A.: Some biologically active lactones of *Allamanda cathartica*. Pahlavi Medical J. 6, 52-62 (1975)

Jolad, S.D., Wiedhopf, R.M., Cole, J.R.: Tumor-inhibitory agent from *Zaluzania robinsonii* (Compositae). J. Pharm. Sci. 63, 1321-1322 (1974)

Jones, J.B., Young, J.M.: Carcinogenicity of lactones III. The reactions of unsaturated γ-lactones with L-cysteine. J. Med. Chem. 11, 1176-1182 (1968)

Kämpf, R.: *Harpagophytum procumbens* DC. Teufelskralle. Schweiz. Apoth. Z. 114, 337-342 (1976)

Karrer, P., Schmid, H.: Über die Konstitution des Aucubins. Helv. Chim. Acta 29, 525-552 (1946)

Kato, Y.: Mechanism of uric acid excretion stimulation by aucubin. Folia Pharmacol. Japon. 42, 37-40 (1946; ref. Chem. Abstr. 47, 1843 (1953)

Khoda, H., Kasai, R., Yamasaki, K., Murakami, K., Tanaka, O.: New sweet diterpene glucosides from *Stevia rebaudiana*. Phytochemistry 15, 981-983 (1976)

Kimura, K., Okuda, T., Takano, T.: Studies on the constituents of *Catalpa ovata* G. DON. Active principles of fruit. Yakugaku Zasshi 83, 635-638 (1963)

Knott, R.P., McCutcheon, R.S.: Phytochemical investigation of a Rubiaceae, *Galium triflorum*. J. Pharm. Sci. 50, 963-965 (1961)

Krueger, G.A.W.: Die Therapie des psychovegetativen Syndroms mit Valmane. Therapiewoche 19, 89 (1969)

Kupchan, S.M.: Recent advances in the chemistry of terpenoid tumor inhibitors. Pure Appl. Chem. 21, 227-246 (1970a)

Kupchan, S.M.: Recent advances in the chemistry of tumor inhibitors of plant origin. Trans. N.Y. Acad. Sci. 32, 85-106 (1970b)

Kupchan, S.M.: Recent advances in the chemistry of tumor inhibitors of plant origin. In: Plants in the Development of Modern Medicine. Swain, T. (ed.). Cambridge (Massachusetts): Harvard Univ. 1972a, pp. 261-278

Kupchan, S.M.: Recent advances in the chemistry of tumor inhibitors of plant origin, Izv. Otd. Chim. Nauki, Bulg. Akad. Nauk 5, 325-340 (1972b)

Kupchan, S.M.: Advances in the chemistry of tumor-inhibitory natural products. In: Recent Advances in Phytochemistry. Runeckles, V.D. (ed.). New York-London: Plenum Press, 1975, Vol. IX, pp. 167-188

Kupchan, S.M., Aynehchi, Y., Cassady, J.M., McPhail, A.T., Sim, G.A., Schnoes, H.K., Burlingame, A.L.: The isolation and structure elucidation of two novel sesquiterpenoid tumor inhibitors from *Elephantopus elatus*. J. Am. Chem. Soc. 88, 3674-3676 (1966)

Kupchan, S.M., Aynehchi, Y., Cassady, J.M., Schnoes, H.K., Burlingame, A.L.: The isolation and structure elucidation of elephantin and elephantopin, two novel sesquiterpenoid tumor inhibitors from *Elephantus elatus*. J. Org. Chem. 34, 3867-3875 (1969c)

Kupchan, S.M., Baxter, R.L.: Mezerein: Antileukemic principle isolated from *Daphne mezereum* L. Science 187, 652-653 (1975)

Kupchan, S.M., Baxter, R.L., Ziegler, M.F., Smith, P.M., Bryan, R.F.: Podolide, a new antileukemic norditerpene lactone from *Podocarpus gracilior*. Experientia 31, 137-138 (1975a)

Kupchan, S.M., Cassady, J.M., Bailey, J., Knox, J.R.: Gaillardin, a new cytotoxic sesquiterpene lactone from *Gaillardia pulchella*. J. Pharm. Sci. 54, 1703-1705 (1965)

Kupchan, S.M., Court, W.A., Dailey, R.G.Jr., Gilmore, C.J., Bryan, R.F.: Triptolide and tripdiolide, novel antileukemic diterpenoid triepoxides from *Tripterygium wilfordii*. J. Am. Chem. Soc. 94, 7194-7195 (1972c)

Kupchan, S.M., Davies, V.H., Fujita, T., Cox, M.R., Bryan, R.F.: Liatrin, a novel antileukemic sesquiterpene lactone from *Liatris chapmanii*. J. Am. Chem. Soc. 93, 4916-4918 (1971a)

Kupchan, S.M., Dessertine, A.L., Blaylock, B.T., Bryan, R.F.: Isolation and structural elucidation of allamandin, an antileukemic iridoid lactone from *Allamanda cathartica*. J. Org. Chem. 39, 2477-2482 (1974)

Kupchan, S.M., Eakin, M.A., Thomas, A.M.: Structurecytotoxicity relationship among the sesquiterpene lactones. J. Med. Chem. 14, 1147-1152 (1971c)

Kupchan, S.M., Fessler, D.C., Eakin, M.A., Giacobbe, T.J.: Reactions of alpha methylene lactone tumor inhibitors with model biological nucleophiles. Science 168, 376-378 (1970a)

Kupchan, S.M., Fujita, T., Maruyama, M., Britton, R.W.: The isolation and structural elucidation of eupaserrin and deacetyleupaserrin, new antileukemic sesquiterpene lactones from *Eupatorium semiserratum*. J. Org. Chem. 38, 1260-1264 (1973a)

Kupchan, S.M., Hemingway, J.C., Cassady, J.M., Knox, J.R.: The isolation and structure elucidation of euparotin acetate, a novel guaianolide tumor inhibitor from *Eupatorium rotundifolium*. J. Am. Chem. Soc. 89, 465-466 (1967)

Kupchan, S.M., Hemingway, R.J., Karim, A., Werner, D.: Vernodalin and Vernomygdin, two new cytotoxic sesquiterpene lactones from *Vernonia amygdalina* Del. J. Org. Chem. 34, 3908-3911 (1969b)

Kupchan, S.M., Hemingway, R.J., Werner, D., Karim, A.: Vernolepin, a novel sesquiterpene dilactone tumor inhibitor from *Vernonia hymenolepis* A. Rich. J. Org. Chem. 34, 3903-3908 (1969a)

Kupchan, S.M., Hemingway, R.J., Werner, D., Karim, A., McPhail, A.T., Sim, G.A.: Vernolepin, a novel elemanolide dilactone tumor inhibitor from *Vernonia hymenolepis*. J. Am. Chem. Soc. 90, 3596-3597 (1968b)

Kupchan, S.M., Karim, A., Marcks, C.: Taxodione and taxodone, two novel diterpenoid quinone methide tumor inhibitors. J. Am. Chem. Soc. 90, 5923-5924 (1968c)

Kupchan, S.M., Karim, A., Marcks, C.: Taxodione and taxodone, two novel diterpenoid quinone methide tumor inhibitors from *Taxodium distichum*. J. Org. Chem. 34, 3912-3918 (1969e)

Kupchan, S.M., Kelsey, J.E., Maruyama, M., Cassady, J.M.: Eupachlorin acetate, a novel chloro-sesquiterpenoid lactone tumor inhibitor from *Eupatorium rotundifolium*. Tetrahedron Lett. 1968a, 3517-3520

Kupchan, S.M., Kelsey, J.E., Maruyama, M., Cassady, J.M., Hemingway, J.C., Knox, J.R.: Structural elucidation of tumor inhibitory sesquiterpene lactones from *Eupatorium rotundifolium*. J. Org. Chem. 34, 3876-3883 (1969d)

Kupchan, S.M., Maruyama, M., Hemingway, R.J., Hemingway, J.C., Shibuya, S., Fujita, T.: Eupacunin, a novel antileukemic sesquiterpene lactone from *Eupatorium cuneifolium*. J. Am. Chem. Soc. 93, 4914-4916 (1971b)

Kupchan, S.M., Maruyama, M., Hemingway, R.J., Hemingway, J.C., Shibuya, S., Fujita, T.: Structural elucidation of novel tumor-inhibitory sesquiterpene lactones from *Eupatorium cuneifolium*. J. Org. Chem. 38, 2189-2196 (1973b)

Kupchan, S.M., Schubert, R.M.: Selective alkylation: A biomimetic reaction of the antileukemic triptolides? Science 185, 791-792 (1974)

Kupchan, S.M., Sigel, C.W., Matz, M.J., Gilmore, C.J., Bryan, R.F.: Structure and stereochemistry of jatrophone, a novel macrocyclic diterpenoid tumor inhibitor. J. Am. Chem. Soc. 98, 2295 (1976b)

Kupchan, S.M., Sigel, C.W., Matz, M.J., Renauld, J.A.S., Haltiwanger, R.C., Bryan, R.F.: Jatrophone, a novel macrocyclic diterpenoid tumor inhibitor from *Jatropha gossypiifolia* L. J. Am. Chem. Soc. 92, 4476-4477 (1970b)

Kupchan, S.M., Sweeny, J.G., Baxter, R.L., Murae, T., Zimmerly, V.A., Sickles, B. R.: Gnididin, gniditrin, and gnidicin, novel potent antileukemic diterpenoid esters from *Gnidia lamprantha*. J. Am. Chem. Soc. 97, 672 (1975b)

Kupchan, S.M., Uchida, I., Branfman, A.R., Dailey, R.G.Jr., Yu Fei, B.: Antileukemic principles isolated from Euphorbiaceae plants. Science 191, 571-572 (1976a)

Lee, K.-H., Anuforo, D.C., Huang, E.-S., Piantadosi, C.: Angustibalin, a new cytotoxic sesquiterpene lactone from *Balduina angustifolia* (Pursh.) Robins. J. Pharm. Sci. 61, 626-628 (1972a)

Lee, K.-H., Cowherd, C.M., Wolo, MacA., T.: Antitumor agents XV: Deoxylephantopin, an antitumor principle from *Elephantopus carolinianus* Willd. J. Pharm. Sci. 64, 1572-1573 (1975b)

Lee, K.-H., Furukawa, H., Kozuka, M.: Molephantin, a novel cytotoxic germacranolide from *Elephantopus mollis*. X-ray crystal structure. J.C.S. Chem. Commun. 1973, 476-477

Lee, K.-H., Huang, H.-C., Huang, E.-S., Furukawa, H.: Eupatolide, a new cytotoxic principle from *Eupatorium formosanum* HAY. J. Pharm. Sci. 61, 629-631 (1972b)

Lee, K.-H., Ibuka, T., Huang, H.-C., Harris, D.L.: Molephantinin, a new potent antitumor sesquiterpene lactone from *Elephantopus mollis*. J. Pharm. Sci. 64, 1077-1078 (1975a)

Lee, K.-H., Imakura, Y., Sims, D.: Structure and stereochemistry of microhelenin-A, a new antitumor sesquiterpene lactone from *Helenium microcephalum*. J. Pharm. Sci. 65, 1410-1412 (1976b)

Lee, K.-H., Imakura, Y., Sims, D., McPhail, A.T., Onan, K.D.: Structure and stereochemistry of microlenin, a novel antitumor dimeric sesquiterpene lactone from *Helenium microcephalum*; X-ray crystal structure. J.C.S. Chem. Commun. 1976a, 341-342

Lee, K.-H., Kimura, T., Okamoto, M., Cowherd, C.M., McPhail, A.T., Onan, K.D.: The structure and stereochemistry of eupahyssopin, a new antitumor germacranolide from *Eupatorium hyssopifolium*. Tetrahedron Lett. 1976c, 1051-1054

Lingen, K.H.: Über die therapeutische Wirksamkeit von Melissengeist bei psychovegetativen Syndromen. Die Heilkunst 87, 36-39 (1974)

Little, J.E., Johnstone, D.B.: Plumericin: an antimicrobial agent from *Plumeria multiflora*. Arch. Biochem. Biophys. 30, 445-452 (1951)

Loomis, W.D.: Biosynthesis and metabolism of monoterpenes. In: Terpenoids in Plants. Pridham, J.B. (ed.). London-New York: Academic Press, 1967, pp. 59-82

Loomis, W.D., Croteau, R.: Biochemistry and physiology of lower terpenoids. In: Terpenoids: Structure, Biogenesis, and Distribution. Runeckles, V.C., Mabry, T.J. (eds.). New York-London: Academic Press, 1973, pp. 147-185

MacMillan, J.: Recent aspects of the chemistry and biosynthesis of the gibberellins. In: The Chemistry and Biochemistry of Plant Hormones. Recent Advances in Phytochemistry. Runeckles, V.C., Sondheimer, E., Walton, D.C. (eds.). New York-London: Academic Press, 1974, Vol. VII, pp. 1-19

Martin-Smith, M., Khatoon, T.: Biological activity of the terpenoids and their derivatives. In: Progress in Drug Research. Jucker, E. (ed.). Basel-Stuttgart: Birkhäuser, 1963, Vol. VI, pp. 279-346

Martin-Smith, M., Sneader, W.E.: Biological activity of the terpenoids and their derivatives. In: Progress in Drug Research. Jucker, E. (ed.). Basel-Stuttgart: Birkhäuser, 1969, Vol. XIII, pp. 11-100

McPhail, A.T., Onan, K.D., Lee, K.-H., Ibuka, T., Huang, H.-C.: Structure and stereochemistry of eupaformonin, a novel cytotoxic sesquiterpene lactone from *Eupatorium formosanum* HAY. Tetrahedron Lett. 1974b, 3203-3206

McPhail, A.T., Onan, K.D., Lee, K.-H., Ibuka, T., Kozuka, M., Shingu, T., Huang, H.-C.: Structure and stereochemistry of the epoxide of phantomolin, a novel cytotoxic sesquiterpene lactone from *Elephantopus mollis*. Tetrahedron Lett. 1974a, 2739-2741

Meier, B.: Die Gehaltsbestimmung von Iridoidglucosiden in Arzneidrogen. Diss. ETH Zürich, in prep.

Meier, B., Sticher, O.: Vortrag über "Gehaltsbestimmung von Iridoidglucosiden in Arzneidrogen mit HPLC". International Congress for Research on Medicinal Plants, München, 6 - 10 September 1976

Milborrow, B.V.: Chemistry and biochemistry of abscisic acid. In: The Chemistry and Biochemistry of Plant Hormones. Recent Advances in Phytochemistry. Runeckles, V.C., Sondheimer, E., Walton, D.C. (eds.). New York-London: Academic Press, 1974, Vol. VII, pp. 57-91

Mills, R.W., Money, T.: Sesquiterpenoids. In: Terpenoids and Steroids. Overton, K.H. (ed.). London: The Chemical Society, 1974, pp. 77-144

Mitschler, L.A.: Antimicrobial agents from higher plants. In: Recent Advances in Phytochemistry. Runeckles, V.C. (ed.). New York-London: Plenum Press, 1975, Vol. IX, pp. 243-282

Miyakado, M., Ohno, N., Hirai, H., Yoshioka, H.: (-)-cis-chrysanthenol O-β-D-glucopyranoside: A new monoterpene glucoside from *Dicoria canescens*. Phytochemistry 13, 2881-2882 (1974)

Money, T.: Sesquiterpenoids. In: Terpenoids and Steroids. Overton, K.H. (ed.). London: The Chemical Society, 1975, pp. 46-92

Münzing-Vasirian, K.: Zur Chemie und Wertbestimmung der Enziandroge. Diss. Ludwig-Maximilians-Universität, München, 1974

Nicholas, H.J.: Terpenes. In: Phytochemistry. Miller, L.P. (ed.). New York-Cincinnati-Toronto-London-Melbourne: Van Nostrand Reinhold, 1973, Vol. II, pp. 254-309

Ogata, A., Nishioji, R.: Seeds of Japanese plantain. J. Pharm. Soc. Japan 514, 1040-1049 (1924); ref. Chem. Abstr. 19, 1726 (1925)

Orzechowski, G.: Biologische Wirkungen von Terpenoiden. Der Deut. Apotheker 18, 43-51 (1966)

Orzechowski, G.: Terpene in der Therapie. Die Heilkunst 87, 170-177 (1974)

Ourisson, G.: Some aspects of the distribution of diterpenes in plants. In: Chemistry in Botanical Classification. Nobel Symposium 25. Bendz, G., Santesson, J. (eds.). Stockholm: Nobel Foundation. New York-London:Academic Press, 1973, pp. 129-134

Pal, R., Kulshreshtha, D.K., Rastogi, R.P.: Antileukemic and other constituents of *Tithonia tagitiflora* Desf. J. Pharm. Sci. 65, 918-920 (1976)

Parker, W., Roberts, J.S., Ramage, R.: Sesquiterpene biogenesis. Q. Rev. Chem. Soc. 21, 331-363 (1967)

Pelletier, S.W., Page, S.W.: Diterpene alkaloids. Alkaloids (London) 3, 232-257 (1973)

Pelletier, S.W., Page, S.W.: Chemistry of the diterpenoid alkaloids. Alkaloids (London) 4, 323-345 (1974)

Petkov, V., Manolov, P.: Pharmacological analysis of the iridoid oleuropein. Arzneim.-Forsch. (Drug Res.) 22, 1476-1486 (1972)

Pettit, G.R., Budzinski, J.C., Cragg, G.M., Brown, P., Johnston La Rea, D.: Antineoplastic agents. 34. *Helenium autumnale* L. J. Med. Chem. 17, 1013-1016 (1974)

Pettit, G.R., Cragg, G.M.: Antineoplastic agents. 32. The pseudoguaianolide helenalin. Experientia 29, 781 (1973)

Pettit, G.R., Herlad, C.L., Judd, G.F., Bolliger, G., Thayer, P.S.: Antineoplastic and cytotoxic components of desert *Baileya*. J. Pharm. Sci. 64, 2023-2024 (1975)

Plouvier, V., Favre-Bonvin, J.: Les iridoides et les secoiridoides: répartition, structure, propriétés, biosynthèse. Phytochemistry 10, 1697-1722 (1971)

Polonsky, J.: Quassinoid bitter principles. In: Progress in the Chemistry of Organic Natural Products. Herz, W., Grisebach, H., Kirby, G.W. (eds.). Vienna-New York: Springer, 1973, pp. 101-150

Poplawski, J., Holub, M., Samek, Z., Herout, V.: Arnicolides - sesquiterpenic lactones from the leaves of *Arnica montana* L. Coll. Czechosl. Chem. Commun. 36, 2189-2199 (1971)

Rauffauf, R.F., Huang, P.-K.C., Le Quesne, P.W., Levery, S.B., Boennan, T.F.: Eremantholide A, a novel tumorinhibiting compound from *Eremanthus eleagnus* Schultz-Bip. (Compositae). J. Am. Chem. Soc. 97, 6884-6886 (1975)

Rideal, E.K., Sciver, A., Richardson, N.E.G.: An investigation into the germicidal powers and capillary activities of certain pure constituents of essential oils. Perfum. Essent. Oil Record 21, 341-344 (1930)
Rombouts, J.E., Links, J.: The chemical nature of the antibacterial substance present in *Aucuba japonica* Thunbg. Experientia 12, 78-80 (1956)
Ronlan, A., Wickberg, B.: The structure of mezerein, a major toxic principle of *Daphne mezereum* L. Tetrahedron Lett. 1970, 4261-4264
Rücker, G.: Sesquiterpene mit cytotoxischen Eigenschaften. Deut. Apoth. Z. 112, 263-266 (1972)
Rücker, G.: Über biologische Eigenschaften von Sesquiterpenen. Deut. Apoth. Z. 113, 1291-1294 (1973)
Ruzicka, L.: History of the isoprene rule. Proc. Chem. Soc. (London) 341 (1959)
Samek, Z., Holub, M., Drozdz, B., Iommi, G., Corbella, A., Gariboldi, P.: Sesquiterpenic lactones of the *Cynara scolymus* L. species. Tetrahedron Lett. 1971, 4775-4778
Samek, Z., Holub, M., Herout, V., Šorm, F.: Revision of the structure of cnicin. Tetrahedron Lett. 1969, 2931-2934
Samek, Z., Holub, M., Vokáč, R., Drozdz, B., Jommi, G., Gariboldi, P., Corbella, A.: The structure of grosheimin. Coll. Czechosl. Chem. Commun. 37, 2611-2629 (1972)
Scheuer, P.J.: Chemistry of Marine Natural Products. New York-London: Academic Press, 1973, pp. 2-22
Schlatter, C., Dürsteler-Meier, A.: Zur Biosynthese des Käferinhaltsstoffes Cantharidin. Chimia 24, 33 (1970)
Schlatter, C., Waldner, E.E., Schmid, H.: Zur Biosynthese des Cantharidins. Experientia 24, 994-995 (1968)
Schmid, W.: Zur Pharmakologie der Bittermittel. In: Pflanzliche Bitterstoffe. Planta Med. Suppl. Schratz, E., (ed.). Stuttgart: Hippokrates, 1966, pp. 34-41
Skopp, K., Hörster, H.: An Zucker gebundene reguläre Monoterpene, Teil I. Thymol- und Carvacrolglykoside in *Thymus vulgaris*. Planta Medica 29, 208-215 (1976)
Standl, R.: Untersuchungen mit einem aus der Baldrianwurzel gewonnenen Wirkstoff zur Sedierung von Zerebralsklerotikern. Z. Gerontologie 1, 188-192 (1968)
Steinegger, E., Hänsel, R.: Lehrbuch der Pharmakognosie, 3rd ed. Berlin-Heidelberg-New York: Springer, 1972
Sticher, O.: Iridoide. Pharm. Acta Helv. 44, 453 (1969)
Sticher, O.: Die Natur als Quelle von Arzneistoffen. Pharm. Acta Helv. 49, 228-234 (1974)
Sticher, O.: Vortrag über "Gehaltsbestimmung von Iridoiddrogen." Internationales Arzneipflanzencolloquium, Graz, 5 - 7 Juli 1976, Pharm. Acta Helv., in press
Sticher, O.: Die aktuelle Droge: *Harpagophytum procumbens*. Deut. Apoth. Z. 117 (1977, in press)
Sticher, O., Junod-Busch, U.: Die Iridoidglucoside und ihre Isolierung. Pharm. Acta Helv. 50, 127-144 (1975)
Stoll, A., Morf, R., Rheiner, A., Renz, J.: Über Inhaltsstoffe aus *Petasites officinalis* Moench. I. Petasin und die Petasolester B und C. Experientia 12, 360-362 (1956)
Straube, G.: Die Bedeutung der Baldrianwurzel in der Therapie. Ther. Gegenwart 107, 555-562 (1968)
Strauch, R., Hiller, K.: Cancerostatisch wirksame Naturstoffe. Pharmazie 29, 656-670 (1974)
Swiatek, L.: Znaczenie lecznicze irydoidow roslinnych. Farm. Pol. 31, 409-414 (1975)
Suzuki, Y.: Diuretic action of the fruit of *Catalpa ovata*. Nippon Yakurigaku Zasshi 60, 544-549 (1964); ref. Chem. Abstr. 62, 15300 (1965)
Tallent, W.H.: Two new antibiotic cyclopentanoid monoterpenes of plant origin. Tetrahedron 20, 1781-1787 (1964)
Teuscher, E.: Pharmakognosie. Braunschweig: Vieweg, 1975, p. 130
Thies, P.W.: Über die Wirkstoffe des Baldrians. Zur Konstitution der Isovaleriansäureester Valepotriat, Acetoxylvalepotriat und Dihydrovalepotriat. Tetrahedron Lett. 1966, 1163-1170

Thies, P.W.: Zur Chemie der Valepotriate. Deut. Apoth. Z. 107, 1411-1412 (1967)

Thies, P.W.: Die Konstitution der Valepotriate. Tetrahedron 24, 313-347 (1968)

Thies, P.W.: Zum chromogenen Verhalten der Valepotriate. Arzneim.-Forsch. (Drug Res.) 19, 319-322 (1969)

Thies, P.W.: Valerosidatum, ein Iridoidesterglycosid aus *Valeriana*-Arten. Tetrahedron Lett. 1970, 2471-2474

Thies, P.W.: Synthesen neuartiger Heterocyclen aus *Valeriana*-Inhaltsstoffen. In: Pharmacognosy and Phytochemistry. Wagner, H., Hörhammer, L. (eds.). Berlin-Heidelberg-New York: Springer, 1971, pp. 41-63

Thies, P.W.: Modification of natural products of modern drug synthesis. Plenary lecture at the International Congress for Research on Medicinal Plants, Munich, 6 - 10 September, 1976

Thies, P.W., Finner, E., Rosskopf, F.: Die Konfiguration des Valtratum und anderer Valepotriate. Tetrahedron 29, 3213-3226 (1973)

Thies, P.W., Funke, S.: Über die Wirkstoffe des Baldrians. Nachweis und Isolierung von sedativ wirksamen Isovaleriansäureestern aus Wurzeln und Rhizomen von verschiedenen *Valeriana*- und *Kenthrantus*-Arten. Tetrahedron Lett. 1966, 1155-1162

Thomas, A.F.: Monoterpenoids. In: Terpenoids and Steroids. Overton, K.H. (ed.). London: The Chemical Society, 1974, pp. 3-76

Thomas, A.F.: Monoterpenoids. In: Terpenoids and Steroids. Overton, K.H. (ed.). London: The Chemical Society, 1975, pp. 3-45

Torrance, S.J., Wiedhopf, R.M., Cole, J.R., Arora, S.K., Bates, R.B., Beavers, W. A., Cutler, R.S.: Antitumor agents from *Jatropha macrorhiza* (Euphorbiaceae). II. Isolation and characterization of Jatrophatrione. J. Org. Chem. 41, 1855-1857 (1976)

Vanhaelen-Fastré, R.: Activités antibiotique et cytotoxique de la cnicine, isolée de *Cnicus benedictus* L. J. Pharm. Belg. 27, 683-688 (1972)

Vanhaelen-Fastré, R., Vanhaelen, M.: Activité antibiotique et cytotoxique de la cnicine et de ses produits d'hydrolyse. Planta Medica 29, 179-189 (1976)

Vokáč, K., Šamek, Z., Herout, V., Šorm, F.: The structure of artabsin and absinthin. Tetrahedron Lett. 1968, 3855-3857

Wagner, H.: Pharmaceutical and economic use of Compositae. In: The Biology and Chemistry of the Compositae. New York-London: Academic Press, in press

Wagner, H., Glasl, H., Huber, G.: Dünnschicht- und gaschromatographische Wertbestimmung der *Petasites*-Droge und Extrakte. Deut. Apoth. Z. 116, 1009-1012 (1976)

Wagner, H., Münzing-Vasirian, K.: Eine chemische Wertbestimmung der Enziandroge. Deut. Apoth. Z. 115, 1233-1239 (1975)

Wagner, H., Sprinkmeyer, L.: Über die pharmakologische Wirkung von Melissengeist. Deut. Apoth. Z. 113, 1159-1166 (1973a)

Wagner, H., Sprinkmeyer, L.: Zur chromatographischen und spektroskopischen Analyse von Drogendestillaten. Arzneim.-Forsch. (Drug Res.) 23, 749-755 (1973b)

Wagner, H., Vasirian, K.: Zur Chromatographie der Enzianbitterstoffe. Deut. Apoth. Z. 114, 1245-1248 (1974)

Waller, G.R.: Metabolism of plant terpenoids. In: Progress in the Chemistry of Fats and other Lipids. Holman, R.T. (ed.). Oxford-London-Edinburgh-New York-Toronto-Sydney-Paris-Braunschweig: Pergamon Press, 1970, Vol. X, pp. 151-238

Walter, W.M.Jr., Fleming, H.P., Etchells, J.L.: Preparation of antimicrobial compounds by hydrolysis of oleuropein from green olives. Appl. Microbiol. 26, 773-776 (1973)

Wani, M.C., Taylor, H.L., Wall, M.E., Coggon, P., McPhail, A.T.: The isolation and structure of taxol, a novel antileukemic and antitumor agent from *Taxus brevifolia*. J. Am. Chem. Soc. 93, 2325-2327 (1971)

Weinheimer, A.J., Matson, J.A.: Crassin acetate, the principal antineoplastic agent in four gorgonians of the *Pseudoplexaura genus*. Lloydia 38, 378-382 (1975)

Weissmann, G.: The distribution of terpenoids. In: Comparative Phytochemistry. Swain, T. (ed.). London-New York: Academic Press, 1966, pp. 97-120

Wheeler, J.W.: Insect and mammalian pheromones. Lloydia 39, 53-59 (1976) and references cited therein

Wildman, W.C., Le Men, J., Wiesner, K.: Monoterpene alkaloids. In: Cyclopentanoid Terpene Derivatives. Taylor, W.I., Battersby, A.R. (eds.). New York: Marcel Dekker, 1969, pp. 239-278

Wittig, K.: Ein therapeutischer Beitrag zur Behandlung von Abstinenzerscheinungen bei Alkohol- und Opiatsuchten. Medizin Heute 18, 49-50 (1969)

Woggon, W.-D.: Zur Biosynthese des Cantharidins. Lecture. Institute of Organic Chemistry, Univ. Zürich, 6th July, 1974 and different papers (Woggon et al., Peter et al.) in preparation

Yamaguchi, K., Fujimoto, N., Kuwanò, S., Inouye, H., Inoue, K.: The mechanism of purgative action of geniposide, an iridoid glucoside of the fruit of *Gardenia*, in mice. Planta Medica 30, 39-47 (1976)

Yamaguchi, K., Sakuragi, R., Kuwano, S., Inouye, H.: Biological and chemical assay of geniposide, a new laxative in the fruit of *Gardenia*. Planta Medica 25, 219-225 (1974)

Yoshioka, H., Mabry, T.J., Timmermann, B.N.: Sesquiterpene Lactones. Tokyo: Univ. Tokyo, 1973

Yoshioka, H., Renold, W., Mabry, T.J.: The structure of salonitenolide and the preferential C-8 relactonization of germacranolides containing C-6 and C-8 lactonizable α-oxygen groups. Chem. Commun. 1970, 148-149

Saponins with Biological and Pharmacological Activity

S. SHIBATA

A. Introduction

Glycosides which produce a foaming aqueous solution are generally named saponins. They also have hemolytic properties and a poisonous effect against fishes and shells. Formation of precipitates with cholesterol in alcohol is also referred to as a characteristic nature of saponins. The crude drugs which contain saponins are generally used for their detergent properties, and some of them which give less irritating effects on oral administration are employed as expectorant and antitussive agents. A great number of species of saponins are distributed in higher plants, while some marine animals, such as seaslug and starfish, also produce saponins. Thus there are many crude drugs which consist of seeds, leaves, stembark, roots and rhizomes of higher plants containing conisderable amount of saponins, whose biological and pharmacological activities, however, have not fully been clarified so far, though the saponins might possibly be playing an important role in such drugs.

Recently antimicrobial activities, especially antifungal activities, have been demonstrated (Tschesche and Wulff, 1965) as one of the characteristic properties of saponins (Tschesche, 1971).

The saponins are classified chemically in two groups: steroidal saponins and triterpenoid saponins on the basis of the chemical structures of their aglycones or sapogenins.

The saponins contained in Liliaceous and Dioscoreaceous plants belong to the former, and those contained in the plants of Araliaceae, Rhamnaceae, Umbelliferae, Leguminosae, Caryophyllaceae, Hippocastanaceae etc. to the latter. The steroidal alkaloids of Solanaceous plants, which contain nitrogen in the steroidal structure show the properties of saponin, and may be designated the basic steroidal saponins.

The structures of numerous sapogenins of both groups have been established, whereas until the 1960s only a few saponins were chemically established. This might be caused by the difficulties in purification of saponins, which have recently been improved by the remarkable developments of various types of chromatographical techniques.

The classical definition of saponins by their physical and biological properties has become obscure. It would, therefore, be more practical to adopt the definition of saponins to the oligoglycosides of spirostans and their biogenetically congenerous steroids and those of triterpenoids.

By the investigation of Guvanov et al. (1970) on 1730 species of 104 families of plants growing in the Central Asia, triterpenoid saponins were found in 627 species, and steroidal saponins in 127 species. About 76 % of plant families so far examined more or less contained saponins (Guvanov et al., 1970). This would suggest a wide distribution of saponins in the plant kingdom.

Tschesche and Wulff referred in 1973 in their review entitled "Chemie und Biologie der Saponine" to 43 steroidal and 110 triterpenoid plant saponins of established chemical structures. In general, steroidal saponins are known to be more important as the starting materials for the syntheses of steroid hormones and related medicines than the direct uses as remedies, whereas some triterpenoid saponins have been shown to possess biological and pharmacological activities which would be developed to some medical uses. Among Chinese drugs there are many herb drugs which contain saponins as their principal constituents, though their biological activities have not yet been studied extensively for cases. In the present article, recent advances in the studies of saponins in the Oriental plant drugs and in western vegetable drugs are discussed.

B. Saponins of Licorice

Licorice (Liquorice), the root of *Glycyrrhiza glabra*, *Glycyrrhiza uralensis*, and their varieties (Leguminosae), is used both in Western and Oriental medicines. In Western medicine, licorice has been used since the ancient Grecian Age as expectorant, antitussive agent and an additive for sweetening. In old Chinese Materia Medica "Shin Nung Pen-T sao Ching," licorice was described as a drug for strengthening muscle and bone, increasing physical strength and curing wounds. It is also employed as an antidote. The main principle of licorice is a sweet tasting saponin, glycyrrhizin, which shows a low hemolytic index. On acid hydrolysis on oleanane-type triterpene, glycyrrhetic acid, and 2 mol of D-glucuronic acid are afforded, the latter each linked with a β-1→2 linkage to the 3-hydroxyl of the sapogenin. Some minor saponins with analogous oleanane-type triterpenes as the aglycones have also been isolated.

Most of these aglycones are characterized by the presence of an αβ-unsaturated C=O system in the C-ring.

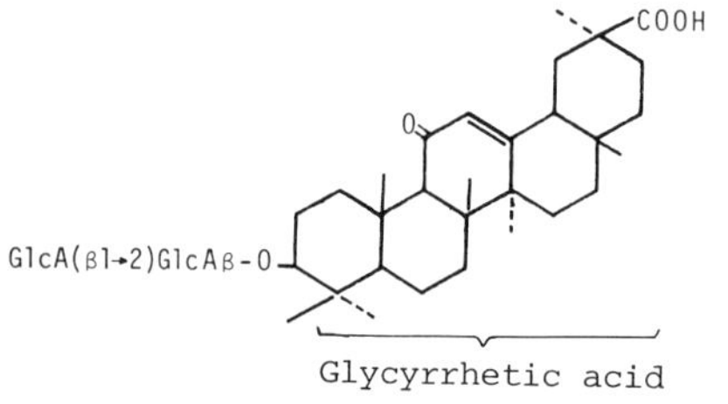

Fig. 1. Glycyrrhizin

I. Corticoidal Activities of Glycyrrhizin

Since Revers reported that licorice extracts were effective clinically for treatment of gastric ulcer, but caused edema and hypertension in 1/5 of the patients treated (Revers, 1946), the physiological and pharmacological studies on glycyrrhizin, the main saponin of licorice, have advanced remarkably. The side effect of licorice extracts was regarded as a mineral corticoid-like action of glycyrrhizin.

Molhuysen found that glycyrrhizin caused retention of Na^+ and Cl^- and excretion of K^+ (Molhuysen et al., 1950). Glycyrrhizin has been noted as a remedy of the Addison disease, but licorice-induced pseudoaldosteronism caused by the excess dosis of glycyrrhizin has also been reported (Conn et al., 1968).

II. Antiinflammatory Activities of Glycyrrhizin

In Chinese medicine administration of Licorice decoctum is used to treat throat inflammation, while in Europe licorice extracts are also used in a form of troche for similar purposes.

Finney and Tarnoky reported that glycyrrhetic acid showed an antiinflammatory activity in 1/8 potency of cortisol by the cotton-pellet method. The acitivity is potentiated to 1/5 of cortisol when "carbenoxolone" (sodium salt of hemisuccinate of glycyrrhetic acid) is used (Finney and Tarnoky, 1960). A glycyrrhizin ointment is employed clinically for aphtha and other inflammatory skin diseases. In these cases glycyrrhizin or its sapogenin, glycyrrhetic acid, potentiates the action of glucocorticoid.

Taking into consideration that glycyrrhizin or glycyrrhetic acid does not produce direct hormonal activities but might react indirectly to enhance the activities of both mineral and gluco-coriticoids in inhibiting the metabolic inactivation of these hormones in liver, Kumagai and Yano and their collaborators incubated cortisol in liver homogenate under the presence of glycyrrhizin in a molar equivalent amout to demonstrate 50 % inhibition of the reduction of Δ^4-3-keto system, and 80 % inhibition of the degradation of the side chain of cortisol. The inhibition of metabolic reduction of Δ^4-3-keto system which has since been proved to be the inhibition of Δ^4-5-β-reductase, has been shown by the liver homogenate incubation method not only for cortisol but also for other steroidal hormones with the same structural system, such as deoxycorticosterone, progesterone and aldosterone (Kumagai et al, 1957; Kumagai, 1968).

Table 1. Effects of glycyrrhizin on the reduction of Δ^4-3-ketone of cortisol

Conc. of cortisol	Conc. of glycyrrhizin	Rate of inhibition
4.5×10^{-4}M	0.75×10^{-4}M	0 %
4.5×10^{-4}	1.5×10^{-4}	33
4.5×10^{-4}	3.0×10^{-4}	62
2.25×10^{-4}	2.0×10^{-4}	59

System: rat liver homogenate. Incubation time: 60 min at 37°C (Kumagai et al., 1957)

Table 2. Effects of glycyrrhizin on the degradation of side-chain of cortisol

Conc. of cortisol	Conc. of glycyrrhizin	Rate of inhibition
4.5×10^{-4}M	0.75×10^{-4}	74 %
4.5×10^{-4}	1.5×10^{-4}	83
4.5×10^{-4}	3.0×10^{-4}	88
2.25×10^{-4}	2.0×10^{-4}	54
0.45×10^{-4}	0.3×10^{-4}	23

System: rat liver homogenate. Incubation time: 60 min at 37°C (Kumagai et al., 1957)

III. Antigastric Ulcer Effects of Glycyrrhizin

Since Revers' report appeared, several clinical observations have been reported on the antigastric ulcer activity of glycyrrhizin or "carbenoxolone" (Ottenjann and Rösch, 1970). Takagi and his coworkers showed that glycyrrhizin inhibits ulcers in Shay rats and also cures experimental gastric ulcers caused by acetic administration. To avoid the side-effects of glycyrrhizin in licorice preparations, such as edema and hypertension, a glycyrrhizin-free fraction of licorice extracts was studied by Takagi and his coworkers, and the so-called FM 100 fraction was found to be effective for gastric ulcers in rats by inhibiting gastric juice secretion. This effect has been confirmed by clinical observation (Takagi et al., 1967, 1969). Shibata, Saitoh and their collaborators isolated several new isoflavonoid and chalcones from the fraction FM 100 (Saitoh et al., 1976).

IV. Metabolic Effects of Glycyrrhizin

Yamamoto found that glycyrrhizin stimulates the biosynthesis of cholesterol in rat liver. However, the total level of cholesterol in blood is decreased by the promotion of excretion of cholesterol by the metabolic effects of glycyrrhizin (Yamamoto et al., 1970b). It is interesting to find such activity in glycyrrhizin-regulating metabolism, which would reasonably coincide with the old Chinese medical use of licorice.

C. The Saponins of Bupleuri Radix and Platycodi Radix

The roots of *Bupleurum falcatum* L. (Umbelliferae) (Chai-hu in Chinese; Saiko in Japanese) is used as an important component of various recipes in Chinese medicine to resolve the tightness and resistance syndrome at the costal margin that might be related to inflammation of the diaphragm and enlargement of liver caused by hepatitis.

The main constituents of this drug are saponins named saikosaponins a,c and d (Kubota and Hinoh, 1968). The genuine sapogenins obtained by the Smith degradation of the sapogenins (saikosaponins E, F and G) were studied independently by Kubota et al., 1968) and Shibata and co-workers (Aimi and Shibata, 1966) almost simultaneously to obtain their oleanane-type structures with a characteristic Δ^{11},13β-28-oxide system.

On acid hydrolysis of saikosaponins, saikogenin A, C and D with a heteroannular diene system in the C and D rings, and saikogenin B with a homoannular diene system in the C ring were obtained first, but it was later confirmed that they are artifacts formed during acid hydrolysis (Shibata et al., 1966; Kubota et al., 1967a,b).

The roots of *Platycodon grandiflorum* DC (Campanulaceae) (Chieh-Keng in Chinese; Kikyo in Japanese) are also used in Chinese medicine as a combined expectorant and antitussive agent. On acid hydrolysis of the crude saponins of Platycodi Radix, platycodigenin was isolated as the main sapogenin (Akiyama et al., 1972a,c) and platycodigenic acids A, B and C (Kubota et al., 1968, 1969; Kubota and Kitawi, 1969) as well as polygalacic acid were obtained as the minor sapogenins (Akiyama et al., 1972b).

On TCL, several saponins, named platycodin A - H, were separated. Among them platycodin D, $C_{57}H_{92}O_{28}$, was isolated as a main saponin of Platycodi Radix to determine the structure in which apiose is present as a sugar component (Tada et al., 1975).

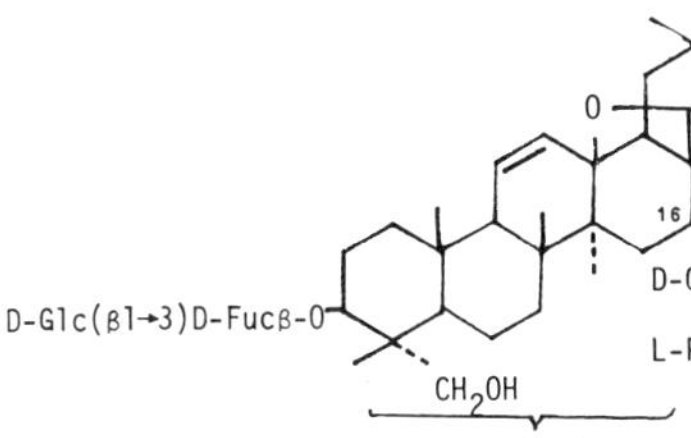

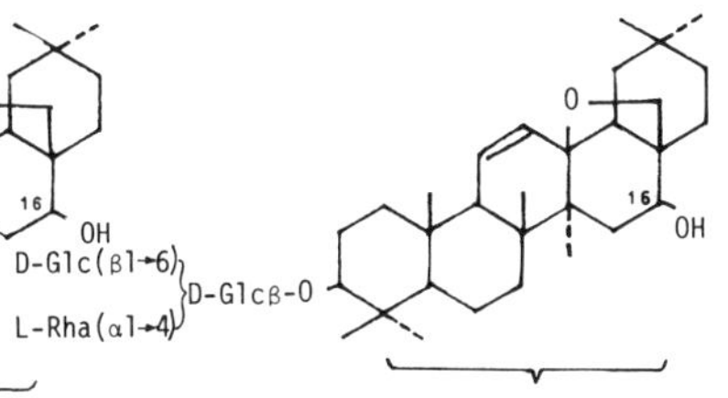

Saikogenin-F

Saikogenin-E

Saikosaponin-a

Saikosaponin-c

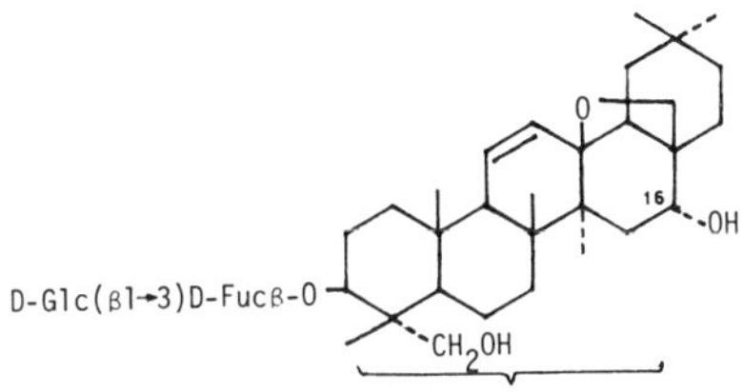

Saikogenin-G

Saikosaponin-d

Fig. 2

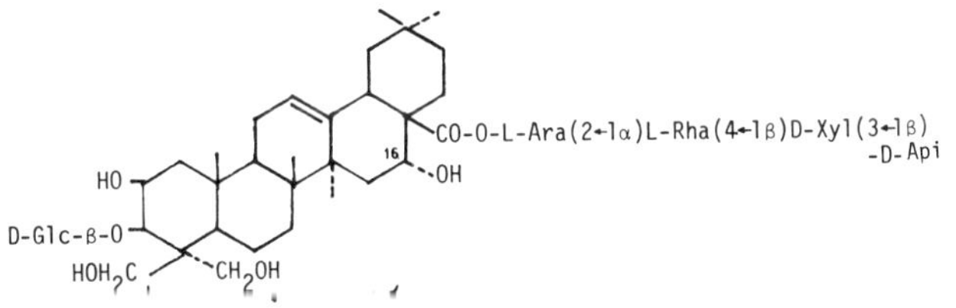

Platycodigenin

Platycodin-D

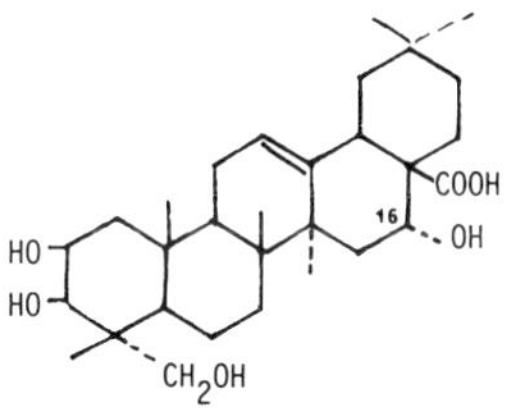

Polygalacic acid

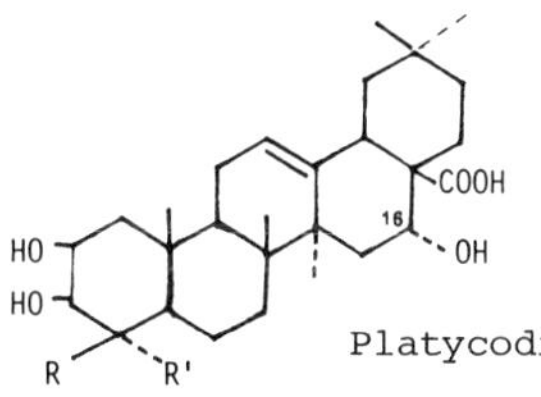

Platycodigenic acid A

R=COOH R'=CH_2OH

Platycodigenic acid B

R=COOH R'=CH_3

Platycodigenic acid C

R=R'=CH_3

Fig. 3

Elyakov isolated platycodiside C for which a structure consisting of platycodigenin, glucose:xylose:rhamnose:arabinose (2:1:1:1) was proposed (Elyakov and Aladjiana, 1972).

Pharmacological studies on the saponins of Bupleuri Radix and Platycodi Radix were carried out by Takagi and this collaborators to give scientific evidence for the use of these drugs in Chinese medicine. By analysing recipes in Chinese medicine containing Bupleuri or Platycodi Radix as the main component, is inflammation the first symptom for this root to be used.

Table 3. Main five therapeutic uses of Bupleuri et Platycodi Radicis in Chinese medicine

Bupleuri Radix		Platycodi Radix	
Inflammation	42 cases	Inflammation	63 cases
Pyrexia	40	Cough	16
Pain	21	Pain	21
Muscle stiffness	21	Hypertension	4
Neurosis	7	Pyrexia	9

Both saikosaponins and platycodins show strong hemolytic activities and local irritation. By means of conditioning animal experiments using the climbing test and the avoiding test, both saponins reveal a central nervous system (CNS)-suppressing effect, while they show analgesic, antipyretic, as well as antitussive action on the animals. The antipyretic action is remarkably demonstrated in saikosaponins.

The antiinflammatory actions of steroidal and nonsteroidal types are clearly revealed by the oral administration of both saponins. Against Shay ulcer, both the saponins are effective; particularly platycodin (Takagi et al., 1969; Takagi and Shibata, 1969; Shibata, 1970; Takagi and Lee, 1972a,b; Kawashima et al., 1972). Yamamoto et al. (1970a) studied the antiinflammatory effects of saikosaponins a, c and d (3:2:2) using the cotton pellet method on rats (results are shown in Table 4).

Table 4. Antiinflammatory effects of saikosaponins

Saponins	No. of rats	Body wt (g)	Cotton pellet wt (mg)	Adrenal gland wt (mg)
Control	5	182 - 188	83	62
Saikosaponin a (0.3 mg/100 g/day x 5)	5	192 - 198	51	61
Saikosaponin c (0.2 mg/100 g/day x 5)	5	180 - 192	75	58
Saikosaponin d	5	184 - 200	45	67

(Yamamoto et al., 1970a)

The results showed that saikosaponins a and d are effective in giving 61 % and 54 % of the weight of cotton pellet in comparison with non-treated control. Saikosaponin c is not effective; it possesses no CH_2OH group in the A ring of sapogenin in contrast to saikosaponin a and d.

In all experiments, the weight of adrenal gland of the animals remains unchanged, which suggests that the administration of saikosaponins has no side-effects such as shrinking of adrenal gland that quite often occurs with the exogeneous administration of predonisolone. Intramuscular administration of saikosaponin mixture reduced cholesterol and triglycerides level in plasma of the cholesterol-diet rats.

In vitro incorporation of acetate-^{14}C into total hepatic lipids and cholesterol was slightly enhanced, whereas elimination of intraperitoneally injected cholesterol-4^{14}C was increased.

Thus, the reduction of cholesterol level in plasma by the administration of saikosaponins would reasonably be explained.

This might give experimental support for the application of Bupleuri Radix in Chinese medicine for hepatobiliary and inflammtory diseases.

D. Saponins of Polygalae Radix and Senegae Radix

Yüan-chi (in Chinese) or Onji (in Japanese), the root of *Polygala tenuifolia* Willd. (Polygalaceae), is used in Chinese medicine as a sedative agent as well as to strengthen the nervous system. In western medicine, an analogous drug, Senegae Radix, the root of *Polygala senega* L., *P. senega* var. *latifolia* Torrey et Gary, is employed as an expectorant for bronchitis and asthma. Fujita and Itokawa reported earlier that the saponins of Chinese Polygalae Radix and Senega are almost identical (Fujita and Itokawa, 1961). Recently, Shoji and his coworkers isolated senegins II, III, and IV from Senegae Radix (Shoji et al., 1971; Tsukitani et al., 1973, Tsukitani and Shoji, 1973), while Sakuma and Shoji isolated onjisaponins A - F from Yüan-chi (Onji) (Sakuma et al., 1975). Comparing the saponins of both drugs, it has been shown that senegin IV is identical with onjisaponin A, while senegin III corresponds to onjisaponin B.

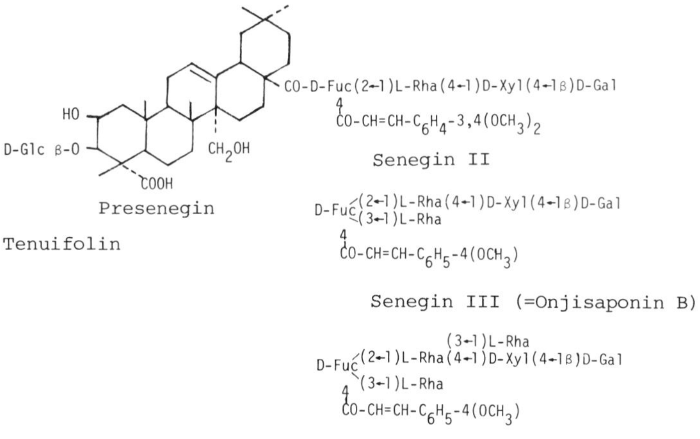

Senegin IV (=Onjisaponin A) Fig. 4

On acid hydrolysis of Senega saponins, a complex rearrangement occurs in the aglycone part, resulting in the formation of several secondary products without giving the genuine sapogenin (Tschesche and Wulff,

1973). Presenegin, 2β, 3β, 27-trihydroxy-olean-23,28-oic acid, a genuine sapogenin of senegins, was obtained by careful treatment in saponification (Dugan et al., 1964; Shimizu and Pelletier, 1966). Yosioka and his collaborators employed soil bacteria to hydrolyze saponins to obtain their genuine sapogenins (Yosioka et al., 1966).

Polygala chinensis L. (Indian Senega) contains a saponin whose aglycone is the same as that of *P. senega* and *P. tenuifolia* (Kumekawa et al., 1974). The sugar moity, however, consists of Glc(1→4)Xyl(1→4)Rha(1→4)Rha

2
↑
1
Glc(1→3)Rha

and is attached only at the 3-OH of the aglycone. The p-methoxycinnamic acid is attached to the carbinol at $C_{(14)}$ of the aglycone (Brieskorn and Kilbingen, 1975).

E. Saponins of Akebiae Vitis

Mu-T'ung (in Chinese) or Mokutsu (in Japanese), the stem-bark of *Akebia quinata* DC (Lardizabalaceae), is used in Chinese medicine as an antiinflammatory agent, diuretic and menses stimulant. From this drug Fujita and co-workers isolated several saponins of oleanolic acid and hederagenin (Fujita et al., 1974a,b). The saponins so far determined are as follows:
Akeboside St-e(=Oleanolic acid 3-O-α-L-rhamnopyranosyl (1→6)β-D-glucopyranosyl(1→2)-α-L-arabinopyranoside),St-b(=Hederagenin 3-O-α-L-arbinopyranoside),St-c (=Hederagenin 3-O-α-L-rhamonopyranosyl(1→2)-α-L-arabinopyranoside),St-d(=Hederagenin 3-O-β-D-glucopyranosyl(1→2)-α-L-arabinopyranoside), and St-f(=Hederagenin 3-O-α-L-rhamonopyranosyl (1→6)-α-D-glucopyranosyl(1→2)-α-L-rhamnopyranoside). Akebosides St-h, St-j and St-k have not yet been established structurally (Kumekawa et al., 1974).

Kawasaki and his collaborators also isolated saponins A - G from the seeds of *Akebia quinata*, whose sapogenin is hederagenin, while saponins P_A-P_H,P_{J1-3} and P_K from the pericarp of the same plant (Higuchi et al., 1972; Higuchi and Kawasaki, 1972, 1976b). The sapogenin of saponins P_A,P_F,P_C,P_D,P_G,P_{J-2}, and P_K is hederagenin, and that of saponins P_B,P_E and P_{J-3} is oleanolic acid. Norarjunolic acid and arjunolic acid are adopted to the sapogenin of saponins P_H and P_{J-1}, respectively (Higuchi and Kawasaki, 1976b).

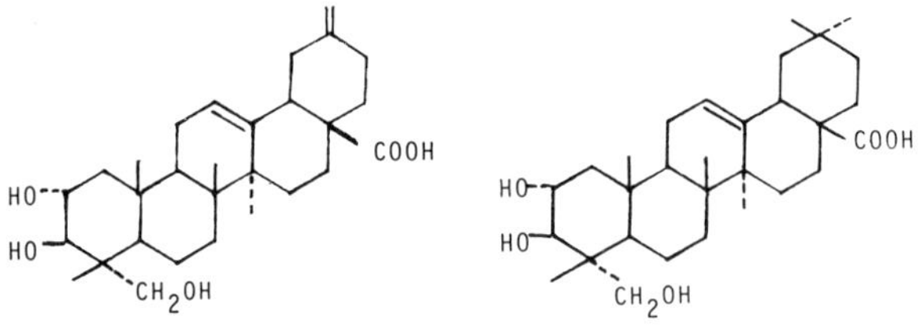

Norarjunolic acid   Arjunolic acid   Fig. 5

F. Aescin, the Saponins of the Seeds of *Aesculus hippocastanum*

The seeds of *A. hippocastanum* L. (Hippocastanaceae) have been used as a folk medicine in France, and the tincture of this drug has been used successfully for hemoroid and venous congestion. The saponin of this drug, aescin, whose yield is about 13 %, is a mixture, though it is obtained in a crystalline form. According to Wulff and Tschesche (1969) the components of "aescin" are shown as follows:

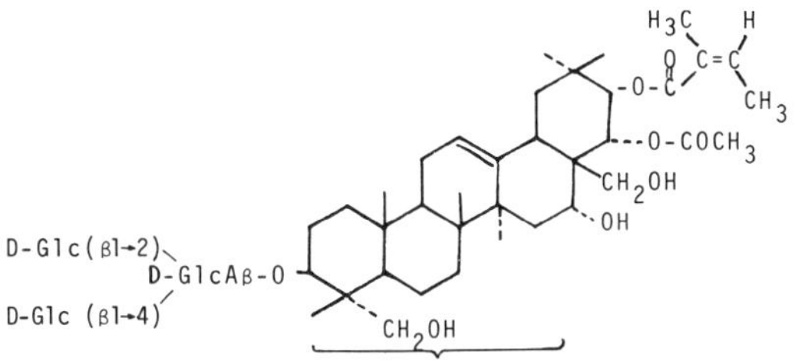

Fig. 6. Main glycoside of "Aescin"

Table 5. The components of main principles of "aescin"

Triterpene	Sugar	Acid	% in Aescin
Proaescigenin	D-GlcA D-Glc D-Glc	Angelic acid Acetic acid	23
	D-GlcA D-Glc D-Glc	Tiglic acid Acetic acid	15
	D-GlcA D-Glc D-Xyl	Angelic acid Acetic acid	9
	D-GlcA D-Glc D-Xyl	Tiglic acid Acetic acid	6
	D-GlcA D-Glc D-Gal	Angelic acid Acetic acid	7
	D-GlcA D-Glc D-Gal	Tiglic acid Acetic acid	5
Barringtogenol	D-GlcA D-Glc D-Glc	Angelic acid Acetic acid	5
	D-GlcA D-Glc D-Glc	Tiglic acid Acetic acid	3

(Tschesche and Wulff, 1973)

Aescin shows an antiinflammatory action, and it is administered orally for clinical use.

G. Saponins of Ginseng

I. Chemical Studies on the Saponins and Sapogenins of Ginseng and its Congeners

Ginseng, the roots of *Panax ginseng* C.A. Meyer (Araliaceae), has been well known among the peoples in East Asian countries since ancient time as a precious drug for longevity or cureall.

Although there were several earlier attempts to discover its effective principle, no remarkable evidence has been obtained until recently.

Petkov in Bulgaria (Petkov, 1959, 1961a,b, 1968) and Brekhman in USSR (Brekhman, 1957; Brekhman et al., 1969a,b) reported in the end of 1950s and early 1960s that the extracts of Ginseng and later the saponin fraction of Ginseng show some stimulation of the central nervous system, antifatigue actions and enhancement of nonspecific resistance.

Shibata and his collaborators reported the isolation of saponins from Ginseng and proposed a structure of panaxadiol as a sapogenin (Fujita et al., 1962; Shibata et al., 1962, 1963) while Elyakov and his coworkers reported their chemical studies on Ginseng saponins named panaxosides A - F and their sapogenin (Elyakov et al., 1962). It was soon found that panaxadiol is an artifact formed by the action of acid on hydrolysis of saponins, and 20-S-protopanaxadiol, a dammarane-type tetracyclic triterpene has been proved to be a genuine sapogenin of Ginseng saponins. The saponins of Ginseng, named ginsenoides R_x (x = o,a,b_1,b_2,b_3,c,d,e,f,20-gluco-f,g_1 and g_2) have been separated by the Silica gel column chromatography. On direct comparison, ginsenoside R_{g-1} is identical with Elyakov's panaxoside A. All the structures of ginsenosides R_x have been established (Shibata, 1974; Nagai et al., 1971; Sanada et al., 1974a,b).

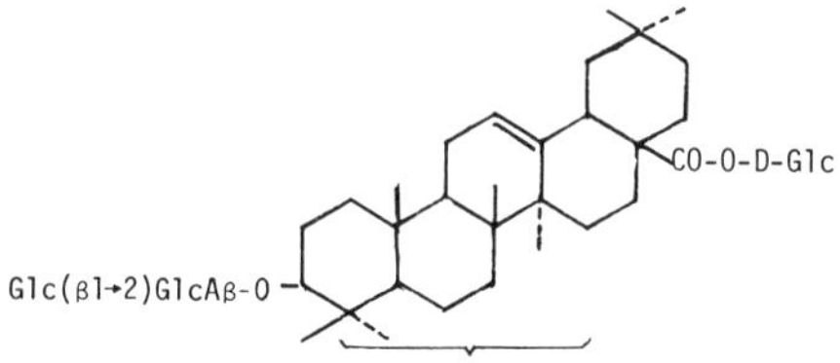

Oleanolic acid

Ginsenoside R_o (= Chikusetsusaponin V)

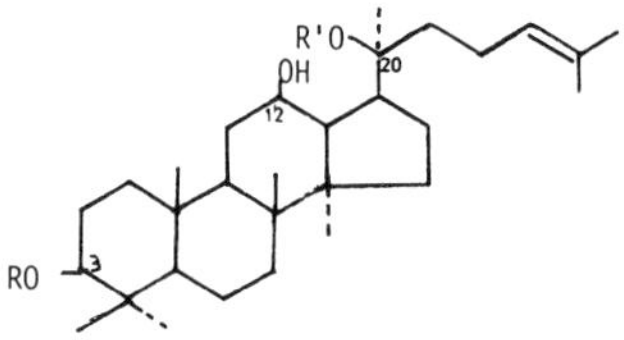

20-S-Protopanaxadiol

Ginsenoside

R_{b-1} R = D-Glc(β1→2)D-Glc
R'= D-Glc(β1→6)D-Glc

R_{b-2} R = D-Glc(β1→2)D-Glc
R'= L-Ara(pyr)(α1→6)D-Glc

R_{b-3} R = D-Glc(β1→2)D-Glc
R'= D-Xyl(β1→6)D-Glc

R_c R = D-Glc(β1→2)D-Glc
R'= L-Ara(fur)(α1→6)D-Glc

R_d R = D-Glc(β1→2)D-Glc
R'= D-Glc

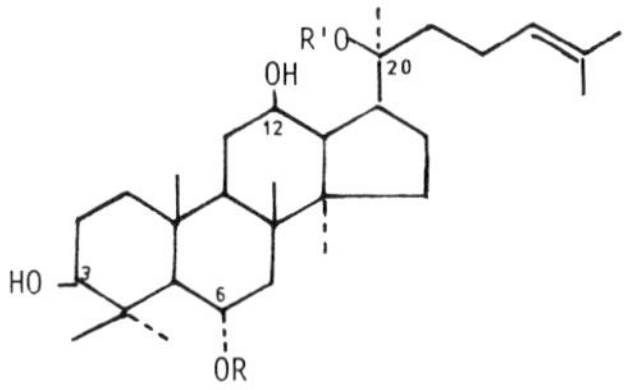

20-S-Protopanaxatriol

Ginsenoside

R_e R = L-Rha(α1→2)D-Glc
R'= D-Glc

R_f R = D-Glc(β1→2)D-Glc
R'= H

20-Gluco-R_f R=D-Glc(β1→2)D-Glc
R'=D-Glc

R_{g-1} R = D-Glc
R'= D-Glc

R_{g-2} R = L-Rha(α1→2)D-Glc
R'= H

(= Chikusetsusaponin I)

Fig. 7

The genuine sapogenin of ginsenosides R_e,R_f, 20-gluco-R_f,R_{g-1} and R_{g-2} is 20-S-protopanaxatriol, which possesses hydrolxyl groups at 3β,6α,12β and 20 positions. The sugar moieties are linked to 6 and 20-hydroxyls, while the 3-hydroxyl remains free.

The stereochemistry of 20-S-protopanaxadiol and -triol was established in relation to dammaranediol I and II and betulafolienetriol. 20-S-sapogenins are readily epimerized into 20-R isomer to form an equilibrium mixture in which the R-form is predominant. Ginsenoside R_o is the only one saponin of Ginseng, which possesses oleanolic acid as the sapogenin.

P. ginseng was initially a wild-growing plant in Northeast China, Korea and the Far-East part of Siberia, and now it is cultivated in Korea and Japan to supply the drug market, but there are several congeners of Ginseng or Korean Ginseng.

The root of *Panax quinquefolium* L. which is either wild-growing or cultivated in the northern part of the U.S.A. is also employed as a drug under the name of American Ginseng for purpose similar to Korean Ginseng.

San-chi Ginseng originated in South-West China, Yun-nan and Kwan-si, and is used as a remedy for bruises and hemorhage. The original plant of San-chi Ginseng is said to be *Panax pseudoginseng* var. *notoginseng* (Burk). Hoo et Tseng or *Panax san-chi* Hoo. Several varieties of *P. pseudoginseng* are found in Asia from the Eastern Himalayas to Southwest China and Japan. The rhizome of *P. pseudoginseng* subsp. *japonicus* Hara (= *P. japonicum* C.A. Meyer), wild-growing in Japan, has been used from olden times as a substitute for Korean Ginseng and according to recent investigations must have different medical effects than Korean Ginseng.

In 1854 Garriques first studied American Ginseng to isolate a saponin fraction named panaquilon. Recent investigation on saponins of American and Sanchi Ginseng revealed some minor differences in TLC and DCC patterns in comparison with Korean Ginseng and each other (Ando et al., 1971). In American Ginseng it is noted that ginsenoside R_{g-1} is not contained and R_{b-1} is dominant. Sanchi Ginseng gives a similar but simpler pattern than that of Korean Ginseng, and ginsenosides R_{b-1}, R_e and R_{g-1} are dominant in the saponin fraction of Sanchi Ginseng. Japanese Pseudo-Ginseng (Chikusetsu-Ginseng) shows an entirely different pattern of saponins in contrast to Korean, American and Sanchi Ginseng, and Chikusetsusaponins I,I_a,I_b,III,IV and V are the characteristic components of the saponins of Chikusetsu-ginseng, whose structure were determined by Shoji and his collaborators (Kondo et al., 1968, 1971, 1973; Lin et al., 1976). They found that oleanolic acid is more dominant as the sapogenins than dammarane-type triterpenes.

II. Pharmacological and Biochemical Studies on Ginseng Saponins

Following chemical studies on Ginseng saponins and sapogenins, several pharmacological and biochemical studies on crude saponins and pure ginsenosides R_x have been reported.

Takagi and his collaborators (Takagi et al., 1972a,b, 1974; Nabata et al., 1973; Saito et al., 1973, 1974; Takagi, 1974) studied the pharmacological properties of Ginseng saponins by the following tests: (1) neuropharmacological observations in mice; (2) effects on respiration and blood pressure in rats; (3) tests on Guinea pig-isolated ileum; (4) effects on writhing induced by intraperitoneally injected

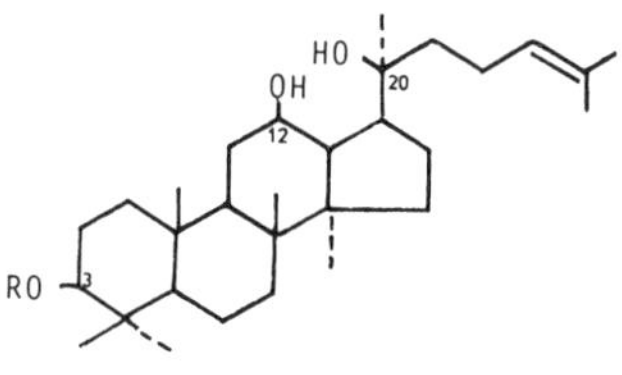

20-S-Protopanaxadiol

Chikustsusaponin

Ia R = D-Xyl(β1→6)D-Glc

III R = D-Xyl(β1→6) } D-Glc
D-Glc(β1→2)

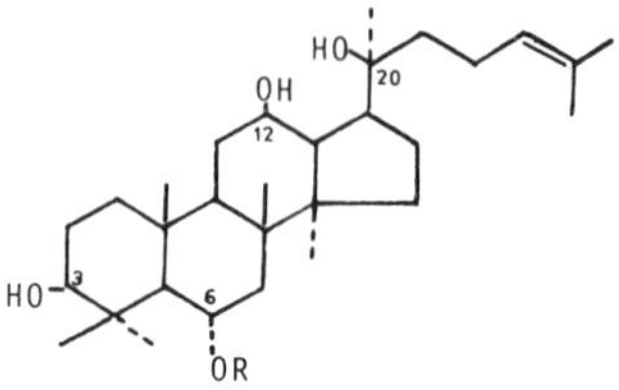

20-S-Protopanaxatriol

Chikusetsusaponin

I R = L-Rha(α1→2)D-Glc
(= Ginsenoside R_{g-2})

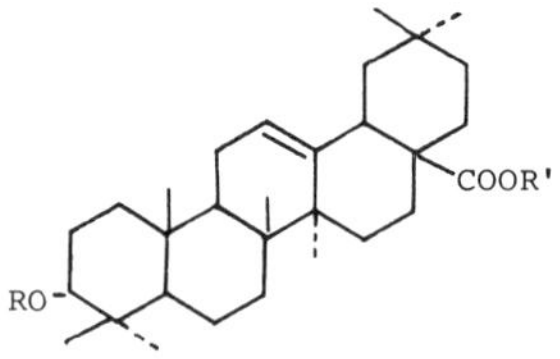

Oleanolic acid

Chikusetsusaponin

Ib R = D-Glc(β1→6) } D-GlcA
L-Ara(α1→4)
R'= H

IV R = L-Ara(α1→4)GlcA
R'= D-Glc

IVa R = D-GlcA
R'= D-Glc

V R = D-Glc(β1→2)D-Glc
R'= D-Glc

Fig. 8

0.7 % acetic acid in mice; (5) effects on the hypnotic action of hexobarbital administered intraperitoneally 70 mg/kg in mice. The results are summarized as follows: (1) slight central nervous system(CNS)-stimulating action and antifatigue action were observed in ginsenoside R_{g-1}; (2) CNS-suppressing effect and tranquillizing action were shown in ginsenoside R_{b-1}.

The CNS activating effect of ginsenoside R_{g-1} was shown from increased discrimination in Y-maze and pole-climbing tests. The antifatigue action of ginsenoside R_{g-1} was revealed in acceleration of recovery from depressed spontaneous and exploratory behaviors, motor incoordination, conditioned avoidance and fighting behavior tests. Ginsenoside R_{b-1} also inhibits stress ulcer in mice. Oura and Hiai (Oura et al., 1975) studied the biochemical properties of the fractions of Korean Ginseng and concluded that the saponin fraction is active to promote RNA and protein biosynthesis in liver cells of rats. An intensive incorporation of ^{14}C-leucine into liver protein and its transference into serum protein were produced by the intraperitoneal administration of ginsenosides R_{b-2},R_c and R_{g-1}, 1 mg/100 g in rats. Incorporation of ^{3}H-thymine into nuclear RNA of bone marrow was also potentiated by the intraperitoneal injection of ginsenosides R_{b-2},R_c and R_{g-1} (Yamamoto, 1973).

These results show some discrepancies with those obtained by Higashi and his co-workers (Sakakibara et al., 1975; Gommori et al., 1976) who carried out the experiments with the following procedure: five mg each saponin was injected intraperitoneally into rats weighing

100 - 120 g. Ginsenoside R_{b-1}, R_c and R_{g-1} were dissolved respectively in saline, and R_d and R_e in 20 % ethanol. Total and free cholesterol in serum and liver were assayed four hours after the injection of saponins. In labeling experiments, 10 μCi of Na acetate-1 ^{14}C/100 g body wt was injected intraperitoneally into normal and saponin-treated rats at a definite time prior to sacrifice. The saponin-treated rats were killed 4 h after the injection of saponins. Incorporation of ^{14}C-acetate into serum cholesterol was measured for the period of 30 min, and that into liver cholesterol was determined for the period of 90 min.

On administration of ginsenoside R_{b-1} into rats, Higashi and his co-workers observed an active acceleration of the incorporation of ^{14}C-acetic acid into liver cholesterol, and ^{14}C-leucine into serum protein. Liver slices prepared from the rats treated with ginsenosides were incubated with ^{14}C-acetate to show the enhancement of cholesterol synthesis, and the highest potency was observed by the administration of ginsenoside R_{b-1} to the rats.

Table 6. Effect of various ginsenosides on cholesterol metabolism

Ginsenoside			R_{b-1}	R_c	R_{g-1}	R_d	R_e
Serum cholesterol	Amount	Total	114	114	96	86	94
		Free	123	75	83	62	62
		F/T[a]	109	67	86	73	66
	Biosynthesis		773	433	133	201	79
Liver cholesterol	Amount	Total	90	81	86	95	108
		Free	100	79	96	123	47
		F/T[a]	113	98	112	130	44
	Biosynthesis		309	155	132	111	176

The values are expressed as percentage of the control.
[a]Free/Total cholesterol x 100. (Lin et al., 1976)

Four hours after intraperitoneal injection of each ginsenoside R_{b-1}, R_c and R_{g-1} at a dose of 5 mg/100 g body wt, incorporation of ^3H-orotic acid into nuclear RNA of rat liver was determined.

The results showed that ginsenoside R_{b-1} increased the incorporation of ^3H into RNA, whereas R_e decreased, while R_{g-1} did not give any remarkable effect.

The effects of ginsenoside R_{b-1} and R_c on the activity of RNA-polymeraze were also observed to show that R_{b-1} enhanced the enzyme activity and R_c repressed it. In vitro both ginsenosides showed any effect on RNA polymerase directly. From these experiments, it has been suggested that the activities of ginsenosides promoting the biosynthesis of RNA, protein and cholesterol would be performed through some intermediate reagents which might include some hormones.

Table 7. Effect of various ginsenosides on serum protein biosynthesis using ^{14}C-leucine as a tracer. Amount and radioactivity of serum proteins fractionated by agar-gel electrophoresis

		Control	Treated with ginsenoside R_{b-1}	R_c	R_{g-1}
Albumin	Amount (mg)	5.6	5.7	5.3	4.1
	Incorporation of radioactivity (cpm)	2720	5410	4720	1880
	Spc. activity (cpm/mg)	485	950	890	460
α-Globulin	Amount (mg)	0.89	0.91	0.90	1.29
	Incorporation of radioactivity (cpm)	710	2120	1770	930
	Spec. activity (cpm/mg)	795	2340	1970	725
β-Globulin	Amount (mg)	0.98	0.98	1.00	0.44
	Incorporation of radioactivity (cpm)	535	1130	1145	270
	Spec. activity (cpm/mg)	545	1155	1145	600
γ-Globulin	Amount (mg)	0.84	1.05	0.60	1.05
	Incorporation of radioactivity (cpm)	160	790	345	340
	Spec. activity (cpm/mg)	190	750	575	325

The sera (0.15 ml) were fractionated by electrophoresis. The gel was sliced in 3 mm-width slots. Each 1/3 was proceeded for Folin determination and 2/3 for radioactivity measurement (Shibata, Y. et al., 1976)

Table 8. Effect of ginsenoside R_{b-1}, R_c and R_{g-1} on incorporation of ^3H-orotic acid into liver nuclear RNA

Rats		^3H-Orotic acid incorporation cpm/unit of OD_{260} (Mean ± S.E.)	
Control	(6)	4666.9 ± 366	100 %
R_{b-1} treated	(6)	5484.6 ± 416	117.5
R_c treated	(6)	3999.7 ± 459	85.7
R_{g-1} treated	(6)	4882.7 ± 535	104.6

Figures in parentheses indicate the number of animals (Iijima et al., 1976)

III. Pharmacological Studies on Japanese Chikusetsu-Ginseng

The pharmacological studies on Japanese Chikusetsu-Ginseng (*Panacis japonici* Rhizoma) carried out by Saito and Takagi and their co-workers (Saito et al., 1976; Lee et al., 1976) showed that chikusetsu-saponin III possesses sedative, antipyretic, antitussive, and expectorant activities, prevents stress ulcers, accelerates intestinal motility and shows antiinflammatory activity; chikusetsu-saponin IV acts as an expectorant and shows prevention of stress ulcers and acceleration of intestinal motility, while chikusetsu-saponin V has an antiinflammatory effect. Chikusetsu-saponins did not demonstrate any of the CNS-stimulant or antifatique agents, which were clearly observed in ginsenoside R_{g-1} of Korean Ginseng.

The description of Ginseng in the oldest Chinese Materia Medica "Shin-Nung Pen T'sao Ching," originating about two thousand years ago is interesting: "Ginseng is effective to calm mental condition, stabilizes spirit, ceases frightened heart, stimulates the mind, extends the memory, makes the sight clear and removes ill-feeling." This suggests not only sedative and tranquillizing but also activating and stimulating effects, both of which have been demonstrated by the pharmacological and biochemical studies on Ginseng saponins, ginsenoside R_{b-1} and R_{g-1} group, respectively. Meanwhile, Yoshimasu-Todo, a Japanese physician in Chinese medicine in the middle of 18th Century wrote a medical text in which he denied the claim of Shin-Nung Pen T'sao Ching to stimulative activities in Ginseng, and emphasized the results for gastroenteric disorder. This would agree with the recent findings on Japanese Chikusetsu-Ginseng as accelerating intestinal motility and preventing stress ulcers. He probably employed Chikusetsu-Ginseng, which might have been more easily available in Japan at that time than the expensive Korean Ginseng.

H. Saponins of Zizyphus Spinosi Semen

The seeds of *Zizyphus jujuba* Mill var. *spinosa* Hu. (Rhamnaceae) are used in Chinese medicine under the name of Suan-Tsao-Jen (Sansonin in Japanese) for strengthening the nervous system as a remedy for insomnia and sometimes for sleepiness, caused both by physical and mental strain.

As the constituents of this drug, Shibata and his co-workers (Shibata et al., 1970; Kawai et al., 1974) isolated saponins named jujubosides A and B. On treatment with snake enzymes jujuboside A is converted into jujuboside B releasing 1 mol of D-glucose. On acid hydrolysis, jujubosides yielded ebelin lactone as the sapogenin and glucose, rhamnose, arabinose and xylose as the sugar components, whose ratio in jujuboside B is 1:1:1:1.

Ebelin lactone was obtained earlier by Eade (Eade et al., 1965) from a saponin of the wood of Australian Rhamnaceous plant, *Emmenospermum aliphitonioides* F. Muell on acid hydrolysis. In later investigations, it has become clear that ebelin lactone is an artifact which is produced by the action of the acid.

Analogous saponins which yield ebelin lactone by acid hydrolysis have been isolated from other plant sources, such as the root-bark of *Hovenia dulcis* whose saponins are named hovenosides, and the whole herb of *Bacopa monniera*, an Indian Ayurvedic drug, Brahmi, from which Rastogi and his co-workers (Chatterji et al., 1963; Kulshreshtha et al, 1973) isolated bacosides.

On Smith-de Mayo's degradation jujubosides A and B and hovenoside G afforded a genuine sapogenin, jujubogenin, for which Shibata and his co-workers (Kawai et al., 1974) proposed a dammarane-type structure. This structure was later confirmed by X-ray analysis of its monobromoacetate. The conversion of jujubogenin into ebelin lactone has been reasonably elucidated, These saponins have now been recognized as the dammarane-type triterpenoid saponins (Otsuka et al., 1976).

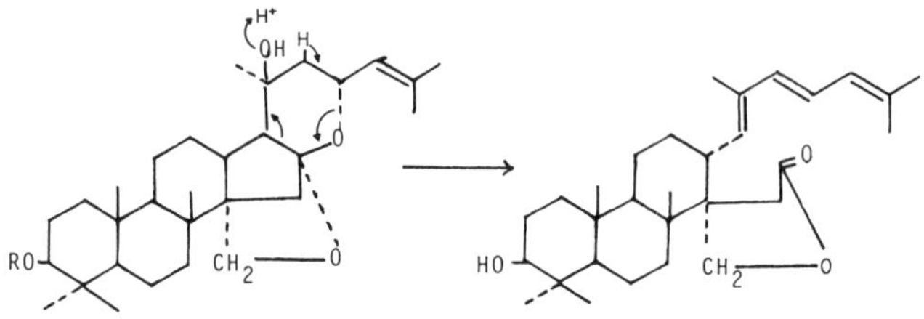

R = H Jujubogenin Ebelin lactone

Jujuboside A:

R = D-Glc(β1→6) D-Xyl(β1→2) | L-Rha(α1→2) D-Glc(β1→3) | L-Ara-

Jujuboside B:

R = D-Xyl(β1→2) L-Rha(α1→2) D-Glc(β1→3) | L-Ara-

Fig. 9

Pharmacological experiments on jujubosides and hobenosides were carried out by Takagi and Saito to reveal sedative and tranquillizing action in animals (Watanabe et al., 1973).

I. Concluding Remarks

It has been shown that the triterpenoid saponins isolated from several plant drugs have remarkable physiological and biochemical activities which enlarge the scope of the classical recognition of saponins. It was noted that a number of drugs traditional in Chinese medicine contain more saponins than alkaloids. It seems then that saponins are responsible for the efficacy of these drugs.

The biochemical investigation referred to in this article suggests that in many cases triterpenoid saponins achieve their biological results through some intermediate mechanisms which are as yet unknown.

Acknowledgements. The author wishes to thank his collaborators, especially Prof. O. Tanaka, now in Hiroshima University, and Prof. J. Shoji, Showa University, who have pursued important parts of the chemical studies which are referred to in the original part of this article. The author also expresses his gratitude to Prof. K. Takagi, now in Tokyo Science University, and Dr. H. Saito, University of Tokyo for their generous cooperation in pharmacological studies on saponins of Chinese drugs. Thanks are also due to Prof. T. Higashi, Showa University, who is engaged in the biochemical studies on Ginseng saponins, for his supply of unpublished data.

References

Aimi, N., Shibata, S.: Saikogenin E, a genuine sapogenin of *Bupleurum* roots. Tetrahedron Lett., 4721 (1966

Akiyama, T., Tanako, O., Shibata, S.: Chemical studies on the oriental plant drugs. XXXII. Sapogenins of the roots of *Platycodon grandiflorum* A.DC. (3). The structure of prosapogenin, 3-O-β-glucoplatycodigenin. Chem. Pharm. Bull. (Tokyo) 20, 1957 (1972a)

Akiyama, T., Tanaka, O., Shibata, S.: Chemical studies on the oriental plant drugs. XXX. Sapogenins of the roots of *Platycodon grandiflorum* A.DC. (1). Isolation of the sapogenins and the stereochemistry of polygalacic acid. Chem. Pharm. Bull (Tokyo) 20, 1945 (1972b)
Akiyama, T., Tanaka, O., Shibata, S.: Chemical studies on the oriental plant drugs. XXXI. Sapogenins of the roots of *Platycodon grandiflorum* A.DC. (2). Structure of platycodigenin. Chem. Pharm. Bull. (Tokyo) 20, 1952 (1972c)
Ando, T., Tanaka, O., Shibata, S.: Chemical Studies on the oriental plant drugs. XXV. Comparative studies on the saponins and sapogenins of Ginseng and related crude drugs. Shoyakugaku Zasshi (J. Jap. Soc. Pharmacognosy) 25, 28 (1971) (in Japanese)
Brekhman, I.I.: "Zhen-Shen" (*Panax ginseng*). Leningrad: Mediz, 1957, 182 pp.
Brekhman, I.I.: Pharmacological investigation of glycosides from Ginseng and Eleutherococcus. Lloydia 32, 46 (1969)
Brekhman, I.I., Dardymov, I.V.: New substances of plant origin which increase nonspecific resistance. Ann. Rev. Pharmacol. 9, 419-430 (1969)
Brieskorn, C.H., Kilbinger, W.: Struktur eines Saponins aus *Polygala chinensis* L. Arch. Pharm. 308, 824 (1975)
Chatterji, N., Rastogi, R.P., Dhar, M.L.: Examination of *Bacopa moniera*. I. Isolation of chemical constituents. Indian J. Chem. 1, 212 (1963)
Conn, J.W., Rovner, D.R., Cohen, E.L.: Licorice-induced pseudoaldosteronism. J. Am. Med. Assoc. 205, 492 (1968)
Dugan, J.J., de Mayo, P., Strratt, A.N.: Senegin. Proc. Chem. Soc. 264 (1964)
Eade, R.A., Rossla, L.P., Simes, H.V., Simes, J.J.H.: Extractives of Australian timbers. VI. Ebelin lactone. Australian J. Chem. 18, 1451 (1965)
Elyakov, G.B., Aladjiana, N.G.: Chemical studies on platycoside C, a glycoside from *Platycodon grandiflorum* (Jacq.) A.DC. Tetrahedron Lett. 1972, 3651
Elyakov, G.B., Strigna, L.T., Khorin, A.Ya., Kochetkov, N.K.: Glycosides from Ginseng roots (in Russian). Isvest. Acad. Nauk USSR 2054 (1962)
Finney, R.S.H., Tarnoky, A.L.: The pharmacological properties of glycyrrhetic acid hydrogensuccinate (disodium salt). J. Pharm. Pharmacol. 12, 49 (1960)
Fujita, M., Itokawa, H.: Studies on saponin-bearing drugs. III. Sapogenins of domestic Senega and Polygala, a Chinese drug "Yuan-chi." Chem. Pharm. Bull. (Tokyo) 9, 1006 (1961)
Fujita, M., Itokawa, H., Kumekawa, Y.: The study on the constituents of *Clematis* and *Akebia* spp. I. Distribution of triterpenes and other components. Yakugaku Zasshi (J. Pharm. Soc. Japan) 94, 189 (1974a)
Fujita, M., Itokawa, H., Kumekawa, Y.: The study on the constituents of *Clematis* and *Akebia* spp. II. On the saponins isolated from the stem of *Akebia quinata* Decne. Yakugaku Zasshi (J. Pharm. Soc. Japan), 94, 194 (1974b)
Fujita, M., Itokawa, H., Shibata, S.: Chemical studies on Ginseng. I. Isolation of saponin and sapogenin from *Radix Ginseng*. Yakugaku Zasshi (J. Pharm. Soc. Japan) 82, 1634 (1962)
Garriques, S.S.: On panaquilone, a new vegetable substance. Ann. Chem. Pharm. 90, 231 (1854)
Gommori, K., Miyamoto, F., Shibata, Y., Higashi, T., Sanada, S., Shoji, J.: Effects of Ginseng saponins on cholesterol metabolism. II. Effect of ginsenosides on cholesterol synthesis by liver slice. Chem. Pharm. Bull. (Tokyo) 24, 2400 (1976)
Guvanov, I.A., Libizov, N.J., Gladkikh, A.S.: Search for saponincontaining plants among the flora of central Asia and southern Kazakhstan. Farmatsiya (Moscow) 19, 23 (1970); Chem. Abstr. 73, 95408 (1973)
Higuchi, R., Kawasaki, T.: Seed saponins of *Akebia quinata* Decne. II. Hederagenin 3,28-O-bisglycosides. Chem. Pharm. Bull. (Tokyo) 20, 2143 (1972)
Higuchi, R., Kawasaki, T.: Pericarp saponine of *Akebia quinata* Decne. I. Glycosides of hederagenin and oleanolic acid. Chem. Pharm. Bull. (Tokyo) 24, 1021 (1976a)
Higuchi, R., Kawasaki, T.: Pericarp saponins of *Akebia quinata* Decne. II. Arjunolic and nor-arjunolic acids and their glycosides. Chem. Pharm. Bull. (Tokyo) 24, 1314 (1976b)
Higuchi, R., Miyahara, K., Kawasaki, T.: Seed saponins of *Akebia quinata*. Hederagenin 3-O-glycosides. Chem. Pharm. Bull. (Tokyo) 20, 1935 (1972)

Iijima, M., Higashi, T., Sanada, S., Shoji, J.: Effect of Ginseng saponins on RNA metabolism. I. Nuclear RNA synthesis in rats treated with ginsenosides. Chem. Pharm. Bull. (Tokyo) 24, 2400 (1976)

Kawai, K., Akiyama, T., Ogihara, Y., Shibata, S.: A new sapongenin in the saponins of *Zizyphus jujuba, Hovenia dulcis* and *Bacopa monniera*. Phytochemistry 13, 2829 (1974)

Kawashima K., Lee, E.B., Hirai, T., Takeuchi, K., Takagi, K.: Effects of crude platycodin on gastric secretion and experimental ulceration. Chem. Pharm. Bull. (Tokyo) 20, 755 (1972)

Kondo, N., Aoki, K., Ogawa, H., Kasai, R., Shoji, J.: Studies on the constituents of *Panacis japonici* Rhizoma. III. The structure of chikusetsu-saponin III. Chem. Pharm. Bull. (Tokyo) 18, 1558 (1973)

Kondo, N., Marumoto, Y., Shoji, J.: Studies on the constituents of *Panacis japonici* Rhizoma. IV. The structure of chikusetsu-saponin IV. Chem. Pharm. Bull. 19, 1103 (1971)

Kondo, N., Shoji, J., Nagumo, N., Komatsu, N.: Studies on the constituents of *Panacis japonici* Rhizoma. I. Isolation and purification of the saponins. (1). Yakugaku Zasshi (J. Pharm. Soc. Japan) 88, 325 (1968) (in Japanese)

Kubota, T., Hinoh, H.: The constitution of saponin isolated from *Bupleurum falcatum* L. Tetrahedron Lett. 1968, 303

Kubota, T., Kitani, H.: Revised structure of triterpene, polygalacic acid: Configuration of the C-16 hydroxyl group. Chem. Commun. 1005 (1968)

Kubota, T., Kitani, H.: The structure of platycodigenin, a 4,4-dihydroxymethyl triterpene. Chem. Commun. 190 (1969)

Kubota, T., Kitani, H., Hinoh, H.: The structures of platycogenic acids A,B and C. Further triterpenoid constituents of *Platycodon grandiflorum* A.DC. Chem. Commun. 1313 (1969)

Kubota, T., Tonami, F., Hinoh, H.: Triterpenoids from *Bupleurum falcatum* L. I. The structures of saikogenins A, C and D. Tetrahedron 23, 3333 (1967a)

Kubota, T., Tonami, F., Hinoh, H.: Triterpenoids from *Bupleurum falcatum* L. II. Isolation of saikogenin B and longispinogenin. Tetrahedron 23, 3353 (1967b)

Kubota, T., Tonami, F., Hinoh, H.: Triterpenoids from *Bupleurum falcatum* L. III. Isolation of genuine sapogenins, saikogenins E, F and G. Tetrahedron Lett. 24, 676 (1968)

Kulshreshtha, D.K., Rastogi, R.P.: Chemical examination of *Bacopa monniera*. V. Identification of ebelin lactone from bacoside A and the nature of its genuine sapogenin. Phytochemistry 12, 887 (1973)

Kumagi, A.: Diuretic and anti-diuretic action of glycyrrhizin, a principle of licorice. Report of 2nd Symp. Japanese-Chinese Drugs. Toyama 1968, pp. 69-79 (Res. Inst. Wakanyaku, Toyama Univ.)

Kumagai, A., Yano, S., Otomo, S.: Studies on the corticoid-like action of glycyrrhizin and the mechanism of its action. Endocrinol. Japonica 4, 17 (1957)

Kumekawa, Y., Itokawa, H., Fujita, M.: The study on the constituents of *Clematis* and *Akebia* spp. III. The structures of akebosides isolated from the stem of *Akebia quinata* Decne. Chem. Pharm. Bull. (Tokyo) 22, 2294 (1974)

Lee, Y.M., Saito, H., Takagi, K., Shibata, S., Shoji, J., Kondo, N.: Pharmacological studies of *Panacis japonici* Rhizoma. II. Japan J. Pharmacol. 26 (1977) in press

Lin, T.D., Kondo, N., Shoji, J.: Studies on the constituents of *Panacis japonici* Rhizoma. V. The structures of chikusetsu-saponin I,I_a,I_b, IVa and glycoside p-1. Chem. Pharm. Bull. 24, 253 (1976)

Molhuysen, J.A., Gerbrandy, J., de Vries, L.A., de Jong, J.C., Lenstra, J.B., Turner, K.P., Borst, J.G.G.: A licorice extract with deoxycortone-like action. Lancet II, 381 (1950)

Nabata, H., Saito, H., Takagi, K.: Pharmacological studies of neutral saponins (GNS) of *Panax ginseng* root. Japan J. Pharmacol. 23, 29 (1973)

Nagai, Y., Tanaka, O., Shibata, S.: Chemical studies on the oriental plant drugs. XXIV. Structure of ginsenoside R_{g-1}, a new saponin of Ginseng root. Tetrahedron 27, 881 (1971)

Otsuka, A., Yamasaki, K., Inoue, O., Ogihara, Y., Shibata, S.: unpublished data (1976)

Ottenjann, R., Rösch, W.: Therapie des Ulcus ventriculi mit Carbenoxolon-Natrium. Ergebnisse eines Doppelblindversuchs. Med. Klin. 65, 74 (1970)

Oura, H., Hiai, S., Odaka, Y., Yokozawa, T.: Studies on the biochemical action of Ginseng saponin. I. Purification from Ginseng extract of the active component stimulating serum protein biosynthesis. J. Biochem. 77, 1057 (1975)

Petkov, W.: Pharmaceutical studies of the drug, *Panax ginseng* C.A. Meyer (in German). Arzneim.-Forsch. 9, 305 (1959)

Petkov, W.: The mechanism of action of *Panax ginseng* C.A. Meyer (in German). I. Arzneim.-Forsch. 11, 288 (1961a)

Petkov, W.: Über den Wirkungsmechanismus des *Panax ginseng* C.A. Meyer. II. Zur Frage einer Pharmakologie der Reaktivität. Arzneim.-Forsch. 11, 418 (1961b)

Petkov, W.: *Panax ginseng*, a reactivity regulator (in German). Pharm. Zeit. 113, 1281 (1968) (C.A. 70, 6521n)

Revers, F.E.: Has licorice juice (*Succus liquiritiae*) a healing action on gastric ulcer? Ned. Tijdschr. Gencesk. 90, 135 (1946)

Saito, H., Lee, Y.M., Takagi, K., Shibata, S., Shoji, J., Kondo, N.: Pharmacological studies of *Panacis japonici* Rhizoma. I. Japan J. Pharmacol. 27 (1977) in press

Saito, H., Morita, M., Takagi, K.: Pharmacological studies of *Panax ginseng* leaves. Japan J. Pharmacol. 23, 43 (1973)

Saito, H., Yoshida, Y., Takagi, K.: Effect of *Panax ginseng* root on exhaustive excersise in mica. Japan J. Pharmacol. 24, 119 (1974)

Saitoh, T., Kinoshita, T., Shibata, S.: Flavonols of licorice root. Chem. Pharm. Bull. (Tokyo) 24, 1242 (1976) (Ref. cit. therein)

Sakakibara, K., Shibata, Y., Higashi, T., Sanada, S., Shoji, J.: Effect of ginseng saponins on cholesterol metabolism. I. The level and synthesis of serum and liver cholesterol in rats treated with ginsenosides. Chem. Pharm. Bull. (Tokyo) 23, 1009 (1975)

Sakuma, S., Sugiura, N., Tanemoto, H., Amakawa, H., Shoji, J.: Studies on the constituents of Polygonaceous plants. IV. Isolation and identification of the glycosides of Polygalae Radix (Onji). Abstr. 95th Ann. Mett. Pharm. Soc. Japan, II p. 247 (Nishinomiya, April, 1975)

Sanada, S., Kondo, N., Shoji, J., Tanaka, O., Shibata, S.: Studies on saponins of Ginseng. I. Structures of ginsenoside R_o,R_{b-1},R_{b-2},R_c and R_d. Chem. Pharm. Bull. (Tokyo) 22, 421 (1974a)

Sanada, S., Kondo, N., Shoji, J., Tanaka, O., Shibata, S.: Studies on the saponins of Ginseng. II. Structures of ginsenoside R_e,R_f and R_{g-2}. Chem. Pharm. Bull. (Tokyo) 22, 2407 (1974b)

Shibata, M.: Pharmacological studies on Bupleuri Radix. III. Relationship between pharmacological actions of crude saikosides and clinical effects of Bupleuri Radix. Yakugaku Zasshi (J. Pharm. Soc. Japan) 90, 398 (1970)

Shibata, S., Fujita, M., Itokawa, H., Tanaka, O., Ishii, T.: The structure of panaxadiol, a sapogenin of Ginseng. Tetrahedron Lett. 419 (1962)

Shibata, S., Fujita, M., Itokawa, H., Tanaka, O., Ishii, T.: The structure of panaxadiol, a sapogenin of Ginseng. Chem. Pharm. Bull. (Tokyo) 11, 759 (1963)

Shibata, S., Kitagawa, I., Fujimoto, H.: Chemical studies on oriental plant drugs. XV. On the constituents of *Bupleurum* spp. (2). The structure of saikogenin A. A sapongenin of *Bupleurum falcatum* L. Chem. Pharm. Bull. (Tokyo) 14, 1023 (1966)

Shibata, S.: Some chemical studies on Ginseng. In: Proc. Intern. Ginseng Symposium. Seoul: Korean Office of Monopoly, 1974, pp. 69-76

Shibata, S., Nagai, Y., Tanaka, O., Doi, O.: A sapogenin of seeds of *Zizyphus jujuba* var. *spinosus*. Phytochemistry 9, 677 (1970)

Shibata, Y., Nozaki, T., Higashi, T., Sanada, S., Shoij, J.: Stimulation of serum protein synthesis in ginsenoside treated rat. Chem. Pharm. Bull. (Tokyo) 24, 2818 (1976)

Shimizu, Y., Pelletier, S.W.: Elucidation of the structures of the sapogenins of *Polygala senega* by correlation with medicagenic acid. J. Am. Chem. Soc. 88, 1544 (1966)

Shoji, J., Kawanishi, S., Tsukitani, Y.: Studies on the constituents of Senegae Radix. I. Isolation and qualitative analysis of the glycosides. Yakugaku Zasshi (J. Pharm. Soc. Japan) 91, 198 (1971)

Tada, A., Kaneiwa, Y., Shoji, J., Shibata, S.: Studies on the saponins of the root of *Platycodon grandiflorum* A.DC. I. Isolation and the structure of platycodin D. Chem. Pharm. Bull. (Tokyo) 23, 2965 (1975)
Takagi, K.: Pharmacological studies on Ginseng. In: Proc. Intern. Ginseng Symposium. Seoul: Korean Office of Monopoly, 1974, pp. 119-127
Takagi, K., Ishii, Y.: Peptic ulcer inhibiting properties of a new fraction from licorice root (FM 100). I. Experimental peptic ulcer and general pharmacology. Arzneim.-Forsch. 17, 1544 (1967)
Takagi, K., Lee, E.B.: Pharmacological studies on *Platycodon grandiflorum* A.DC. I. Acute toxicity and central depressant activity of crude platycodin. Yakugaku Zasshi (J. Pharm. Soc. Japan) 92, 951 (1972a)
Takagi, K., Lee, E.B.: Pharmacological studies on *Platycodon grandiflorum* A.DC. II. Antiinflammatory activity of crude platycodin. Its activities on isolated organs and other pharmacological activities. Yakugaku Zasshi (J. Pharm. Soc. Japan) 92, 961 (1972b)
Takagi, K., Okabe, S., Saziki, R.: A new method for the production of chronic gastric ulcer in rats and the effect of several drugs on its healing. Japan J. Pharmacol. 19, 418 (1969)
Takagi, K., Saito, H., Nabata, H.: Pharmacological studies of *Panax ginseng* root. Japan J. Pharmacol. 22, 245 (1972a)
Takagi, K., Saito, H., Tsuchiya, M.: Pharmacological studies of *Panax ginseng* root. Pharmacological properties of a crude saponin fraction. Japan. J. Pharmacol. 22, 339 (1972b)
Takagi, K., Saito, H., Tsuchiya, M.: Effect of *Panax ginseng* on continuous movement and exercize in mice. Japan J. Pharmacol. 24, 41 (1974)
Takagi, K., Shibata, M.: Pharmacological studies on Bupleuri Radix. I. Toxicity and CNS-suppressing action of crude saikosides. Yakugaku Zasshi (J. Pharm. Soc. Japan) 89, 712 (1965)
Takagi, K., Shibata, M.: Pharmacological studies on Bupleuri Radix. II. Antiinflammatory action and some other pharmacological activities of crude saikosides. Yakugaku Zasshi (J. Pharm. Soc. Japan) 89, 1367 (1969)
Tschesche, R.: Advances in the chemistry of antibiotic substances from higher plants. In: Pharmacognosy and Phytochemistry. Wagner, H., Hörhammer, L. (eds.). Berlin-Heidelberg-New York: Springer 1971, pp. 274
Tschesche, R., Wulff, G.: Über die antimikrobielle Wirksamkeit von Saponinen. Z. Naturforsch. 20b, 543 (1965)
Tschesche, R., Wulff, G.: Chemie und Biologie der Saponine. In: Fortschr. d. Chemie d. organ. Naturstoffe. Herz, W., Griesenbach, H., Kirby, G.W. (eds.). Vienna-New York: Springer, 1973, pp. 462-606
Tsukitani, Y., Kawanishi, S., Shoji, J.: Studies on the constituents of Senagae Radix II. The structure of senegin. II. A saponin from *Polygala senega* L. var. *latifolia* Torry et Gray. Chem. Pharm. Bull. (Tokyo) 21, 791 (1973)
Tsukitani, Y., Shoji, J.: Studies on the constituents of Senegae Radix. III. The structure of senegenin III and IV. Saponins from *Polygala senega* var. *latifolia* Torry et Gray. Chem. Pharm. Bull. (Tokyo) 21, 1564 (1973)
Watanabe, I., Saito, H., Takagi, K.: Pharmacological studies of Zizypus seeds. Japan J. Pharm. 23, 563 (1973)
Wulff, G., Tschesche, R.: Über Triterpene. XXVI. Über die Struktur der Rosskastaniensaponine und die Aglykone verwandter Glykoside. Tetrahedron 25, 415 (1969)
Yamamoto, M.: Biochemistry of *Panax ginseng*. Biochemical effect on bone marrow, testes and cancer cells. Metabolism 10, 581 (Nakayamashoten, Tokyo (1973)) (in (Japanese)
Yamamoto, M., Takeuchi, N., Kotani, S., Kumagai, A.: Effects of glycryyrhizin and cortisone on cholesterol metabolism in the rat. Endocrinol. Japon. 17, 339 (1970b)
Yamamoto, M., Yamamura, Y., Kumagai, A.: Antiinflammatory and metabolic actions of saikosaponins a, c and d. Rep. Sympl. Japan. Chinese Drugs. 4. 41 (1970a) (Toyama University)
Yosioka, I., Fujio, M., Osamura, M., Kitagawa, I.: A novel cleavage method of saponin with soil bacteria intending to the genuine sapogenin: On Senega and Panax saponins. Tetrahedron Lett. 1966, 6303

Dimeric Natural Compounds with Pharmacological Activity

A. E. SCHWARTING

A. Definitions and Classification

The term "dimer" is from the Greek *dimeres*, meaning "of two parts." In chemical terms, a dimer is a compound representing a covalently bonded pair of like molecules. In the strictest sense the two moieties are identical, the compound is produced without loss of atoms, and it is bonded through "equivalent" carbon atoms. Such compounds do exist; nordihydroguairetic acid (Formula 1), for example, must originate

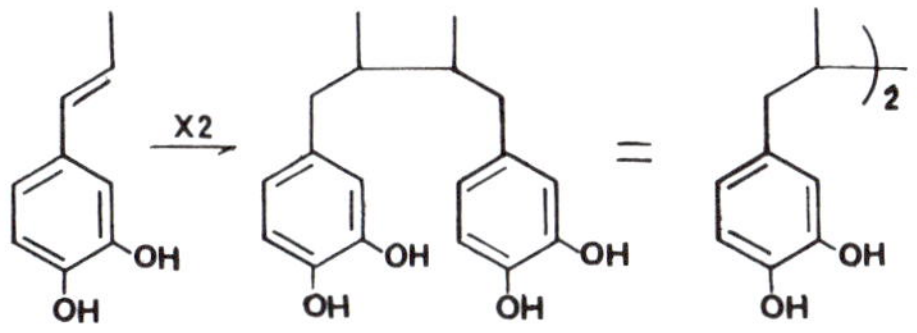

Formula 1

from two identical cinnamyl precursors, is bonded through "equivalent" carbon atoms, and the dimer is at the same oxidation level as the precursor. In a less restrictive definition a dimer may be (a) a compound of two similar, rather than identical parts, as in bixin (Formula 2) or (b) a compound bonded through dissimilar carbon atoms, as in diosyprin (Formula 3), or (3) a compound produced with loss of protons of the progenitor(s) as in both Formulas 2 and 3 as well as in

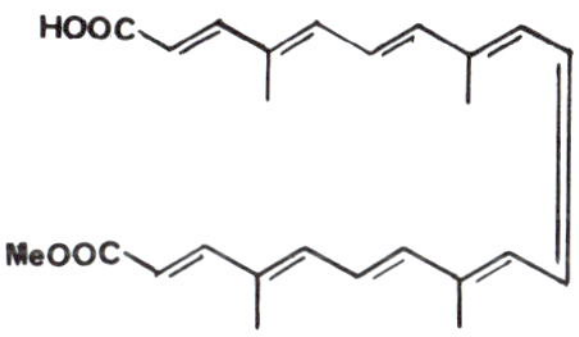

Formula 2

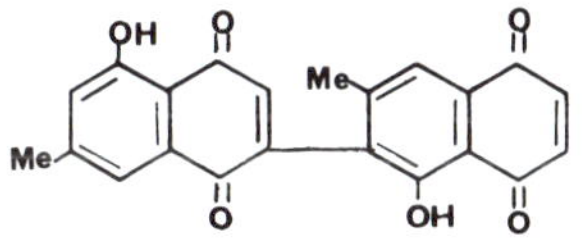

Formula 3

the biphenyl compound, ellagic acid (Formula 4) and in the ether, libocedrol (Formula 5) and the acetal, maltose (Formula 6). A single co-

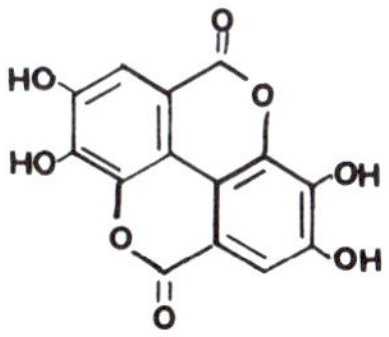

Formula 4

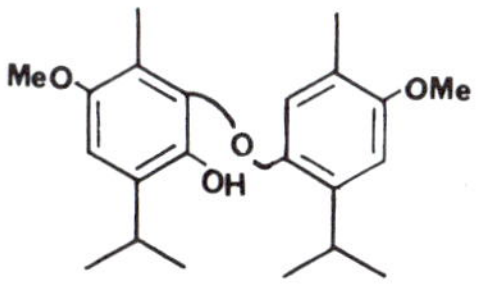

Formula 5

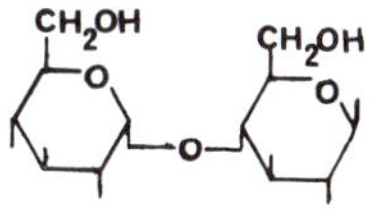

Formula 6

valent bond between the components is typical of many dimers, but additional bonds arise as in hypericin (Formula 7), elsinochrome A (Formula 8) and in duclauxin (Formula 9). But not all of these dimers are

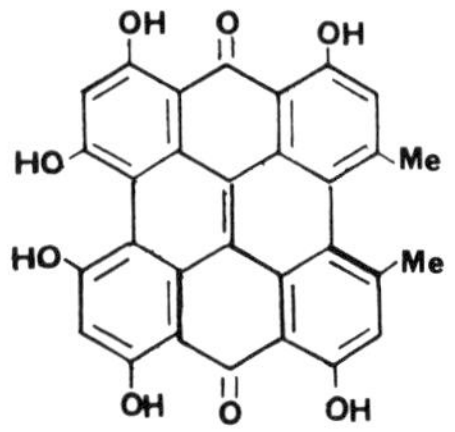

Formula 7

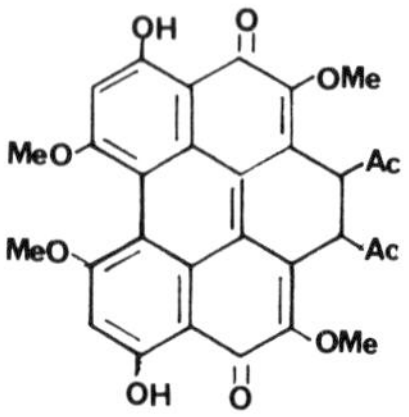

Formula 8

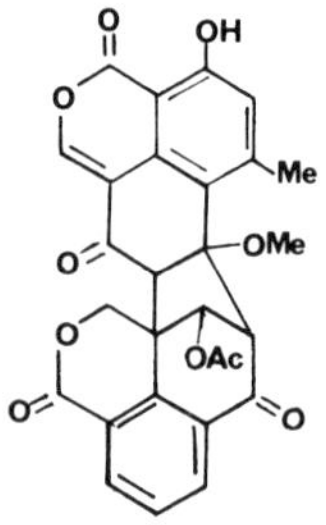

Formula 9

ordinarily double- or triple-bonded; sennoside A (Formula 10) is an example of a bisanthraquinone in which the monomer units are united through a single bond. Finally, not all uniting bonds are C-C; cubebin (Formula 11) possesses both C-C and C-O-C bonds. A bisquinolizidine

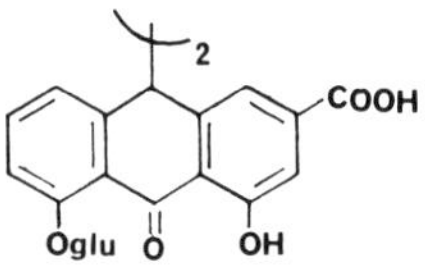

Formula 10

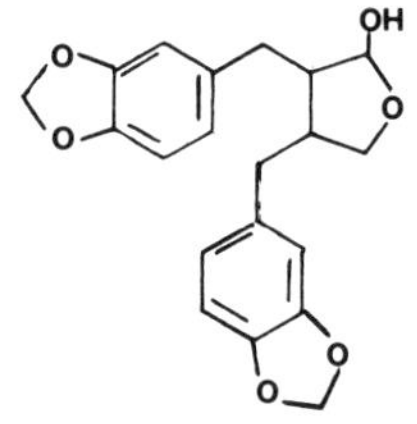

Formula 11

alkaloid (see Formula 40) is a single example of a dimeric molecule containing a sulfur bridge, uniting the monomer units, and C-toxiferine I (see Formula 35) exemplifies a group of dimeric alkaloids where a pair of carbon bridges unite nitrogen and carbon elements of the monomer units.

Among the preceding examples only Formula 1 is a "true" dimer. The others, Formulas 2 to 11, and among the known natural compounds, the majority are not "perfect" according to the criteria established for dimers. These, and other molecules like them, must be labeled as dimeric compounds. The terms "dimer" and "dimeric compound" are used in this context throughout this manuscript.

Formulas 1 to 11 provide a preliminary view of different nonnitrogenous dimers and dimeric compounds. These different structures, are representatives of types or classes of compounds, as follows: *lignans* (Formulas 1, 11), *carotenoid* (Formula 2), *binaphythyls* (Formula 3, 8), *biphenyl* (Formula 4), *bismonoterpene* (Formula 5), *disaccharide* (Formula 6), *bisanthraquinones* (Formulas 7, 10), and *biphenalenone* (Formula 9).

Other natural nonnitrogenous dimeric compounds include the following classes with individual examples in each case. The dimeric flavonoids are found linked at a number of positions in the ring system of the monomeric units. In the *biflavonoids* (Formula 12) the C-C bonds are at 6-4, 8-3, 8-3', 8-4, 8-6 and 8-8. *Bixanthyl* compounds are represented by secalonic acid A (Formula 13). Gossypol (Formula 14) is an example of the *disesquiterpene* type and microlenin (Formula 15) is a *disesquiterpene-lactone* type. The *terphenyl* type is represented by atromentin (Formula 16), a class which may be regarded as a type of lignan. Dicoumarol (3,3'-methylenebis[4-hydroxy-coumarin]) (Formula 17) is a dimeric compound in which the monomer components are united through a methylene bridge. This *biscoumarin* is not, however, a "normal" metabolite. It arises in "spoiled" sweet clover hay; the carbon of the methylene bridge is derived from "atmospheric" formaldehyde. But other biscoumarins occur without the "extra" carbon, bicoumol (Formula 18), candicanin (Formula 19) and thamnosin (Formula 20) are examples of

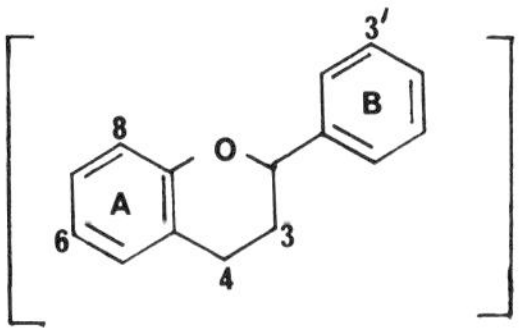

Formula 12

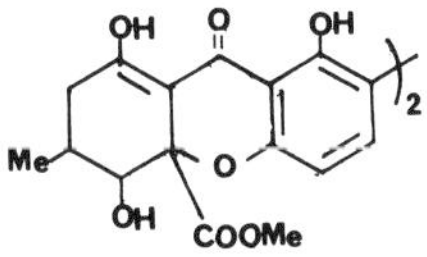

Formula 13

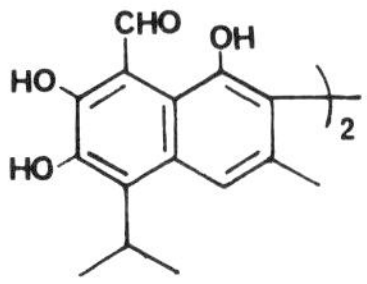

Formula 14

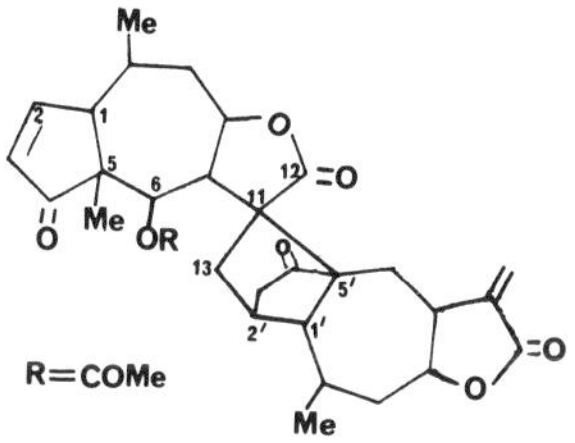

Formula 15

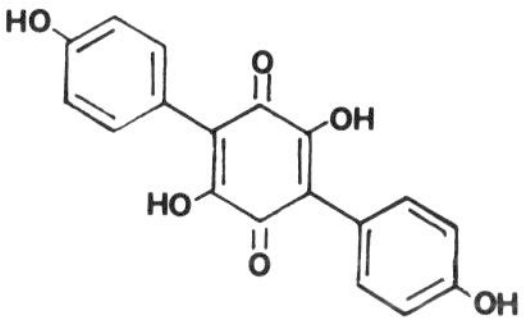

Formula 16

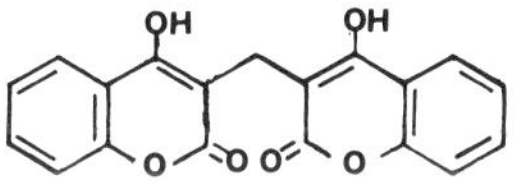

Formula 17

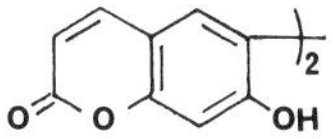

Formula 18

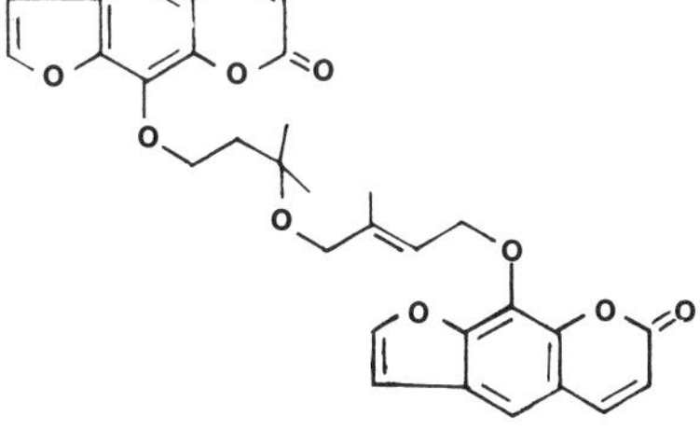

Formula 19

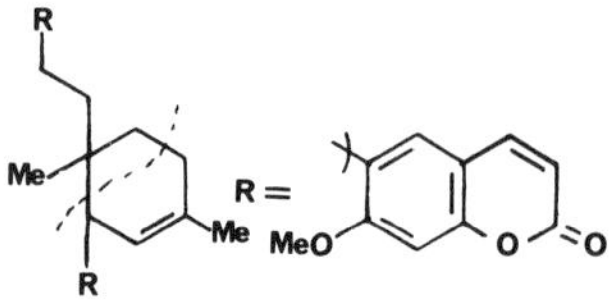

Formula 20

this small but diverse group. Anemonin (Formula 21), a 2-carbon bridged *bisfurane*, is a representative of a small group of naturally,occurring dimeric furans and pyrones. The 1-carbon bridge of Formula 17 and the 2-carbon bridge of Formula 21 are not especially unique among dimeric compounds. The *benzophenones* (Formula 22), *stilbenes* (Formula 23), and *rotenoids* (Formula 24) are ostensibly dimeric compounds, showing 1- or

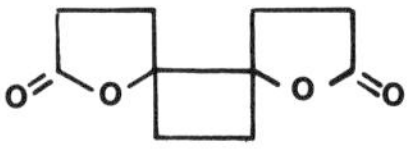

Formula 21

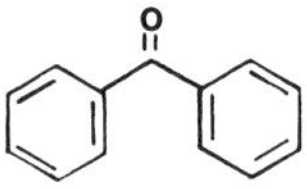

Formula 22

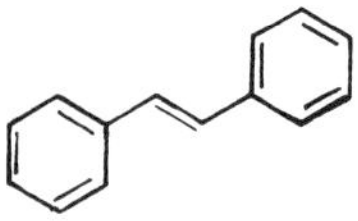

Formula 23

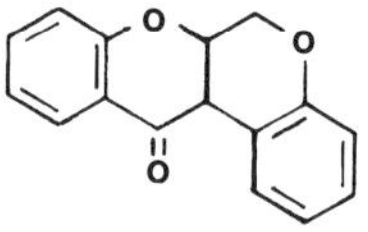

Formula 24

2-carbon "connectors" of aromatic rings. These compounds, however, like the monomeric flavonoids (see Formula 12) are shikimate/acetate derived molecules and are not truly dimeric. In Formula 22 to 24, one ring originates via the shikimate pathway and the other is of acetate origin via a polyketide precursor. The union of the two parts is thus of a C-6/C-3 (see also Formula 12, ring B), or of a C-6/C-2, or a C-6/C-1 unit of shikimate origin, and of another aromatic unit which originates from acetate. The carbon bridge of α-kosin (Formula 25) and related *methylenebisphloroglucinols*, like the bridge of the *methylene-biscoumarins*, is an "extra" carbon, originating in this case, however, from methionine. Coupling of a *methylphloracetophenone* pair, however, produces a different *biphloroglucinol*, for example, usnic acid (Formula 26). In this type of compound the two halves are joined, without a

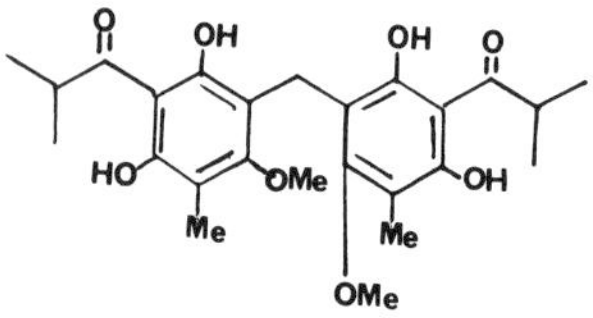

Formula 25

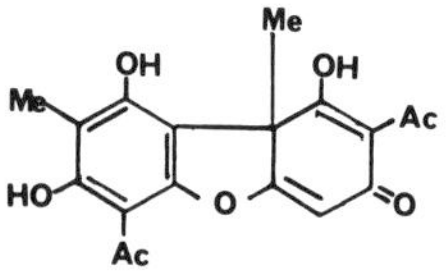

Formula 26

bridge, by a covalent bond. This "family" also includes the *bisbenzo-quinones*, like oosporein (Formula 27). Several other natural dimeric benzoquinones are linked through a bridge of two or more carbon atoms.

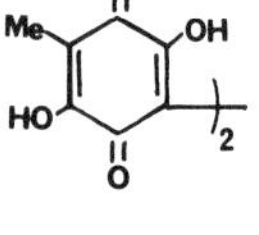

Formula 27

In the above presentation, a consideration of biogenesis, as well as of molecular structure, has been applied in establishing the dimeric nature of some compounds. In some cases it is quite necessary that both characteristics be considered in establishing the dimeric or nondimeric nature of individuals as well as classes of compounds. Evidence for the need for such consideration is clearly shown in determining the nature of ellagic acid (Formula 4) and of alternariol (Formula 28). Both are clearly biphenyl compounds but only Formula 4 is truly dimeric; Formula 28 arises from a polyketide chain, whereas Formula 4 arises by the bonding of two aromatic nuclei of shikimate origin.

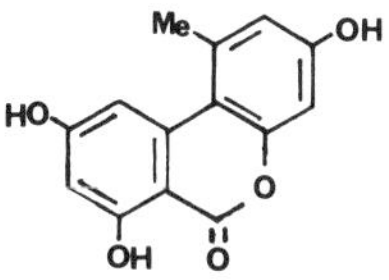

Formula 28

Finally, in any consideration of dimerization one must deal with other questions of structure and biogenesis. The structures of cantharidin (Formula 29) and of cannabinol (Formula 30) illustrate other parameters relating to the dimerization phenomenon. Cantharidin may be viewed as a dimer of an isoprenoid precursor - but so also are a whole group of linear and cyclic terpenoids. The dissimilarity, both structurally as well as biogenetically, of the bonded units of cannabinol - a p-menthane and an orcinol derivative - precludes the classification of such a molecule as dimeric.

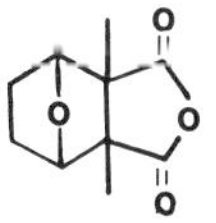

Formula 29

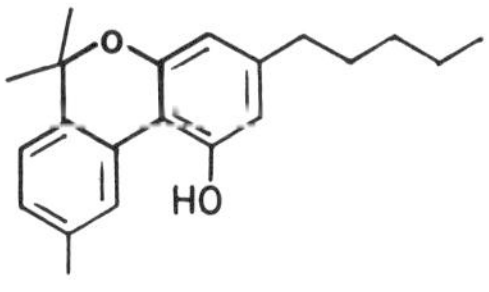

Formula 30

The number of classes of natural compounds of carbon and of carbon and oxygen, which include dimeric molecules, is thus relatively small. Moreover, the number of dimeric compounds within each of these classes is also relatively small. Among the compounds of nitrogen, several classes of alkaloids include dimeric representatives. One of these classes, the *bisbenzylisoquinolines* is the largest group of known alkaloids. This large group is divided (1) into 21 subgroups on the basis of aromatic substituents and on the position and nature of the uniting bond(s). Two of these subgroups include proven or potentially useful pharmacological agents. Tubocurarine (Formula 31) of the *curine-chondocurine* subgroup and (+)-cepharanthine (Formula 32) of the *oxycanthine* subgroup are noteworthy examples. Thalicarpine (Formula 33) is an *aporphinebenzylisoquinoline* dimer and vincaleucoblastine (Formula 34) is a dimer of the *indolic* group. C-Toxiferine (Formula 35) is one of the potent dimeric indole alkaloid isolated from Calabash curare. This structure is a typical representative of a group of bases structurally related to the Wieland-Gumlich aldehyde. Presecamine (Formula 36) also is an indolic dimer of the *presecamine* group, but the molecule also embodies a pair of piperidine analogs. Carpaine (Formula 37) is a unique dimeric *piperidine* alkaloid and 2,3'-bipyridyl (Formula 38) is a natural dimeric *pyridine* base, and each of these are known to occur in single species.

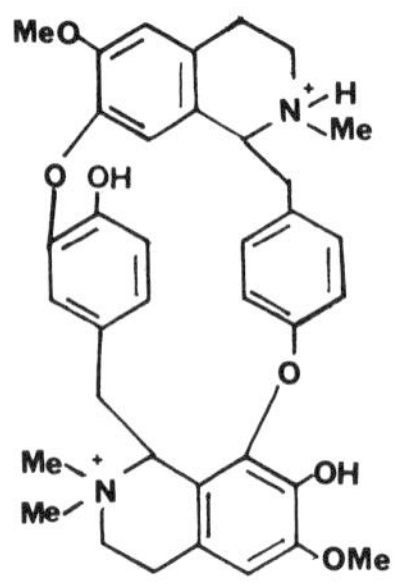

Formula 31

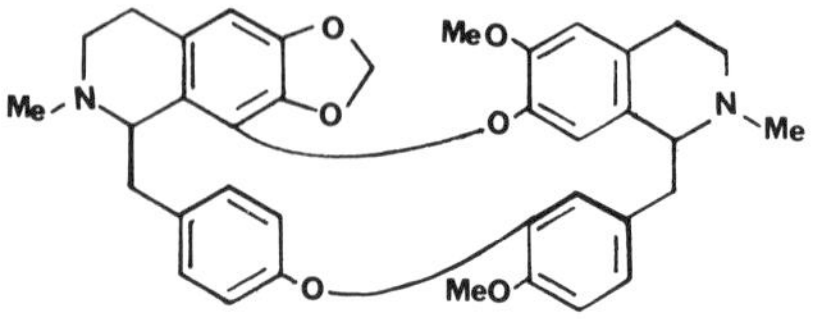

Formula 32

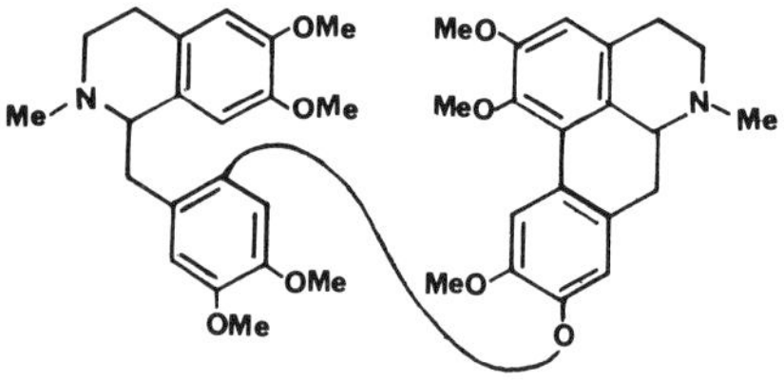

Formula 33

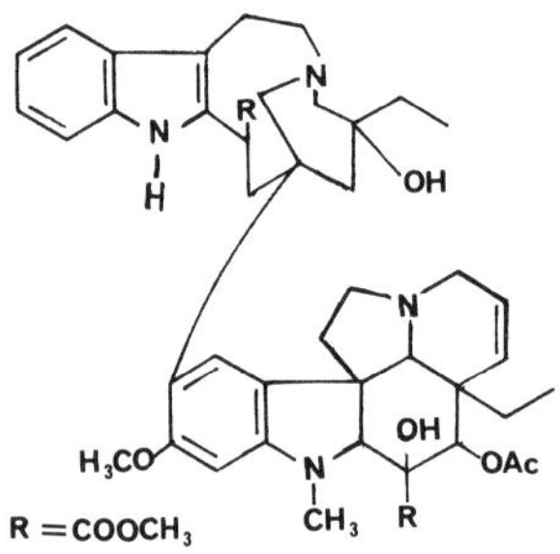

Formula 34

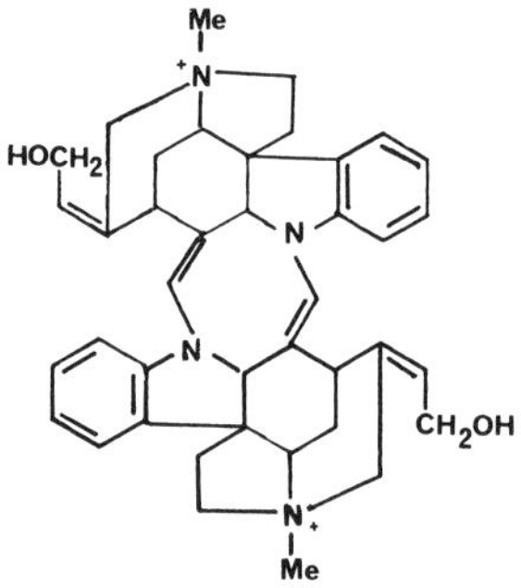

Formula 35

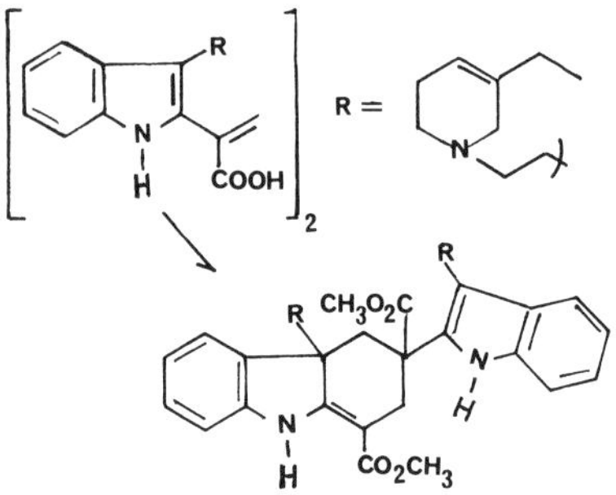

Formula 36

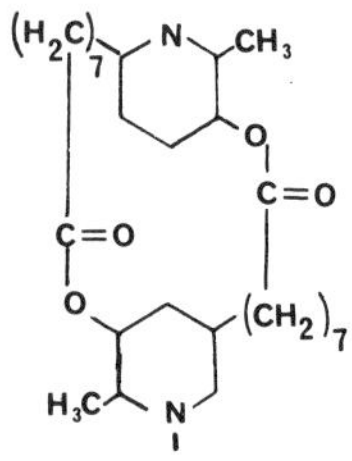

Formula 37

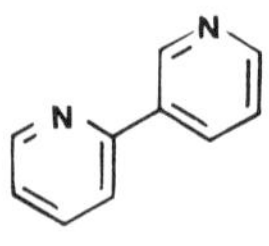

Formula 38

The *biacridone* alkaloid ataline (Formula 39) is an example of the only known dimer in a large class of alkaloids. The position of the ether link was not established with certainty but it is biogenetically reasonable. 6,6'-Dihydroxythiobinupharidine (Formula 40) is uniquely different from the majority of dimeric compounds. Its sulfur bridge is one of the two bond structures which join the monomer units. Finally, among the amines, the *spermine* derived base, homaline (Formula 41) is an apparent dimer in which the base units are joined by a 4-carbon bridge.

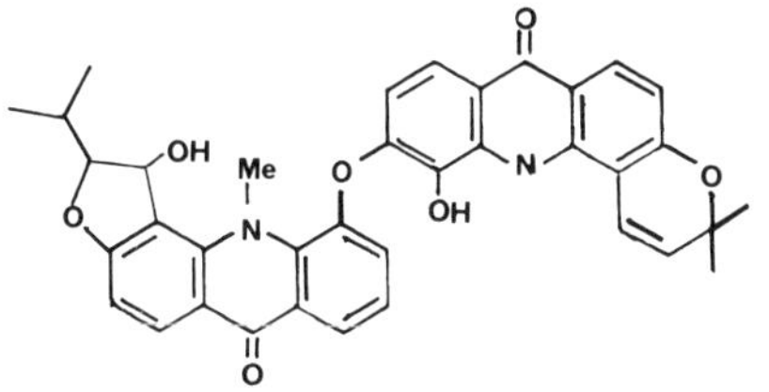

Formula 39

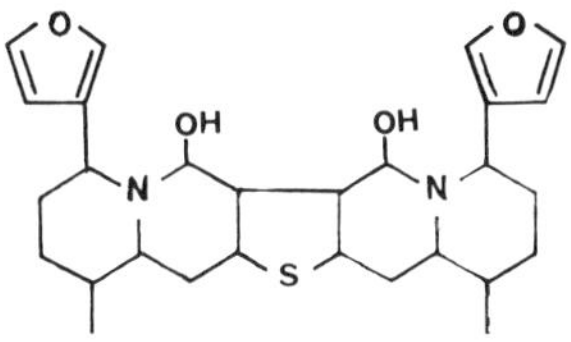

Formula 40

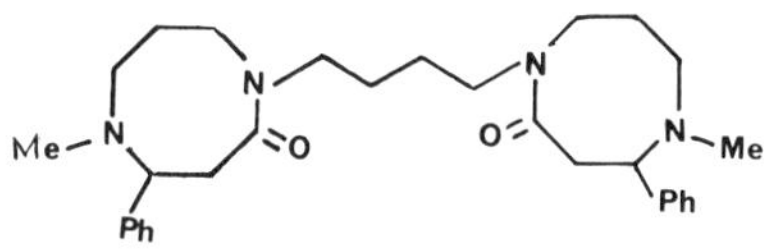

Formula 41

Like the carbocyclic and oxygen heterocyclic compounds, the alkaloids include a number of compounds whose apparent dimeric nature must be viewed from both structural and a biogenetic characteristics. Cuscohygrine (Formula 42) and anaferine (Formula 43) probably originate from two ring units, one of which, in its intermediate development, bears the 3-carbon substituent which ultimately separates the pyrrolidine and piperidine rings. The final bond formation, creating the molecule, is between two dissimilar moieties. Anabasine (Formula 44) likewise is generated from two moieties of dissimilar biosynthetic paths. Finally, in this regard, the monomeric units of the benzylisoquinoline alkaloids (see Formulas 31 to 33), even though they originate from a pair of phenylalanine-derived units, are not truly dimeric; one of the monomer units undergoes nitrogen loss in the biosynthetic sequence.

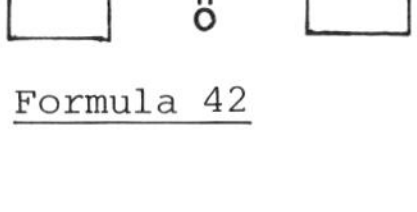

Formula 42

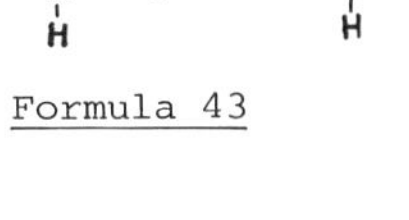

Formula 43

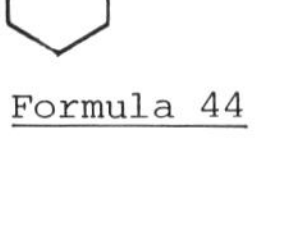

Formula 44

B. The Formation of Dimeric Compounds

The formation of a large number of dimeric compounds may be explained in terms of oxidative coupling of two phenolic units. Loss of a proton from a phenol or removal of an electron from a phenolate anion would produce the radical which would, in turn, give rise to a stable molecule, by intermolecular coupling. In Formula 45, the abstraction of an electron from the phenol at the left yields the radicals shown to the right. This "family" of phenylpropenoid radicals would provide all of the monomeric units necessary to form the known C-C and C-O-C, oxidatively produced, bonds of the lignans. These samples, extended to other phenolic molecules, would explain the basis for their dimerization.

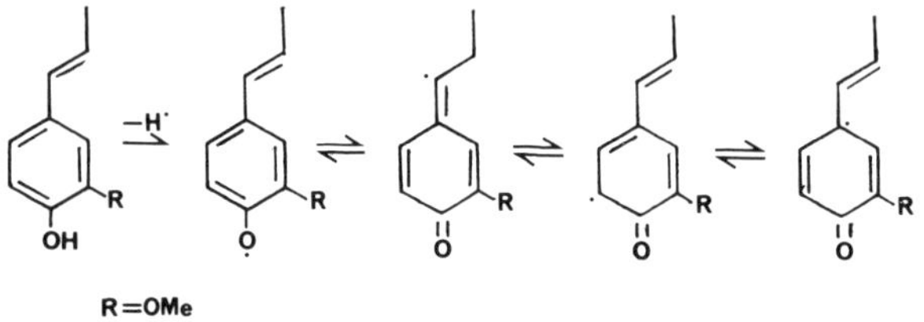

Formula 45

A small number of dimeric compounds appear to arise via a Diels-Alder type reaction - an addition reaction of a four-π, with a two-π electron system. In thamnosin (Formula 46) an origin may be viewed as occuring

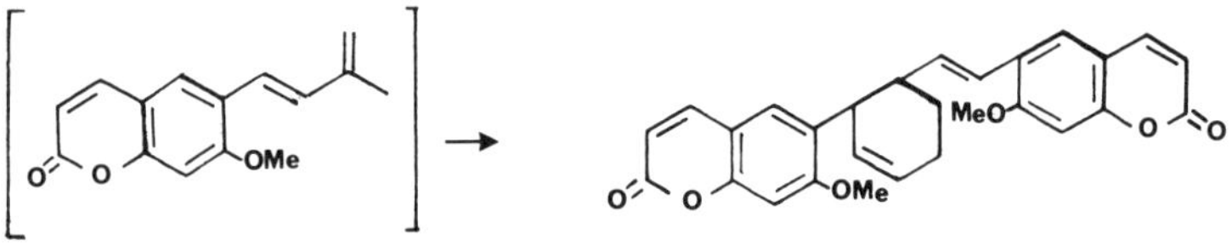

Formula 46

via such a cycloaddition reaction of the diene shown in brackets in the scheme. In microlenin (Formula 15) the condensation would require a 11, 13-double bond in the precursor and the enol form of the cyclopentanone ring would be necessary. Helenalin, a monomeric sesquiterpene, occurs with microlenin in a *Helenium* sp. and it possesses the required methylene carbon. It is not impossible that compounds such as thamnosin and microlenin are artifacts generated in extraction-purification procedures.

A biomimetic approach to the coupling of indole and dihydroindole alkaloids (2) portrays another possible biosynthetic route, in this case, for the biosynthesis of the bisindole alkaloid vincaleucoblastine. A fragmentation of the N-oxide system of the cartharanthine monomer generates the required intermediate for the electrophilic attack of vindoline, to provide the bisindole product (Formula 47) shown in the scheme (see also Formula 34).

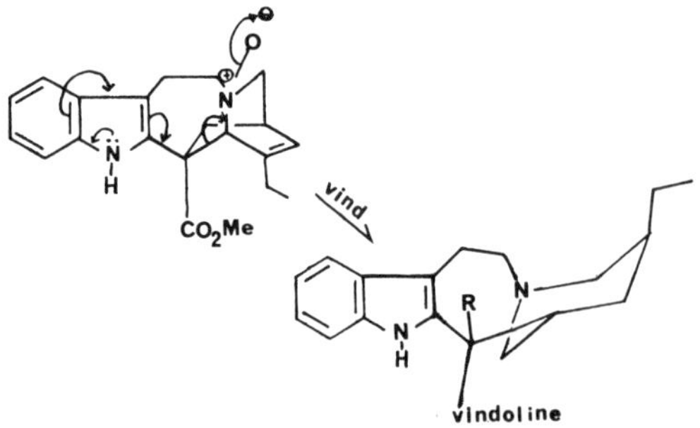

Formula 47

The monomer precursor to the dimeric indole bases such as C-toxiferine I (Formula 35) is structurally related to the Wieland-Gumlich aldehyde (the carbonyl functions are the methylene bridge carbons of Formula 35). The dimerization process is evidently a Schiff-base condensation.

C. Pharmacological and Physiological Activity

Differences, qualitatively or quantitatively, in the physiological and pharmacological activity, or in the relative toxicity, of monomeric and dimeric compounds have been recorded for a small number of such pairs. Dimeric compounds, quite regularly, exceed the potency or possess therapeutic values which are superior to those of their monomeric counterparts. But this dogma may not be stated unequivocally; broad generalizations about structure-activity relationships may not be made. Moreover, a substantial number of the known dimeric compounds and their monomeric progenitors have not been studied for their specific or relative activity, and many studies are very preliminary in nature or are incomplete.

A view of contrasts in activity in this group may be seen in the following examples. Antitumor activity resides in certain dimeric indole and in several aporphine-benzylisoquinoline alkaloids and is not present, or weakly so, in the monomeric counterparts. On the other hand, both monomeric and dimeric sesquiterpene lactones show promising antitumor activity in test systems. The provitamin A substances are a group of structurally related C_{40} polyenes derived from aliphatic hydrocarbon monomeric units; neither the monomer nor the dimer possesses vitamin activity. But in vivo conversion of the dimer by "central" fission - a retro dimerization process - and oxidation produces a "monomeric" derivative which is active (see Formula 48; β-carotene → vitamin A_1).

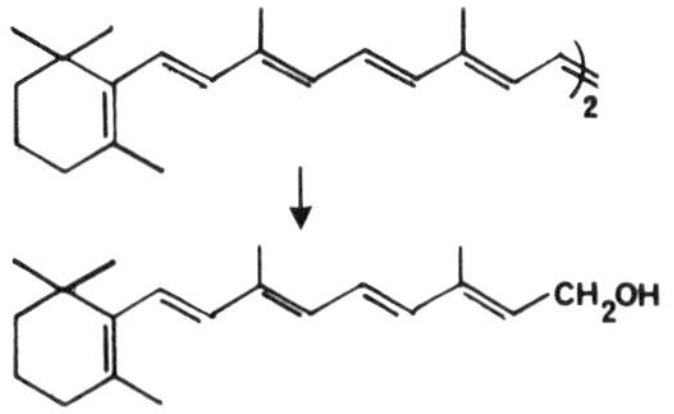

Formula 48

In general, one would expect a loss in hydrophilic character with dimerization and subtle changes in dissociation constants have been noted in dimeric-monomeric pairs. But neither of these changes may be viewed as contributing appreciably to changes in biological transport sufficient to cause a two-fold, or as in some cases a multitudinous, increase in activity resulting from dimerization.

In the investigations of antineoplastic activity it is thought that some planar polycyclic drugs are firmly bound to DNA in a process called intercalation. In this event the drug molecule becomes inserted between adjacent pairs in the DNA helix. An interpretation of the antitumor activity of dimeric proanthocyanidins (see Formula 12) has been proposed (3). It is also possible, however, that the polyhydroxy composition of the flavonoid/catechin group may be responsible for a weaker ionic reaction with the DNA molecule.

Nonplanar dimeric molecules offer greater associations and relationships of their functional groups simply by virtue of the increased numbers of groups over their monomeric counterparts. Molecular models (4) have revealed that there is a common atomic arrangement in the structures of a number of antileukemic drugs. Three electronegative atoms, containing at least one lone pair of electrons, form a triangle whose dimensions are illustrated in Formula 49. The N-O-O triangular pattern is the dotted line in the structure presentation of vincaleucoblastine. It is to be especially noted that the nitrogen atom of one monomeric unit and that the two oxygen atoms of the other monomeric unit are implicated. The triangular structure may be involved in receptor site binding on certain vital cellular biopolymers or be a basis of transport control.

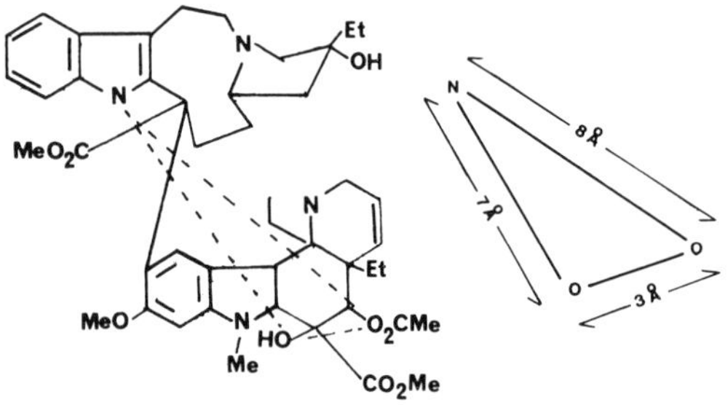

Formula 49

Historically, the first attempts to establish structure-activity relationships of drugs were made with curaremimetic drugs and d-tubocurarine became the model for intense study. The bis-nitrogen structure, and particularly the bisquarternary ammonium structure, of the curare alkaloids and their derivatives appeared to be a major factor contributing to curaremimetic potency. The inter-nitrogen distance, 12.5Å, became a template for synthetic approaches, but this feature in other curaremimetic molecules is not essential.

Examples of the physiological or pharmacological activity of a number of dimeric compounds are presented in Table 1. This presentation excludes the lignans, coumarins and the photosensitizing dianthrones, and related compounds. These compounds will be given more detailed consideration in the concluding section of this manuscript since the detail about their activities is greater and more complete. While this attention could also have been given the dimeric indole alkaloids, the fact that they are being given attention in other papers of this symposium suggested abbreviated attention in this presentation.

I. Lignans

The cytotoxic lignans include three natural compounds and a variety of synthetic analogs. A summation of test system studies on podophyllotoxin, burseran and deoxypodophyllotoxin is presented in Table 2. Podophyllotoxin (Formula 50) and its cogeners have long been used in the treatment of veneral warts (condylomata acuminata) and also against plantar warts. Its cytotoxicity in this regard was the basis for extensive testing in tumor systems. A revival of interest in this group is again manifest. The activity represents studies directed towards more fundamental inquiry into the site and mechanism of action. Both podophyllotoxin and 4'-dimethylepipodophyllotoxin-β-O-glucoside inhibit cellular uptake of thymidine and uridine by inhibiting the

Table 1. Examples of physiologically active dimeric compounds

Compounds class and individual	Physiological and/or pharmacological activity Physiological and/or	Remarks
Bisanthraquinone		
Sennoside A	Cathartic	Both monomeric and dimeric compounds are active. Preparations are mixtures
Bisbenzyl		
Ellagic Acid	Cytotoxic	Inhibits in sarcoma test systems (a characteristic activity of tannins)
Bisbenzylisoquinoline		
(+)-Cepharanthine	Antimicrobial (5)	Effective in vitro against human tuberculosis and leprosy
(+)-Tubocurarine	Neuromuscular blocking	Blocks transmission of nerve impulses at the myoneural junction
(+)-Thalicarpine	Cytotoxic (6)	In Phase II clinical studies as an oncolytic agent
Biflavanoid/bicatechin		
Procyanidin compounds	Cytotoxic (7)	Compounds isolated from *Ouratea* and *Persea* spp. are effective in sarcoma test systems
Procyanidin isomers	Positive inotropic (8)	Extracts of the leaves and fruits of *Crataegus oxycantha* dilate the coronary artery in pharmacological test systems. Preparations are devoid of monomeric compounds
Dimeric procyanidin-flavanoid mixture	Cardiovascular (9)	A standardized extract of the leaves *Ginkgo biloba* (Tebonin® is used in cardiovascular disorders
Bisindole		
Vincaleucoblastine	Cytotoxic	Therapeutic agent via mitotic blockade
C-Toxiferine I	Muscular relaxant	In clinical use
Bispiperidine		
Carpaine	Digitalis-like and amebicidal	In need of further study
Bispyridyl		
2,3-Bipyridyl	Nicotine-like (10)	Isolated from a phylum of carniverous marine worms
Bisquinolizidine		
6,6'-Dihydroxythiobinupharadine	Fungicidal (11)	In vitro activity against *Histoplasma*, *Microsporum*, and *Trichophyton* spp.

Table 1. (Continued)

Bisesquiterpene		
Gossypol	Antiviral and cytotoxic (12)	Effective in herpes simplex and in lymphocytic leukemia test system
Microlenin	Cytotoxic (13)	Effective in Walker 256 test system

Table 2. Cytotoxic lignans[a]

Compound	Tumor system[b]	Dose range tested (mg/kg)	Response (mg/kg)			Evaluation	
			MTD[c]	MED[d]	TWI (%)[e]	ILS (%)[f]	ED_{50}[g]
Podophyllo-toxin	SA	0.175-15	∿ 0.50	-	29	-	-
	CA	0.13-1.1	∿ 1.1	-	24	-	-
	LL	1-4	∿ 2	2	64	-	-
	LE	0.14-2.70	∿ 1.62	-	-	20	-
	FV	0.135-1.1	0.55	-	17	-	-
	MM	1-10	∿ 2.7	-	33	-	-
	PI	1.85-3.70	∿ 3.70	-	15	-	-
	HI	0.0012-5	∿ 0.0048	-	1	-	-
	LZ	5-180	23	-	-	9	-
	PS	1-16	∿ 10	∿ 2	-	71	-
	8P	0.9-4	∿ 2.2	-	20	-	-
	WM	0.9-13	∿ 6	6	73	-	-
	KB	-	-	-	-	-	0.01
Burseran	WM	11-67	67	-	12	-	0.026
Deoxypodo-phyllotoxin	SA	4-75	4	-	0	-	-
	LL	5.15	∿ 5	-	10	-	-
	LE	6.25-400	200	∿ 100[h]	-	27	-
	PS	1.5-80	∿ 10	5	-	48[i]	-
	WM	2.5-160	20	-	41	-	-
	KB	-	-	-	-	-	0.0012

[a]Taken from Hartwell, J.L. and Abbott, B.J.: Adv. Pharmacol. Chemotherapy, Vol. VII. Academic Press, New York, 1969, pp. 117-211. [b]CA: Adenocarcinoma 755. Mouse; FV: Friend virus leukemia. Mouse; H1: HS1 human sarcoma; KB: Human epidermoid carcinoma of the nasopharynx. Cell culture; LE: Leukemia L-1210. Mouse (intraperitoneal); LL: Lewis lung carcinoma. Mouse; LZ: Leukemia L-1210. Mouse (subcutaneous). Delayed treatment; MM: Melanotic melanoma. Hamster; PI: Plasmacytoma No. 1. Hamster; 8P: P-1798 lymphosarcoma. Mouse; PS: P-388 lymphocytic leukemia. Mouse; SA: Sarcoma 180. Mouse; WM: Walker carcinosarcoma 256. Rat (intramuscular). [c]MTD: Maximum tolerated dose at approximately the LD_{10}. [d]MED: Minimum effective dose. [e]TWI: Tumor weight inhibition. [f]ILS: Increase in life span. [g]ED_{50}: Dose level in µg/ml at which 50 % inhibition of growth of cells (in vitro) is noted vs. untreated controls. [h]Single injection procedure; inactive in chronic test. [i]Results not reproducible

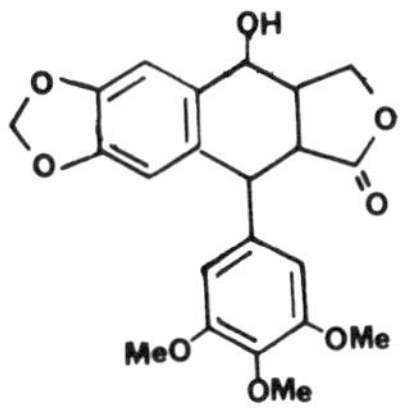

Formula 50

facilitated diffusional component of nucleoside transport. The former prevents microtubule formation in vitro and the latter induce single stranded breaks in *Hela* cell DNA.

Podophyllotoxin and the related lignans form the active components of resin of podophyllum (podophyllin), a cathartic of extensive use in proprietary drugs. The structural similarity of podophyllotoxin to phenophthalein should be noted.

Finally, a number of lignans are effective antimicrobial agents and possess antioxidant activity. Nordihydroguaiaretic acid possesses both of these properties. The minimum inhibitory concentration in an agar test system was 10 µg/ml for *Streptococcus*, *Staphylococcus* and *Bacillus* spp. and it is extensively used as an antioxidant in the preservation of lipids, but the bis-structure is not an essential requirement for these activities.

II. Dimeric Photosensitizers

The hypericins, of *Hypericum* spp. the elsinochromes of *Elsinoe* spp., and duclauxin of *Penicillium* spp., are dimeric compounds which sensitize cells of other organisms to wavelengths of light of sunlight. These are photooxidative sensitizers, requiring the presence of oxygen, and they act as an exogenous photosensitizer for colorless cells which are then injured or killed by strong visible light.

The sunlight provoked irritation and endematous eruption sometimes followed by necrosis, in unpigmented areas of skin of range animals, has been long known and is associated with the ingestion of *Hypericum* spp. plants. The etiology of the disease has been followed in white rabbits and the action spectrum corresponds roughly with the absorption spectrum of extracts of a *Hypercium* sp. The effects are mediated in wavelengths longer than 320 nm.

The monomeric units of the hypericins, elsinochromes and duclauxin have not been implicated in photosensitization. Therefore, the nature of the chromophore of the bi-molecule and its absorption spectrum must be related to this unusual activity. But photosensitization is not limited to these natural compounds. Chlorophyll and other porphyrins and the psoralens - of the furanocoumarins - are also exogenous photosensitizers.

III. Coumarins

More is known about the biological activity and the metabolism of the coumarins than any group of monomeric-dimeric compounds. Moreover, it is a large group - more than 1000 compounds have been described. Included in the panorama of activity are such topics as (a) growth effect in plants, (b) toxicity from "chronic" ingestion as a food flavor additive, particularly the hepatic toxicity, (c) carcinogenecity, particularly associated with the aflatoxins, (d) the antibiotic activity, particularly associated with novobiocin, and

(e) the anticoagulant activity. But this is only a small list since some coumarins are diuretic, increase photosensitivity, are molluscocidal, have an anticholerostatic activity, are oestrogenic, hypnotic, antispasmodic, rodenticidal, antiatherosclerotic and are vasodilators.

Among all of these activities the bis-arrangement of the molecule is a structural requirement for effective prolongation of the anticoagulent effect (Table 3) and is the most formidable coumarin structure in

Table 3. Anticoagulant activity of coumarins[a]

Compound	Action (days) Onset	Peak	Duration	Peak plasma prothrombin level %
Coumarin	1	2	5	55
3-OH-Coumarin	—	inactive	—	100
3-MeO- Coumarin	2	3	4	82
4-OH-Coumarin	1	2	5	40
4-OH-7,8-$(MeO)_2$-"	2	4	5	15
Dicoumarol	1	6	12	10
7,8-$(MeO)_2$-"	1	4	5	20

[a]Taken from Arora, R.B., Mathur, C.N.: Brit. J. Pharmacol. 20, 29 (1963)

hypoprothombinemic activity. It is not essential for antagonizing the action of vitamin K. Dicoumarol is viewed as a compound which is readily absorbed, possesses a slow metabolism and its effects are slow after the initial dosage. Other coumarins act more rapidly, are easier to control and are more rapidly excreted, but dicoumarol was and is the prototype molecule.

This essay portrays elements of the chemical and pharmacological characteristics of natural dimeric molecules. A great diversity of structure types and of pharmacological activity is obvious. The basis for dimerization is readily predictable or is understood; the biological processes have served as a model for synthesis in a number of instances. An explanation of the relative pharmacological activity of monomeric and dimeric compounds is not understood in most cases and the observed action of dimers is not predictable. The relatively small group of dimeric compounds, however, include a few important therapeutic agents and clinical developments and understanding about several compounds hold high interest at this time.

References

1. Shamma, M.: The isoquinoline alkaloids: chemistry and pharmacology. New York: Academic Press, 1972, p. 115
2. Kutney, J.P., Hibino, T., Jahngen, E., Okutani, T., Ratcliffe, A.H., Treasurywala, A.M., Wunderly, S.: Total synthesis of indole and dihydroindole alkaloids. IX. Studies on the synthesis of bisindole alkaloids in the vinblastine-vincristine series. The biogenetic approach. Helv. Chim. Acta 59, 2858-2882 (1976)

3. Marini Bettolo, G.B., Delle Monache, F.: Dimeric proanthocyanidins: structure and biological activity. Pontif. Acad. Sci. 2, 1-13 (1972)
4. Zee-Cheng, K.-Y., Cheng, C.C.: Common receptor-complement feature among some antileukemic compounds. J. Pharm. Sci. 59, 1630-1634 (1970)
5. Lewis, A., Shepherd, R.G.: Antimycobacterial agents. In: Medicinal Chemistry 3rd ed. Burger, A. (ed.). New York: Wiley, 1970, p. 409; see also Büchi, J., Schweiz. Apoth. Z. 83, 198 (1945)
6. Kupchan, S.M., Liepa, A.J.: Tumor-inhibiting thalicarpines. Brit. Pat. 1,373, 399 (1974); through Chem. Abstr. 83, 59135
7. DeOliveira, M.M., Sampaio, M.R.P., Simon, F., Gilbert, B., Mors, W.B.: Antitumor activity of condensed flavanols. Ann. Acad. Bras. Cienc. 44, 41-44 (1972)
8. Rewerski, W., Lewak, S.: Einige pharmakologische Eigenschaften der aus Weisdorn (*Crataegus oxyacantha*) isolierten Flavan-Polymeren. Arzneim.-Forsch. 17, 490-491 (1967); and Rewerski, W., Piechocki, T., Rylski, M., Lewak, S.: Einige pharmakologische Eigenschaften der aus Weisdorn (*Crataegus oxyacantha*) isolierten oligomeren Procyanidine. Arzneim.-Forsch. 6, 886-887 (1971)
9. Hemmer, R., Tzavellas, O.: Cerebral activity of an herbal preparation (Tebonin) from *Ginkgo biloba*. Arzneim.-Forsch. 17, 491-493 (1967); and Ramaswamy, A.: Pharmacological action of the biflavonoids from gymnosperms with special reference to *Ginkgo biloba*. J. Indian Med. Assoc. 55, 163-165 (1970)
10. Kem, W.R., Scott, K.N., Duncan, J.H.: Hoplonemertine worms - a new source of pyridine neurotoxins. Experientia 32, 684-686 (1976)
11. Cullen, W.P., LaLonde, R.T., Wang, C.J., Wong, C.F.: Isolation and in vitro antifungal activity of 6,6'-dihydroxythiobinupharidine. J. Pharm. Sci. 62, 826-827 (1973)
12. Dorsett, P.H., Kerstine, E.E., Powers, L.J.: Antivinal activity of gossypol and apogossypol. J. Pharm. Sci. 64, 1073 (1975)
13. Lee, K.-H., Imakura, Y., Sims, D.: Structure and stereochemistry of microlenin; a novel antitumor dimeric sesquiterpene lactone from *Helenium microcephalum*; X-ray crystal structure. J.C.S. Chem. Comm., p. 341-342 (1976)

Chemical and Biological Investigations on Indian Medicinal Plants

T. R. GOVINDACHARI

A. Introduction

A large part of the population in India depends even at the present time on the Indian systems of medicine, Ayurveda, Unani and Siddha. Although mineral and animal products are used to some extent, the greater part of indigenous drugs are from plants. It was estimated by Col. R.N. Chopra, the pioneer in the investigation of Indian drugs using Western methodology, that about 2300 plants were used in the traditional medicine practiced in the various regions of the country.

The chemical investigation of plants has been a favourite area of research in India, leading to the isolation of several hundred new compounds and elucidation of structure of many novel and complex molecules. Notable work has been done during the past two decades at the National Chemical Laboratory, Poona, the Regional Research Laboratory, Jammu and the Chemistry Department at Presidency College, Madras and the Delhi and Calcutta Universities. However, this review will deal mainly with work carried out at the Ciba-Geigy Research Centre, Bombay and the Central Drug Research Institute, Lucknow, two centres where teams of chemists and biologists have worked in close cooperation on plants with a view to discover active principles of potential therapeutic value. At the former, over 1300 extracts from 500 species, belonging to over 100 genera have been tested during the last twelve years. At the latter, some 2000 extracts from 1700 species belonging to 1000 genera have been put through much wider biological screening (1) which included anticancer testing under a collaborative programme with the C.C.N.S.C., U.S.A. In keeping with the objectives of this symposium only compounds showing some kind of biological activity or other, or those isolated from plants of reputed medicinal value will be included. The approach is selective rather than all-inclusive and the presentation is based on a classification according to chemical structure.

B. Alkaloids

I. Tylophora Alkaloids

The phenanthroindolizidine alkaloids isolated from *Tylophora asthmatica* Wight et Arm. (syn. *Tylophora indica*) and other species of the genus Tylophora, as well as *Cynanchum vincetoxicum* L. Pers. of the same family and from *Ficus septica* (Moraceae) constitute an interesting series of biologically active compounds. Earlier work has been adequately summarized (2). The absolute configuration of tylophorine (Formula 1) has now been rigorously established by exhaustive ozonolysis, which gave S-pyrrolidine-2-acetic acid, characterized through its N-trifluoracetyl(-)-(S)prolyl derivative (Formula 2) identified by gas chromatography (3). The absolute configuration of all other phenanthroindolizidine alkaloids at C_{13a} can be assigned by comparison of their optical rotatory dispersion (o.r.d.) curves with that of tylophorine.

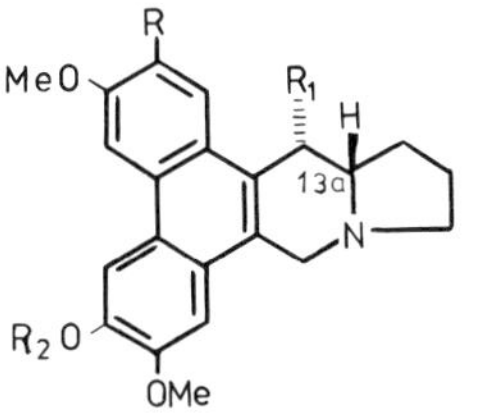

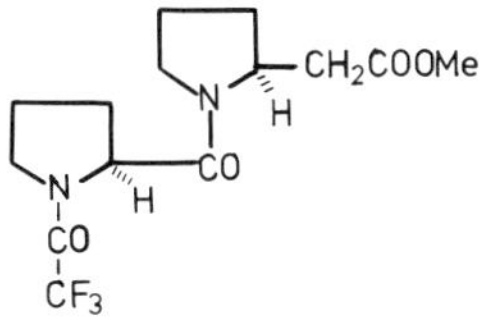

Formula 1. R = OMe; R_1 = H; R_2 = Me   Formula 2

Formula 3. R = H; R_1 = OH; R_2 = H

Fig. 1

The structure (4) and stereochemistry (5) of the minor alkaloid tylophorinidine (Formula 3) has been established and confirmed (6) by X-ray analysis of its diacetate methiodide.

Tylophorine has a paralyzing action on the heart muscle, but a stimulating action on the muscles of the blood vessels (7). Tylophorine, tylophorinine and tylocrebrine (8) and some other related minor alkaloids (9) all show significant anticancer activity, which has been fully recorded (10).

The leaves of *T. asthmatica* are used widely in India for treatment of asthma. The careful clinical studies of Shivpuri (11) using not only the leaves, but also the total alkaloids and pure tylophorine indicate their beneficial effects in providing relief to patients suffering from allergic rhinitis and/or asthma and more extended studies with the pure alkaloids would be worth while.

II. Ancistrocladus Alkaloids

Examination of *Ancistrocladus heyneanus* Wall, the only species of the genus Ancistrocladaceae occurring in India led to the isolation of four new alkaloids. The structures of ancistrocladine (Formula 4; ref. 12), ancistrocladinine (Formula 5; ref. 13), ancistrocladisine (Formula 6; ref. 14) and ancistrocladidine (Formula 7; ref. 15) were established by a combination of chemical and spectroscopic methods, as well as by X-ray analysis in the case of ancistrocladine (16). X-ray analysis indicated that the naphthalene and isoquinoline rings were at an angle of 87° due to restricted totation about the bond joining the two nuclei, introducing an element of dissymmetry at this bond. The absolute configurations at C_3 were found to be S in all the alkaloids, since perozonolysis yielded (+) L-β-aminobutyric acid. The application of the exciton chirality method (17) enabled a depiction of the absolute configuration around the bond joining the naphthalene and isoquinoline rings (16, 18).

Of the four alkaloids, ancistrocladidine showed spasmolytic activity on the isolated guinea pig ileum at a concentration of 5 μg/ml. comparable with that of papaverine.

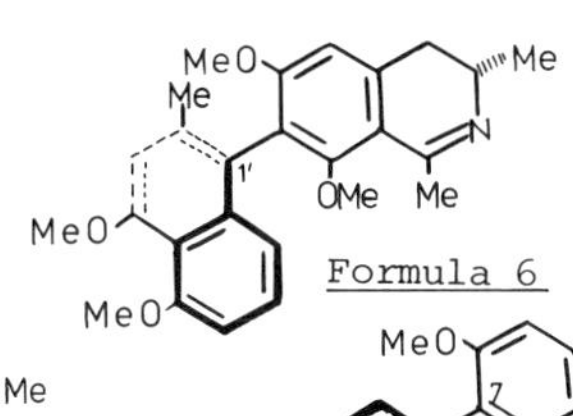

Formula 6

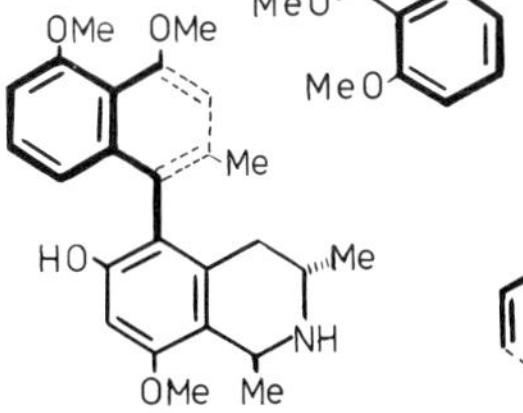

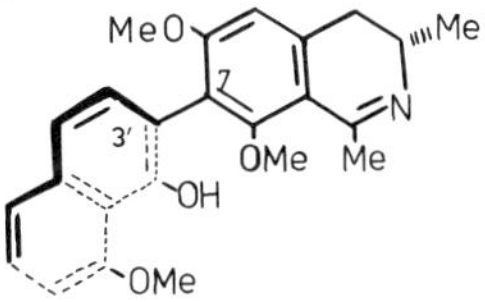

Formula 4

Formula 5. 1,2-dehydro   Formula 7

Fig. 2

III. Alkaloids of *Croton sparsiflorus* Morong

C. sparsiflorus Morong, a weed of common occurrence in the plains of India yielded three proaporphine bases, crotsparine (Formula 8), N-methylcrotosparine, O,N-dimethylcrotosparine, two dihydroproaporphines, crotosparinine (Formula 9), N-methylcrotosparinine and the aporphine sparsiflorine (19). The absolute configuration of these alkaloids has been determined (20). Biosynthetic studies showed that the alkaloids are derived from tyrosine and coclaurine (21).

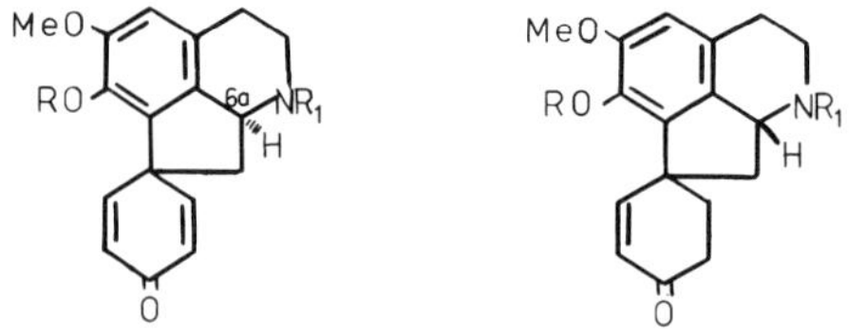

Formula 8. $R = R_1 = H$ Formula 9. $R = R_1 = H$ Fig. 3

N-Methylcrotosparine exhibited significant hypotensive activity in cats, an i.v. dose of 5 - 15 mg producing a lowering of blood pressure by 50 - 70 % for 1 - 3 h (22). The hypotensive activity appears to be mainly due to α-adrenergic blockade associated with a negative ionotropic effect and direct suppression of supraspinal vasomotor loci (23).

IV. Alkaloids of *Mappia foetida* Miers

The value of random screening of plants was well demonstrated when extraction of *M. foetida* Miers, for which no medicinal properties has been attributed, yielded (24) over 0.1 % of camptothecine, which has attracted wide attention as an anticancer drug (25), available earlier only in low yield (0.005 %) from *Camptotheca acuminata*. Besides camptothecine (Formula 10) and 9-methxycamptothecine (Formula 11), mappicine (Formula 12) was also isolated from the plant (26). The structure of mappicine was established by a partial synthesis from camptothecine.

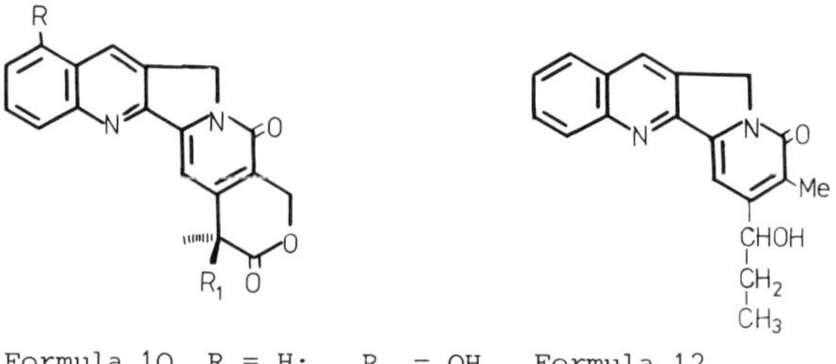

Formula 10. $R = H$; $R_1 = OH$ Formula 12
Formula 11. $R = OMe$; $R_1 = OH$ Fig. 4

9-Methoxycamptothecine showed anticancer activity (145 %) in P-388 lymphocytic leukemia (mouse) at a dose of 0.5 mg/kg as compared to the activity of campthothecine (161 %) at a dose of 1 mg/kg.

V. Alkaloids of *Piper trichostachyon* C.Dc.

From *P. trichostachyon* C.Dc. four new alkaloids piperstachine (Formula 13; ref. 27), cyclostachine-A (Formula 14), cyclostachine-B (Formula 15) and cyclopiperstachine (Formula 14a) were isolated and their structures determined (28). Confirmation of the structure of cyclostachine-A was obtained by X-ray analysis (29). Cyclostachines A and B evidently arise by an internal Diels-Alder reaction of the amide (Formula 13a) and cyclopiperstachine from piperstachine. These compounds are, however, not artefacts but exist in the plant.

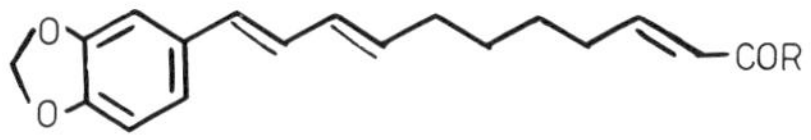

Formula 13. R = $NHCH_2CHMe_2$

Formula 13a. R = 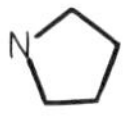

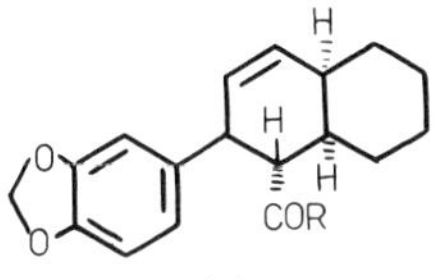

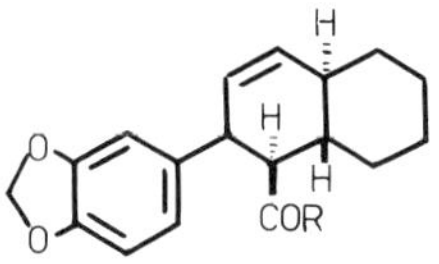

Formula 14. R = 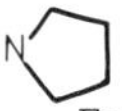

Formula 14a. R = $NHCH_2CHMe_2$

Formula 15. R = 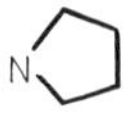

Fig. 5

Cyclostachine-A showed sedative and anticonvulsant activity at 250 mg/kg per oral (p.o.). It also showed weak antibacterial, antifungal and anti-TB activities.

VI. Alkaloids from some Menispermaceae Plants

1. *Alkaloids from Tiliacora racemosa Colebr.*

Essential features of the structures of tiliacorine, its diastereoisomer tiliacorinine and the mono-N-nor bases corresponding to the latter, nortiliacorinine A and nortiliacorinine B, isolated from *T. racemosa* Colebr. were established some years ago (30) and confirmed by a total synthesis of dl-O-methyltiliacorine (31). It was only recently that the position of the phenolic hydroxyl group in tiliacorine could be established as in Formula 16, by a selective cleavage at one of the benzylic carbon atoms (32). The determination of the absolute configuration at the two assymetric centres and the position of the N-methyl group in the two *nor*-bases await solution.

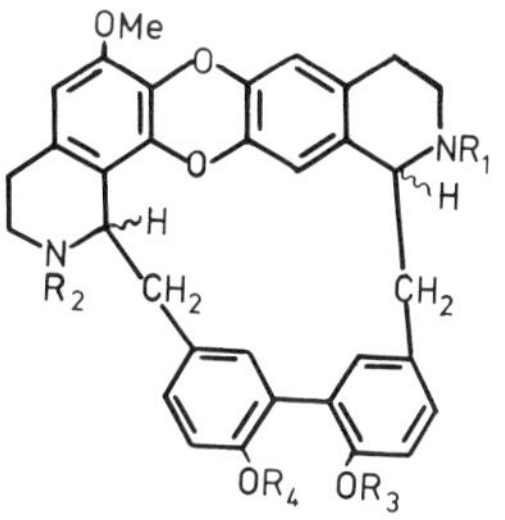

Formula 16. R_3 = H; R_1, R_2, R_4 = Me

Fig. 6

T. racemosa roots are used in Indian medicine against a variety of skin infections. The total alkaloid fraction fraom *T. racemosa* showd significant hypotensive activity, due perhaps to some minor constituents, since none of the four pure alkaloids was active.

2. Alkaloids of Cocculus pendulus (Forsk) Diels and Cocculus laurifolius Dc.

Six biscoclaurine alkaloids were isolated from *C. pendulus* (Forsk) Diels (33) of which cocculinin (Formula 17) showed activity against human epidermoid carcinoma of the nasopharynx in tissue culture (KB) at a concentration of 4.7 ν/ml.

From the related species *C. laurifolius* D.c. isococculidine (Formula 18) was isolated and its structure established (34). It has a powerful neuromuscular blocking action, the 50 % inhibitory concentration to acetyl choline-induced contraction of the frog rectus being 6 x 10^{-6}M (35).

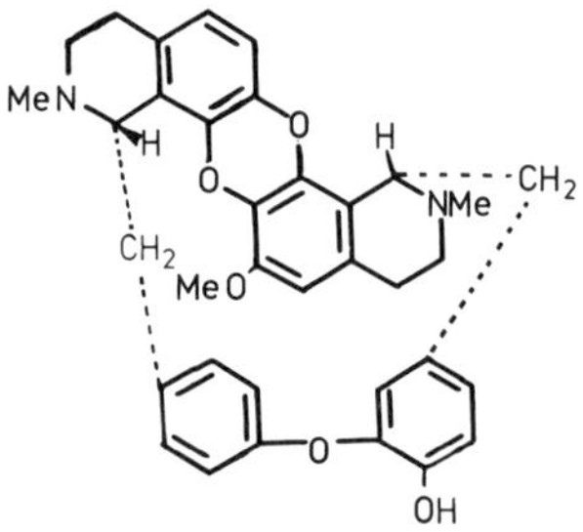

Formula 17

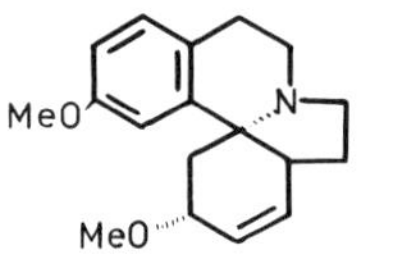

Formula 18

Fig. 7

3. Alkaloids of Cissampelos pareira Linn.

From the roots of *C. pareira* Linn. a reputed drug in Ayurvedic medicine, several bisbenzylisoquinoline alkaloids were isolated, many of them of known structure (36). Extensive pharmacological studies (37) have been carried out on hayatin (dl-bebeerine) metho salts. Hayatin is a major component of the alkaloidal fraction in roots collected from Kashmir. Clinical studies carried out in hayatin dimethiodide showed that it was about one third as potent as tubocurarine and the duration of activity was of equal extent at equipotent doses.

C. Oxygen Heterocycles

I. Cryptocaryalactone and Cryptocaryone

From the roots of *Cryptocarya bourdilloni* Gamb (Lauraceae) cryptocaryalactone (Formula 19; ref. 38) and cryptocaryone (Formula 20; ref. 39) were isolated and their structure established.

Cryptocaryone undergoes a remarkable rearrangement to a compound of structure (Formula 21) on warming with 1N NaOH, perhaps by the mechanism depicted alongside.

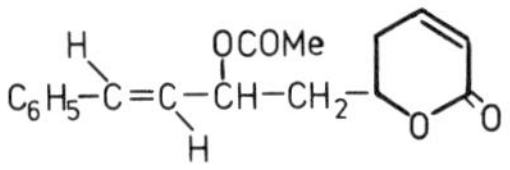

Formula 19

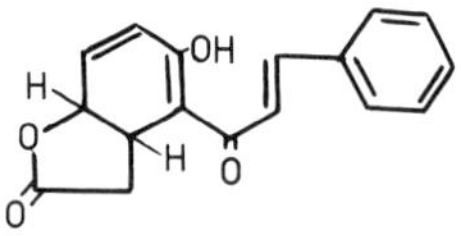

Formula 20

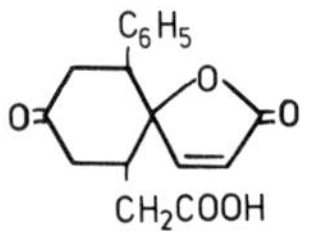

Formula 21

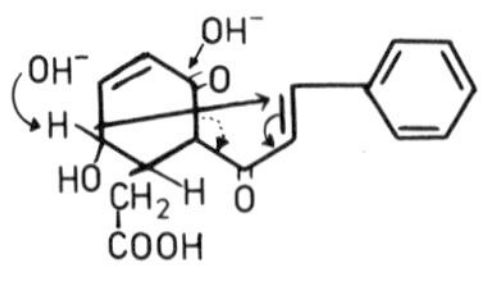

Fig. 8

Cryptocaryalactone shows moderate antifungal activity *(Candida albicans)* at 62.5 ν/ml in vitro and has slight sedative activity in mice lasting up to 320 h at 250 mg/kg. Cryptocaryone produces a prolonged fall of blood pressure (b.p.) at 9 mm/kg in the dog.

II. Surangin A and B

From the roots of *Mammea longifolia* (Wight) Planch and Triana (Guttiferae) two new coumarins surangin A and surangin B were obtained by hexane extraction. Their structures were established (40) entirely by spectroscopic methods as Formulas 22 and 22a. Surangin A showed antistaphylococcal activity at 7.8 ν/ml in vitro. Surangin B was active against neurovaccinia but toxic (LD_{50} 50 mg/kg i.p. in the mouse). It was active against mosquito larvae, mustard beetle and housefly at 0.05 ν/ml.

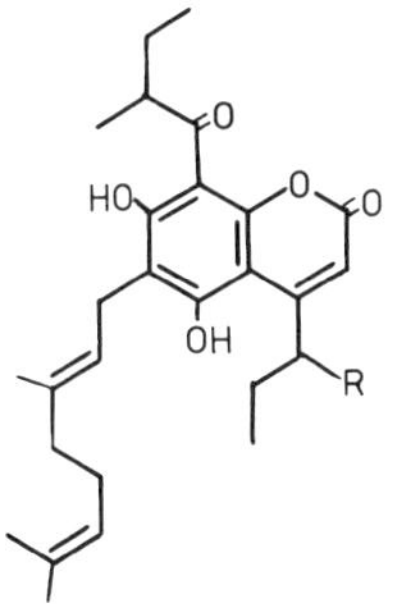

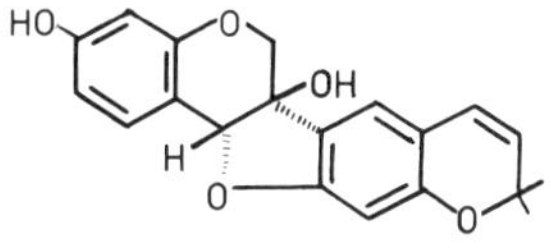

Formula 22. R = H
Formula 22a. R = OCOMe

Formula 23

Fig. 9

III. Tuberosin

Extracts of *Pueraria tuberosa* DC gave indications of antitubercular activity. From the benzene extract of the tubers, a new pterocarpan tuberosin was isolated whose structure was established as Formula 23 (41). Tuberosin showed antistaphylococcal activity at 250 ν/ml, antitubercular activity at 125 ν/ml, and antifungal activity at 31.2 ν/ml.

D. Terpenoids

I. Sesquiterpenes of *Cedrus deodara* Loudon

Five sesquiterpene alcohols were isolated from *C. deodara* of which himachalol (Formula 24; ref. 42) and centdarol (Formula 25; ref. 43) exhibited pronounced spasmolytic activity (44). The ED_{50} (μM) against $BaCl_2$-induced spasm in isolated guinea pig ileum eas himachalol (1.1), centdarol (14.13) compared to papaverine (4.55). The percent antagonism against carbachol-induced spasm in anaesthetized cat was himachalol (60), centdarol (72) compared to papaverine (60). This observation is of interest, since such activity has not been noted for sesquiterpenes earlier.

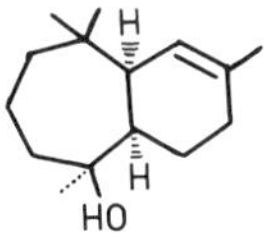

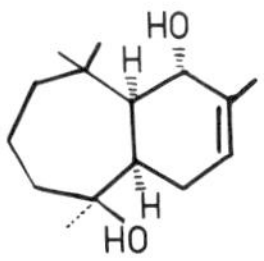

Formula 24 Formula 25 Fig. 10

II. Enhydrin

The highly oxygenated germacranolide enhydrin (Formula 26) was isolated from *Enhydra fluctuans* Lour. and its structure established (45). This was also confirmed by X-ray analysis (46).

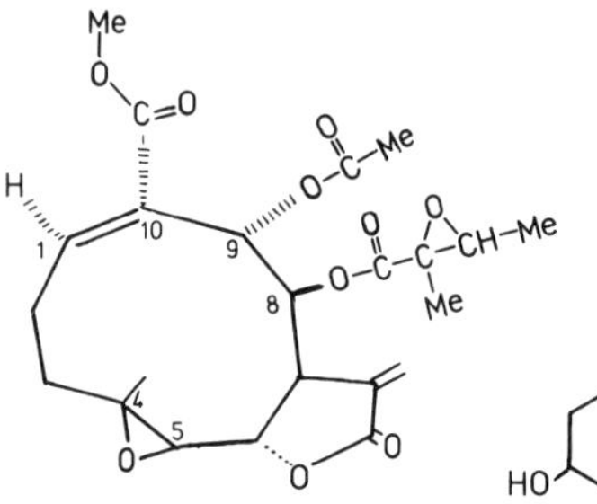

Formula 26

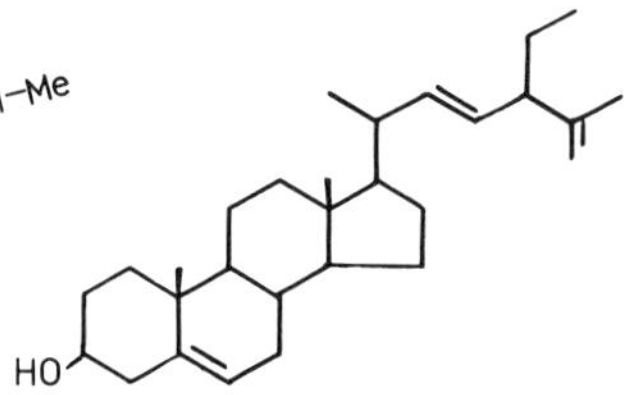

Formula 27

Fig. 11

Enhydrin produced a 40 mm fall of b.p. at an i.v. dose of 9 mg/kg. The accompanying sterol (Formula 27) which has been isolated from *Clerodendron campbelli* (47) produced a 80 mm fall of b.p. at 3 mg/kg i.v. of short duration.

III. Tagitinins A and F

A number of germacranolides were isolated (48) from *Tithonia tagetiflora* of which tagitinin F (Formula 28; ref. 49) displayed significant anti-cancer activity (KB system, 7.8 ν/ml).

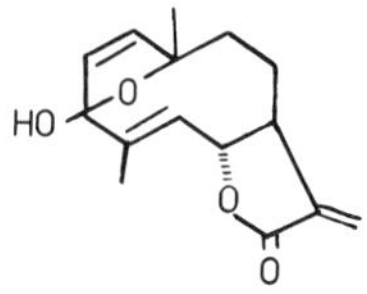

Formua 28

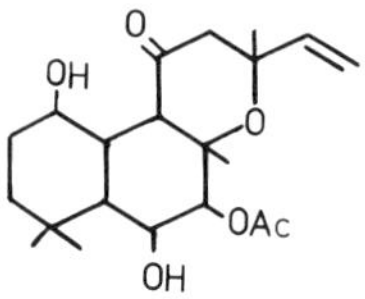

Formula 29

Fig. 12

IV. Coleonol

The diterpene alcohol, coleonol (Formula 29) isolated from *Coleus barbatus* Benth. exhibited good hypotensive activity, causing a 60 mm fall of b.p. lasting 80 min in cats at a dose of 0.5 mg/kg i.v. (50).

V. Diosbulbine

The report that tubers of *Dioscorea bulbifera* Linn. have hunger-suppressing properties led to the chemical examination of the material. A crystalline compound diosbulbine was obtained by chloroform extraction of the tubers. On the basis of spectroscopic and degradative evidence, diosbulbine was shown to be a norditerpene lactone of structure (Formula 30; ref. 51). It did not show biological activity of any kind.

VI. Dysobinin

The modified triterpene dysobinin (Formula 31; ref. 52) isolated from *Dysoxylum binectriferon* HK. 7 showed significant CNS-depressant activity (53).

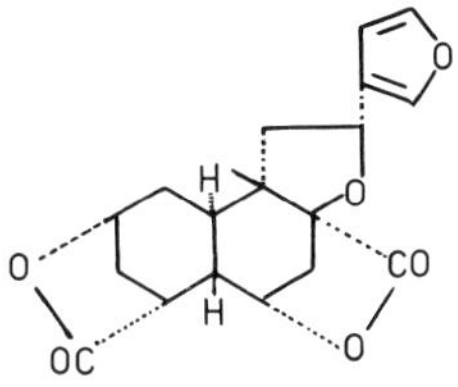

Formula 30

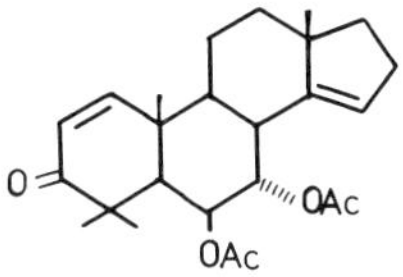

Formula 31

Fig. 13

VII. Triterpenes of *Salacia prinoides* DC

The roots and bark of *S. prinoides* are used widely in Indian medicine for the treatment of diabetes. Recently, two groups in Bombay and Delhi have investigated this plant in detail.

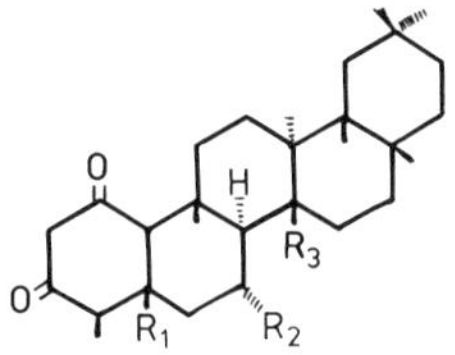

Formula 32. P: R_1=R_3=Me; R_2=H
Q: R_1=Me; R_2=H; R_3=CHO
S: R_1=R_3=Me; R_2=OH
T: R_1=Me; R_2=H; R_3=CH_2OH
U: R_1=Me; R_2=H; R_3=COOH

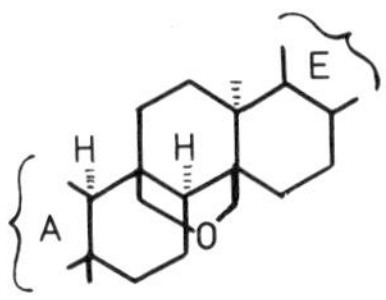

Formula 33. R

Fig. 14

Six closely related triterpenes have been isolated from this plant and shown to be 1,3-diketofriedelane derivatives (54a,b). The structures of substances Q, T and U were revised (54c) recently by the aid of X-ray analysis to compounds having functionalities at C_{26} instead of at C_{24} as originally proposed (54a), (Formula 32). The correct position of the ether linkage in substance R could be established only by X-ray analysis (Formula 33; ref. 55).

E. Glycosides

I. Cleistanthin

From the leaves of *Cleistanthus collinus* Roxb. Benth and Hook F. ellagic acid, diphyllin (56) and two new lignan lactones collinusin (57) and cleistanthin were isolated. The structure of cleistanthin was shown to be Formula 34 (58).

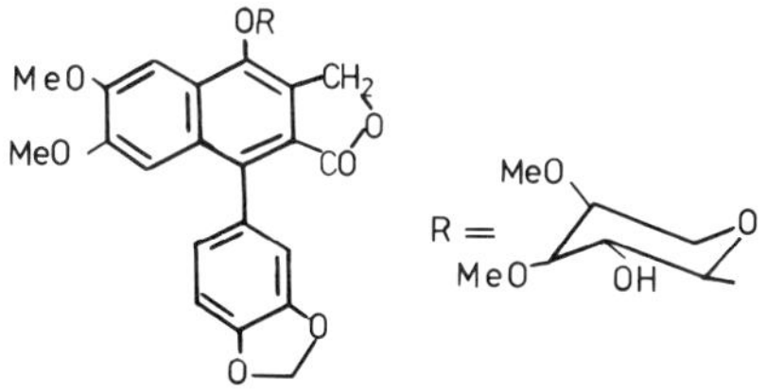

Formula 34

Fig. 15

Cleistanthin induces significant increase in neutrophilic granulocyte count (NGC) in rats, mice, cats and monkeys when administered by oral, intraperitoneal, intraveneous, intramuscular and subcutaneous routes. A dose of 0.25 mg/kg/day maintained increased levels of NGC for one month in rats (59).

II. Ipolearoside

A glycoside with the structure depicted (Formula 35) was isolated from *Ipomoea leari* Paxt. (60). This showed activity against Walker carcinosarcoma 250 (rats) at 10 mg.

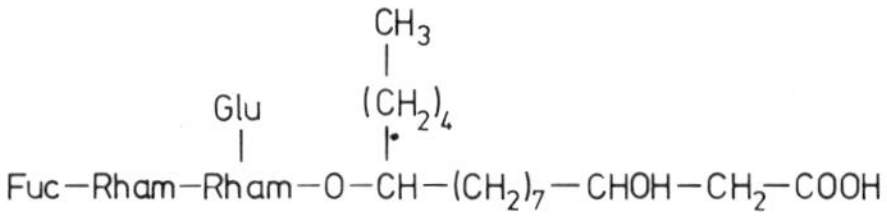

Formula 35 Fig. 16

III. Stigmasta-7, 22-diene-3β-O-glucoside

The above glucoside was isolated from *Vittadenia australis* A. Rich. (61). It possessed diuretic activity comarable to chlorthiazide (62).

IV. Scuttelarein-5-glucuronide

This compound (Formula 36) isolated from *Millingtonia hortensis* L.F. was half as active as a diuretic relative to chlorthiazide (63).

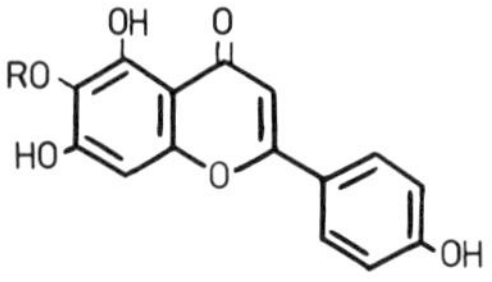

Formula 36. R = Glucuronyl

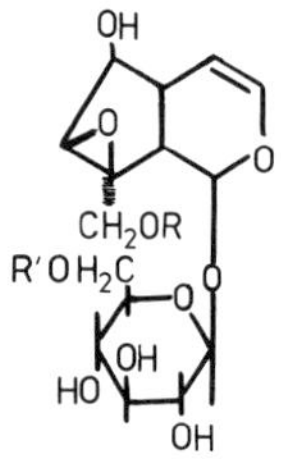

Formula 37. R = H; R' = Cinnamoyl
Formula 38. R = Vanilloyl; R' = H

Fig. 17

V. Glycosides of *Picrorhiza kurrooa* Benth.

In a reinvestigation of this reputed medicinal plant, two C9 iridoid glycosides picroside I (Formula 37) and kutkoside (Formula 38) have been isolated and their structures determined (64). Kutkin (65) which is a stable mixed crystal of these two glycosides shows weak diuretic activity, about a sixth of that chlorthiazide.

VI. Asclepin

Examination of *Asclepia currasavica* Linn. collected from Dehra Dun yielded results (66) differing from the plant of Brazilian origin (67). The principal glycoside was asclepin (3'-O-acetyl-calotropin) (Formula 39). Asclepin showed excellent cardiotonic activity. The oral absorption in cats was 22.5 % in 5 h similar to digoxin. A single dose of asclepin persisted up to 96 h (digoxin, 72 h) and the cumulative toxicity was lower than that of digoxin (68).

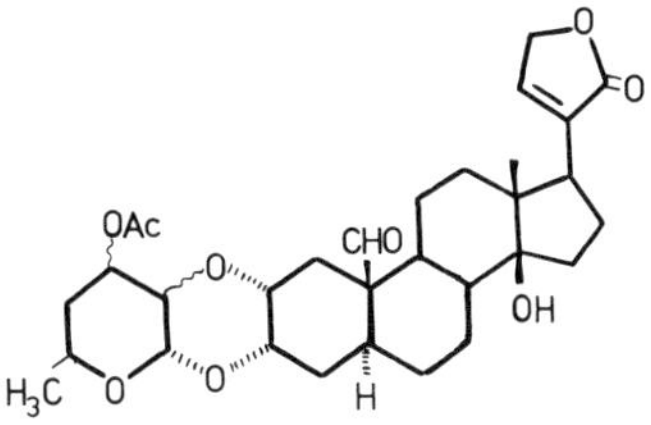

Formula 39 Fig. 18

VII. Shatavarins I - IV

Four new glycosides, named shatavarin I - IV were isolated from the medicinal plant *Asparagus racemosus* Willd. The structure of shatavarin IV has been elucidated (Formula 40) it being a glycoside of sarsaspogenin, the sugar moieties being rhamnose (2) and glucose (1) (69). Shatavarin I has an additional glucose unit, whose position has not been determined. It exhibited significant antioxytoxic activity (70).

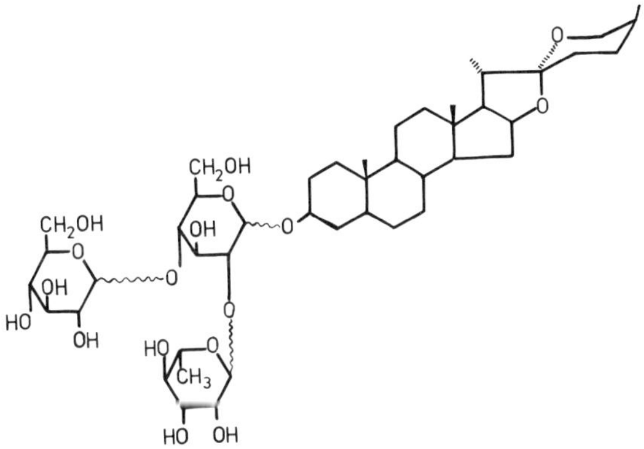

Formula 40 Fig. 19

VIII. Glycosides of *Carissa* Species

The glycosidic fraction from *Carissa carandas* Linn. showed good cardiotonic activity (71). This was shown to be due to the presence of glucosides of odoroside H (72). *Carissa spinarum* Linn. yielded five cardiac glycosides, three of which have been identified as odoroside H, evomonoside and odoroside G (73).

IX. Peruvoside

This cardiac glycoside was isolated from *Thevetia nerifolia* Juss. in 1959 (74) and its structure was established (75). Extensive biological work has been done both in India and in Germany on peruvoside (76). The compound has undergone extensive clinical trials and has been introduced in Germany under the trade name Encordin. From their reports it appears that peruvoside is a rapidly effective drug, with dependable absorption from the gastrointestinal tract and has a relatively high therapeutic index compared to digoxin (77).

F. Miscellaneous

I. Curcumine

Curcumine (Formula 41) is a major constituent of *Curcuma longa* which is said to possess local as well as systemic antiinflammatory property. The antiinflammatory property of curcumine was evaluated in several models and compared favourably with phenylbutazone (78). It is now undergoing clinical trials.

II. Arnebin

From the roots of *Arnebia nobilis* Rachinger six naphthogquinones were isolated, five of these being derivatives of alkanin (79). Of these arnebin (Formula 42) showed good anticancer activity (80). (KB. 25.0 μg/ml, WM 6 mg; PS 3 mg).

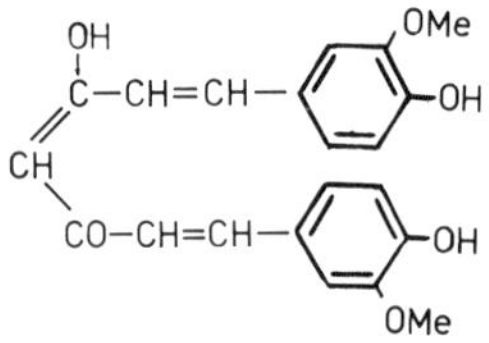

Formula 41

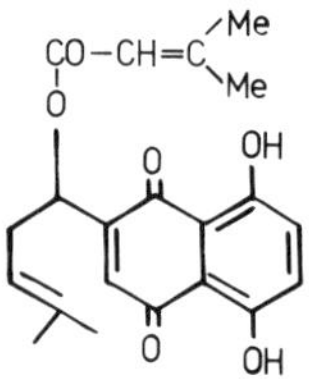

Formula 42

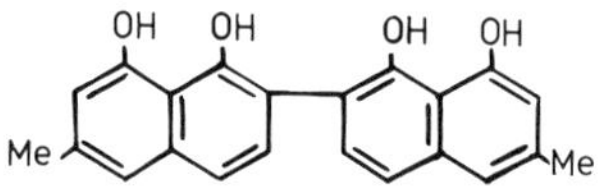

Formula 43

Fig. 20

III. Diospyrol

Extracts of the fresh fruits of *Diospyros mollis* Griff. are widely used in Thailand as an anthelmintic, particularly against hookworm. The active principle was recognized to be diospyrol (Formula 43; ref. 81), but no pharmacological or clinical work has been carried out on the pure substance. The LD_{50} of diospyrol is over 3000 mg/kg in several species of experimental animals. Tests carried out recently (82) showed that in hamsters infected with human hookworm *Necator americanus*, a dose of 200 mg/kg for three days cured 80 % of the infected hamsters (non-patent infection) while a single dose of 500 mg/kg effected 100 % cure of the patent infection. Diospyrol was also effective against *Hymenolopis nana* and *Nematospiroides dubius* parasites in mice (82). Thus there is sound basis for the use of the juice of fresh fruits of *D. mollis* against parasitic infections.

IV. Steroidal Constituents of *Commiphora mukul*

The gum resin exudate from the tree *C. mukul* (Hook, ex. Stocks) Engl. is highly rated in Ayurvedic medicine for the treatment of rheumatoid arthritis, obesity and several other disorders (83). Pharmacological studies on the crude drug as well as some of its fractions and pure constituents revealed significant antiinflammatory, antirheumatic and hypocholesteremic activity, providing support to the ancient claims (84). The active constituents are present in the steroid fraction which yielded the three new sterols, guggulusterol -I, guggulusterol -II and guggulusterol -III which are formulated as Formulas 44, 45 and 46 respectively (85).

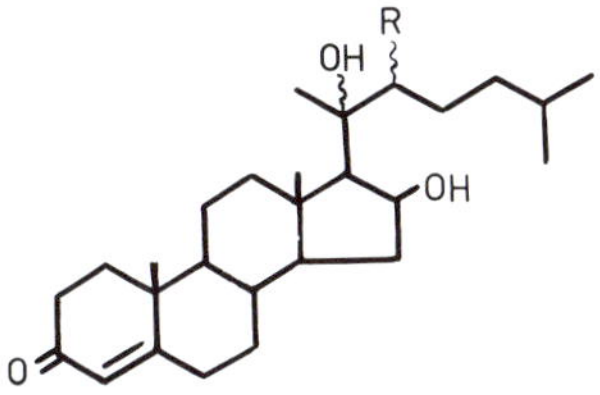

Formula 44. R = OH
Formula 46. R = H

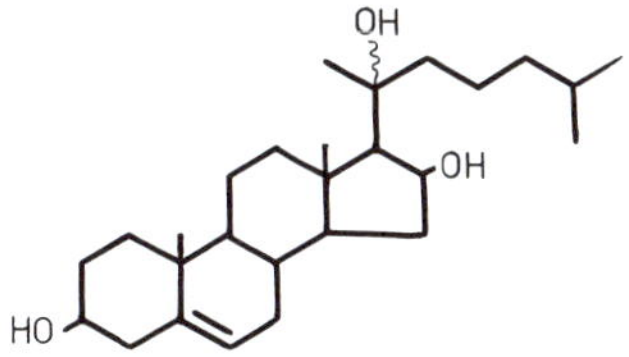

Formula 45

Fig. 21

This brief review does poor justice to the vast amount of chemical work done on medicinal plants in India. It has been circumscribed by the condition that the review should deal with natural products possessing biological activity. Practically, all the better known medicinal plants of India have been investigated at the Central Drug Research Institute, Lucknow during the past two decades and at the Ciba-Geigy Research Centre, Bombay during the past twelve years. A large proportion of the extracts from these plants, or the pure compounds of fascinatingly complex structure isolated from them have usually proved inert in the biological test systems conventionally employed in drug research. Perhaps this approach of testing extracts from plants with a view to evaluating their effectiveness is unsuitable and a better system has to be devised. As a case in point, I would cite an experience with *Mucuna pruriens* Baker. The seeds of this plant have been used in the treatment of nervous disorders since ancient times. Some years ago, it was shown that the seeds contain 5 - 6 % of L- Dopa (86). In a carefully-designed clinical trial conducted in one of the leading hospitals in Bombay, the seed powder, up to 60 g in three to four divided doses was administered to patients with Parkinsons disease. A substantial and statistically significant therapeutic response was observed and the side effects were infrequent and mild. The therapeutic benefit cannot be ascribed to the L-Dopa content alone (87). Efforts to discover whether there are any other active compounds responsible for the degree of effectiveness observed in treatment of Parkinsonism have not succeeded.

A few years ago, the Indian Council of Medical Research launched a new scheme with the object of evaluating the claims of efficacy of a large number of plant drugs. It set up nine 'circuits' in different parts of India, each staffed by a team comprising pharmacognosists, chemists, biologists and clinicians of both Indian and Western medicine. A vast amount of work has been done under this scheme, but the study is still incomplete. If taken to its logical conclusion the study will be helpful in evaluating the effectiveness of a large number of commonly used Indian plant remedies.

The chances of discovering new drugs from old plant remedies seem to be meagre, but so are the chances of discovering new drugs from purely synthetic compounds. In a country like India with its vast flora numbering nearly 20.000 species of higher plants, investigation not only of plants which have been termed 'medicinal,' but also of those collected in systematic botanical surveys in different regions of the country would be well worthwhile.

Acknowledgements. My grateful thanks are due to Drs. R.S. Grewal, B.S. Joshi, N. Viswanathan and P.C. Parthasarathy of the Ciba-Geigy Research Centre and Drs. Nitya Anand, M.M. Dhar, B.N. Dhawan and R.P. Rastogi of the Central Drug Research Institute, Lucknow for making available all the chemical and biological data from the investigations on plants in their respective laboratories and to Dr. B.R. Pai for valuable help in preparation of this article.

References

1. Dhar, M.L., Dhar, M.M., Dhawan, B.N., Mehrotra, B.N., Ray, C.: Indian J. Expl. Biol. 6, 233 (1968; Bhakuni, D.S., Dhar, M.L., Dhar, M.M., Dhawan, B.N., Mehrotra, B.N.: Indian J. Expl. Biol. 7, 250 (1969); Bhakuni, D.S., Dhar, M.L., Dhar, M.M., Dhawan, B.N., Gupta, B., Srimal, R.C.: Indian J. Expl. Biol. 9, 91 (1971); Dhar, M.L., Dhar, M.M., Dhawan, B.N., Mehrotra, B.N., Srimal, R.C., Tandon, J.S.: Indian J. Expl. Biol. 11, 43 (1973); Dhar, M.L., Dhawan, B.N., Prasad, C.R., Rastogi, R.P., Singh, K.K., Tandon, J.S.: Indian J. Expl. Biol. 12, 512 (1974)
2. Govindachari, T.R.: J. Indian Chem. Soc. 50, 1 (1973); Wiegrebe, W.: Pharm. Z. 117, 1509 (1972)
3. Govindachari, T.R., Rajagopalan, T.G., Viswanathan, N.: J.C.S. Perkin I, 1161 (1974)
4. Govindachari, T.R., Viswanathan, N., Radhakrishnan, J., Pai, B.R., Natarajan, S., Subramanian, P.S.: Tetrahedron 29, 891 (1973)
5. Govindachari, T.R., Viswanathan, N., Pai, B.R.: Indian J. Chem. 12, 886 (1974)
6. Wadhawan, V.K., Sikka, S.K., Mulchandani, N.B.: Tetrahedron Lett. 1973, 5091
7. Chopra, R.N., Ghosh, N.N., Bose, J.B., Ghosh, S.: Arch. Pharm. 275, 236 (1937)
8. Gellert, E., Govindachari, T.R., Lakshmikantham, M.V., Ragade, I.S., Rudzate, R., Viswanathan, N.: J. Chem. Soc. 1008 (1962)
9. Rao, K.V., Wilson, R., Cummings, B.: J. Pharm. Sci. 59, 1501 (1970)
10. Hartwell, J.L., Abbot, B.J.: Advan. Pharm. Chemother. 7, 117 (1969)
11. Shivpuri, D.N., Menon, M.P., Prakash, D.: J. Assoc. Physicians, India 16, 9 (1968); Shivpuri, D.N., Menon, M.P., Prakash, D.J.: Allergy (U.S.A.) 43, 145 (1969); Shivpuri, D.N.: Lecture at V Convention of I.C.A.I., Jaipur, 1971
12. Govindachari, T.R., Parthasarathy, P.C.: Tetrahedron 27, 1013 (1971); Govindachari, T.R., Parthasarathy, P.C., Desai, H.K.: Indian J. Chem. 9, 931 (1971)
13. Govindachari, T.R., Parthasarathy, P.C., Desai, H.K.: Indian J. Chem. 9, 1421 (1971)
14. Govindachari, T.R., Parthasarathy, P.C., Desai, H.K.: Indian J. Chem. 10, 1117 (1972)
15. Govindachari, T.R., Parthasarathy, P.C., Desai, H.K.: Indian J. Chem. 11, 1190 (1973)
16. Govindachari, T.R., Nagarajan, K., Parthasarathy, P.C., Rajagopalan, T.G., Desai, H.K., Kartha, G., Sow-mei Lai Chen, Nakanishi, K.: J.C.S. Perkin I, 1413 (1974)
17. Harada, N., Nakanishi, K.: Acc. Chem. Res. 5, 257 (1972)
18. Govindachari, T.R., Parthasarathy, P.C., Rajagopalan, T.G., Desai, H.K., Ramachandran, K.S.: J.C.S. Perkin I, 2134 (1975)
19. Bhakuni, D.S., Satish, S., Dhar, M.M.: Phytochemistry 9, 2573 (1970)
20. Bhakuni, D.S., Satish, S., Dhar, M.M.: Tetrahedron 28, 4579 (1972)
21. Bhakuni, D.S., Satish, S., Uprety, H., Kapil, R.S.: Phytochemistry 13, 2767 (1974)

22. Dubey, M.P., Srimal, R.C., Dhawan, B.N.: Indian J. Pharmacology 1, 73 (1969)
23. Dubey, M.P., Srimal, R.C., Dhawan, B.N.: Indian J. Pharmacology 3, 18 (1971)
24. Govindachari, T.R., Viswanathan, N.: Indian J. Chem. 10, 453 (1972); Govindachari, T.R., Viswanathan, N.: Phytochemistry 11, 3529 (1972)
25. Schultz, A.G.: Chem. Rev. 73, 385 (1973); Danieli, B., Palmisano, G.: Fitoterpia 45, 87 (1974)
26. Govindachari, T.R., Ravindranath, K.R., Viswanathan, N.: J.C.S. Perkin I, 1215 (1974); Agarwal, J.S., Kulshrestha, D.K., Rastogi, R.P.: Indian J. Chem. 13, 758 (1975)
27. Joshi, B.S., Viswanathan, N., Gawad, D.H.: Helv. Chim. Acta. 58, 1551 (1975); Viswanathan, N., Balakrishnan, V., Joshi, B.S., Phillipsborn, W.: Helv. Chim. Acta 58, 2026 (1975)
28. Joshi, B.S., Viswanathan, N., Gawad, D.H., Balakrishnan, V.: Helv. Chim. Acta 58, 2295 (1975)
29. Joshi, B.S., Viswanathan, N., Gawad, D.H., Balakrishnan, V., Phillipsborn, W., Quick, A.: Experientia 31, 880 (1975)
30. Anjaneyalu, B., Govindachari, T.R., Sathe, S.S., Viswanathan, N.: Tetrahedron 25, 3091 (1969)
31. Anjajeyalu, B., Govindachari, T.R., Viswanathan, N.: Tetrahedron 27, 439 (1971)
32. Shamma, M., Foy, J.E., Govindachari, T.R., Viswanathan, N.: J. Org. Chem. 41, 1293 (1976)
33. Bhakuni, D.S., Joshi, P.P.: Tetrahedron 31, 2575 (1975)
34. Dhar, M.M.: Pers. Comm.
35. Kar, K., Mukerjee, K.C., Dhawan, B.N.: Indo-Soviet Symp. on Natural Products. Lucknow, India: Central Drug Research Instituts, 1976
36. Bhatnagar, A.K., Popli, S.:.: Indian J. Chem. 5, 102 (1967); Bhatnagar, A.K., Bhattachargji, S., Roy, A.C., Popli, S.P., Dhar, M.L.: J. Org. Chem. 32, 819 (1967)
37. Patnaik, G.K., Pradhan, S.N., Vohra, M.M.: Indian J. Exp. Biol. 11, 89 (1973) and references cited therein
38. Govindachari, T.R., Parthasarathy, P.C.: Tetrahedron Lett. 1971, 3401; Govindachari, T.R., Parthasarathy, P.C., Mody, J.D.: Indian J. Chem. 10, 149 (1972)
39. Govindachari, T.R., Parthasarathy, P.C., Desai, H.K., Shanbag, M.N.: Tetrahedron 29, 3091 (1973)
40. Joshi, B.S., Kamat, V.N., Govindachari, T.R., Ganguly, A.K.: Tetrahedron 25, 1453 (1969)
41. Joshi, B.S., Kamat, V.N.: J.C.S. Perkin I, 907 (1973)
42. Bisarya, S.C., Dev, S.: Tetrahedron 24, 3869 (1968)
43. Kulshrestha, D.K., Rastogi, R.P.: Phytochemistry 15, 557 (1976)
44. Kar, K., Puri, V.N., Patnaik, G.K., Sur, R.N., Dhawan, B.N., Kulshrestha, D.K., Pastogi, R.P.: J. Pharm. Sci. 64, 258 (1975)
45. Joshi, B.S., Kamat, V.N.: Indian J. Chem. 10, 771 (1972)
46. Kartha, G., Go, K.T., Joshi, B.S.: J.C.S. Chem. Commun. 1327 (1972)
47. Bolger, L.M., Rees, H.H., Ghisalberti, E.L., Goad, L.J., Goodwin, T.W.: Tetrahedron Lett. 1970, 1883
48. Pal, R., Kulshresta, D.K., Rastogi, R.P.: Indian J. Chem. 14B, 259 (1976)
49. Tandon, J.S., Dhar, M.M., Venkatesan, K.: Unpubl. work
50. Dubey, M.P., Srimal, R.C., Dhawan, B.N.: Indian J. Pharmacol. 6, 15 (1971)
51. Joshi, B.S., Rane, D.F.: Indian J. Chem. 7, 452 (1969); Komovi, T., Arita, M., Ida, Y., Fujukura, T., Kawasaki, T., Sekine, K.: Justus Liebigs Annalen der Chemie, 978 (1973)
52. Dhar, M.M.: Pers. Comm.
53. Prasad, C.R., Chak, I.M., Dhawan, B.N.: Unpubl. work
54a. Joshi, B.S., Kamat, V.N., Viswanathan, N.: Tetrahedron 29, 1365 (1973)
54b. Tewari, N.C., Ayengar, K.N.N., Rangaswamy, S.: J.C.S. Perkin I, 146 (1974)
54c. Rogers, D., Philips, F.L., Joshi, B.S., Viswanathan, N.: Unpubl. work
55. Rogers, D., Williams, D.J., Joshi, B.S., Kamat, V.N., Viswanathan, N.: Tetrahedron Lett. 1974, 63
56. Horii, Z., Ohkawa, K., Kim, S., Momon, T.: J.C.S. Chem. Commun. 653 (1968)
57. Govindachari, T.R., Sathe, S.S., Viswanathan, N.: Tetrahedron Lett. 1967, 4183

58. Govindachari, T.R., Sathe, S.S., Viswanathan, N.: Tetrahedron 25, 2815 (1969)
59. Rao, R.R., Nair, T.B.: Pharmacology 4, 347 (1970)
60. Sarin, J.P., Garg, H.G., Khanna, N.M., Dhar, M.M.: Phytochemistry 12, 2461 (1973)
61. Sarin, J.P.S., Garg, H.G., Khanna, N.M., Dhar, M.M.: Indian J. Chem. 13, 199 (1975)
62. Kar, K., Sarin, J.P.S., Khanna, N.M.: Unpubl. work
63. Kar, K., Singh, S., Khanna, N.M.: Indian J. Pharm. 38, 26 (1976)
64. Singh, B., Rastogi, R.P.: Indian J. Chem. 10, 29 (1972)
65. Rastogi, R.P., Sharma, V.N., Siddiqui, S.: J. Sci. Ind. Res. 8B, 173 (1949); 18B, 219 (1959)
66. Singh, B., Rastogi, R.P.: Indian J. Chem. 7, 1105 (1969)
67. Tschesche, R., Forstmann, D., Rao, V.K.M.: Chem. Ber. 91, 1204 (1958); Tschesche, R., Snatzke, G., Grimmer, G.: Naturwissenschaften 46, 263 (1959)
68. Patnaik, G.K., Dhawan, B.N.: Indian J. Pharmacol. 3, 8 (1973)
69. Sukh Dev: Pers. Comm.
70. Gaitonde, B.B., Jetmalani, M.H.: Arch. Intern. Pharmacodyn. 179, 121 (1969)
71. Rastogi, R.C., Vohra, M.M., Rastogi, R.P., Dhar, M.L.: Indian J. Chem. 4, 132 (1966)
72. Rastogi, R.C., Rastogi, R.P., Dhar, M.L.: Indian J. Chem. 5, 215 (1967)
73. Rastogi, R.C., Kulshrestha, D.K., Rastogi, R.P.: Indian J. Chem. 7, 1102 (1969)
74. Rangaswamy, S., Venkat Rao, E.: J. Sci. Ind. Res. 18B, 445 (1959)
75. Bisset, N.G., Von Euw, J., Frerejacque, M., Rangaswamy, S., Schindler, O., Reichstein, T.: Helv. Chim. Acta. 45, 938 (1962)
76. Kohli, J.D., Vohra, M.M.: Arch. Internal. Pharmacodyn. 126, 412 (1960); Arora, R.B., Sharma, J.N., Bhatia, M.L.: Indian J. Exp. Biol. 5, 31 (1967); Schorscher, Von E., Sommer, S., Wild, A.J.N., Block, A.: Arzneim. Forsch. 12, 1582 (1968) and following papers
77. Arora, R.B., Rangaswamy, S.: 'Peruvoside and other Cardiotonic glycosides of *Thevetia nerifolia*,' C.C.R.I.M.H. (New Delhi) Monograph - 1 (1972)
78. Srimal, R.C., Dhawan, B.N.: J. Pharm. Pharm. Pharmacol. 25, 447 (1973)
79. Shukla, Y.N., Tandon, J.S., Dhar, M.M.: Experientia 25, 357 (1969); Phytochemistry 10, 1909 (1971)
80. Gupta, S.K., Mathur, I.S.: Indian J. Cancer 9, 50 (1972)
81. Loder, J.W., Mongolsuk, S., Robertson, A., Whalley, W.B.: J. Chem. Soc. 2233 (1957); Yoshira, K., Natori, S., Kanchanapee, P.: Tetrahedron Lett. 4857 (1967); Yoshira, K., Tezuka, M., Kanchanapee, P., Natori, S.: Chem. Pharm. Bull. (Tokyo) 19, 2271 (1971)
82. Sen, H.G., Joshi, B.S., Parthasarathy, P.C., Kamat, V.N.: Arzneim. Forsch. 24, 2000 (1974)
83. Nadkarni, A.K.: The Indian Materia Medica. Popular Book Depot. Bombay, India, 1954, pp. 167-170
84. Nitya Anand, S., Kapoor, N.K.: Indian J. Exptl. Biol. 9, 376 (1971)
85. Patil, V.D., Nayak, U.R., Dev, S.: Tetrahedron 28, 2341 (1972)
86. Damodaran, M., Rangaswamy, R.: Biochem. J. 31, 2149 (1937)
87. Vaidya, A.B., Rajagopalan, T.G., Mankodi, N.A., Antarkar, D.S., Purohit, A.V., Wadia, N.H.: To be published

Chemistry of Neolignans with Potential Biological Activity

O. R. GOTTLIEB

A. Introduction

The two classes of naturally occurring dimeric lignoids (58) comprise the lignans (34) and the neolignans (29), generated, respectively, by the oxidative coupling of cinnamic acids (Formula 1.1) and/or cinnamyl alcohols (Formula 1.2) and of propenylphenols (Formula 1.3) and/or allylphenols (Formula 1.4). Examples of lignans are podophyllotoxin (Formulas 1.5, ex 1.1 and 1.2) (33), pinoresinol (Formulas 1.7, ex 1.2 and 1.2) (56), steganacin (Formulas 1,9, ex 1.1 and 1.2) (39) and hordatine (Formulas 1.11, ex 1.1 and 1.1) (51); examples of neolignans are otobain (Formulas 1.6, ex 1.3 and 1.3) (27), nor-dihydroguaiaretic acid (Formulas 1.8, ex 1.3 and 1.3) (55), schizandrin (Formulas 1.10, ex 1.3 and 1.3) (38) and piperenone (Formulas 1.12, ex 1.3 and 1.4) (41).

These compounds are clearly connected with the defense mechanism of their host species: otobain (Formula 1.6) and hordatine (Formula 1.11) are antifungal factors, and piperenone (Formula 1.12) is the insect antifeeding factor, respectively of otoba butter (ex *Myristica otoba*), used in Columbia in veterinary practice (1), barley seedling (51) and *Piper futokadzura* (41). Pharmacological activity was reported for the remaining compounds. Schizandrin (Formula 1.10) is one of the active principles (40, 44, 52) of *Schizandra chinensis* (50, 53), long used in the Orient as a stimulant (37). Steganacin (Formula 1.9) (ex *Steganotaenia araliacea*) showed activity in vivo against leukemia in mice and in vitro against cells derived from human carcinoma of the nasopharynx (39). Podophyllotoxin (Formula 1.5) is the major constituent of extracts from the Himalayan shrub *Podophyllum emodi* which have been used in the treatment of malignant diseases for over 2000 years (36). Being responsible for the antimitotic and antineoplasic activities of Pinaceae and Burseraceae species, it is so much in demand in the drug trade that *Podophyllum peltatum* (may apple) was considered a potential new cash-crop plant of eastern North America (43). Two derivatives of podophyllotoxin have been used in the treatment of human malignancies (36). Nor-dihydroguaiaretic acid (Formula 1.8), also implicated in cancer therapy (47), was described as the most potent anticancer metabolite in vitro (19). It shows astoundingly varied pharmacological, antimicrobial and biochemical activities. Industrial applications include use as antioxidant for food materials (46).

Clearly, lignoids would merit attention as potentially useful medicinal products. The quoted examples are representative, however, of only four skeletal types, represented by Formulas 2.1 (pinoresinol, NDGA), 2.2 (podophyllotoxin, otobain), 2.3 (steganacin, schizandrin) and 2.7 (hordatine, piperenone). This (Formula 2.7) and the additional types portrayed in Fig. 2, comprising about 85 compounds, have recently been discovered. It is hoped that this report on some pertinent chemical aspects will stimulate interest in their pharmacological evaluation.

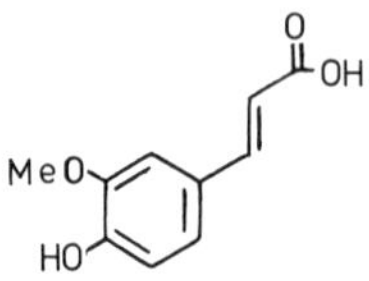

Formula 1.1

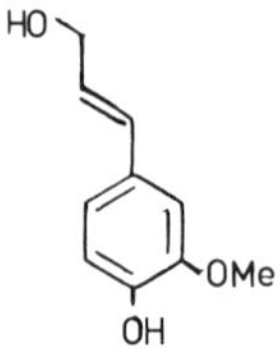

Formula 1.2

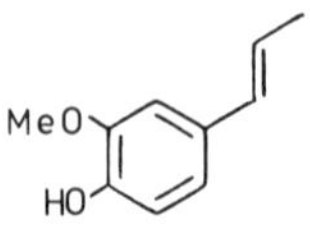

Formula 1.3

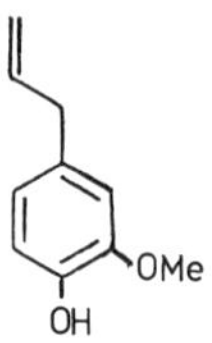

Formula 1.4

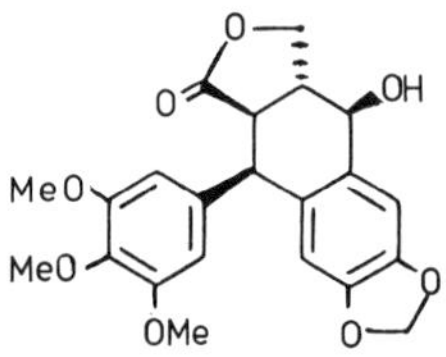

Formula 1.5

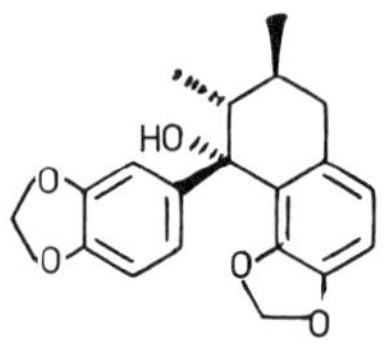

Formula 1.6

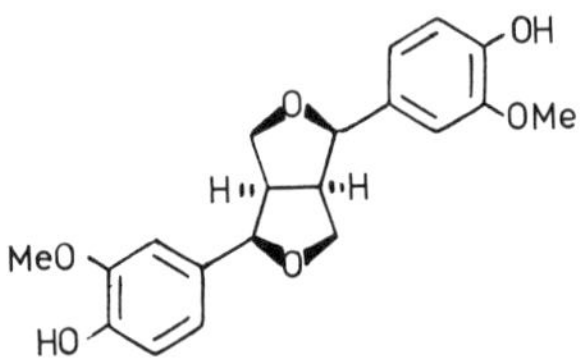

Formula 1.7

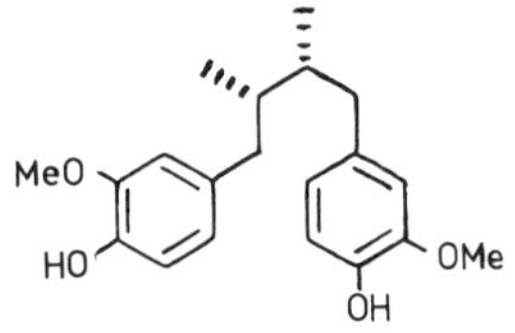

Formula 1.8

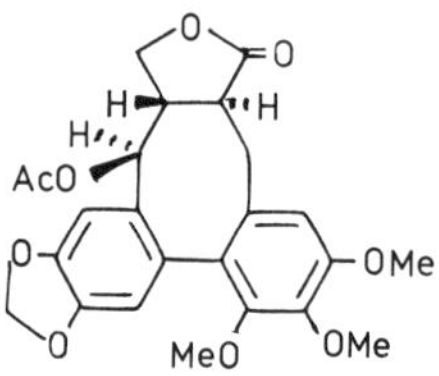

Formula 1.9

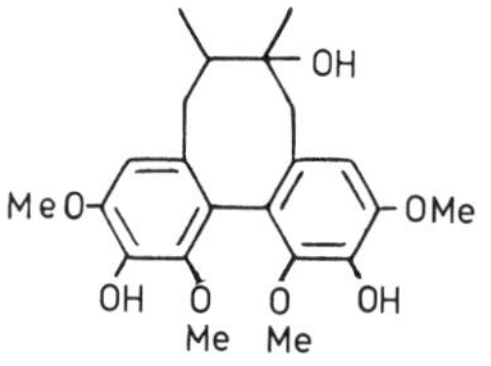

Formula 1.10

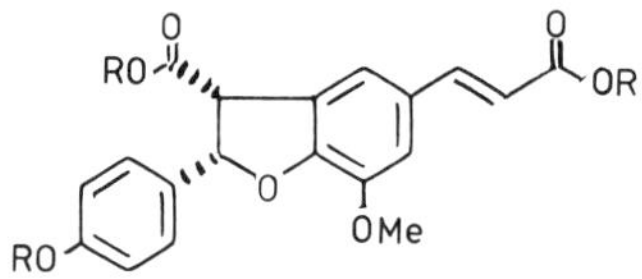

Formula 1.11

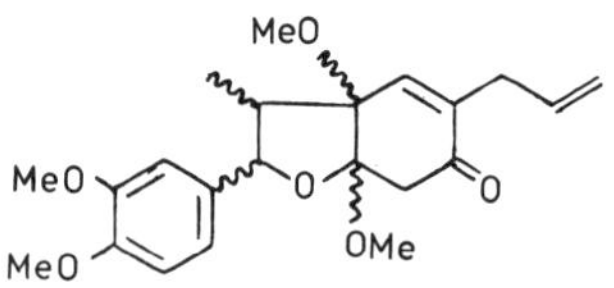

Formula 1.12

Fig. 1. Examples of two classes of dimeric lignoids: lignans (Formulas 1.5, 1.7, 1.9, 1.11), derived from cinnamic acids (e.g. Formula 1.1) and/or cinnamyl alcohols (e.g. Formula 1.2); and neolignans (Formulas 1.6, 1.8, 1.10, 1.12), derived from propenylphenols (e.g. Formula 1.3) and/or allylphenols (e.g. Formula 1.4)

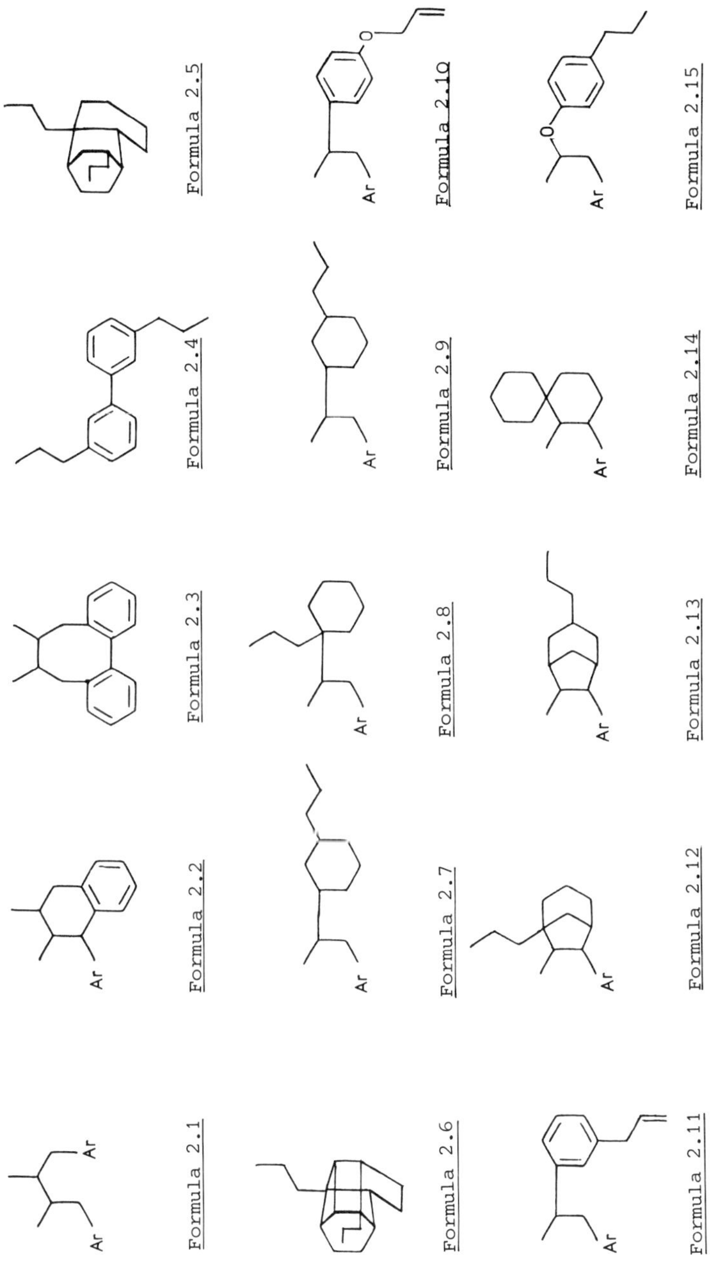

Fig. 2. Carbon skeleta of dimeric lignoids (Formulas 2.9, 2.10 and 2.11 possibly formed by rearrangement of Formula 2.8; in this and the subsequent Figures, Ar stands for one or more phenyls substituted by 4-OH; 4-OMe; 3,4-diOH; 4-OH-3-OMe; 3,4-diOMe; 3,4-O_2CH_2; 2,4-diOH; 4-OH-2-OMe; 3,4,5-triOMe; or 3-OMe-4,5-O_2CH_2 groups)

B. Benzofuranoid Neolignans

I. Di- and Tetrahydrobenzofurans

Work concerning a series of benzofuran neolignans (14, 48) will not be considered.

The constitutional proposals for the di-, tetra- and hexa-hydrobenzofuran neolignans (Formulas 2.7 - 2.11) were deduced by spectral means (3, 4, 7, 8, 12, 15, 24, 32), and for some 2,3-trans-dihydrobenzofurans (Formulas 3.2, 3.4) confirmed by synthesis involving the abnormal Claisen rearrangement of potential cinnamyl aryl ethers (Formulas 3.1, 3.3) (5). Only the arguments which led to their absolute configuration will be discussed in the present lecture (31).

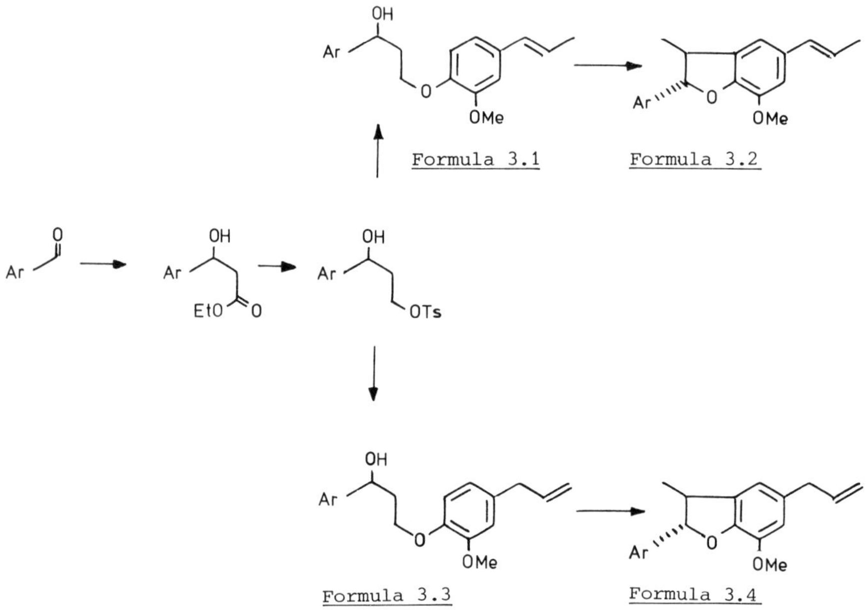

Formula 3.1 Formula 3.2 Formula 3.3 Formula 3.4

Fig. 3. Synthesis of 2,3-trans-dihydrobenzofuran neolignans

The relative configurations of the 2,3-bonds were established by ^{1}H NMR, substitution by Ar/Me trans (as in Formulas 4.1 - 4.5) and cis (as in Formula 4.6) leading to ^{1}H Me-resonances respectively < 9.1 and > 9.1 τ. Conformation of the heterocycles were revealed by $J_{H-2,H-3}$. In the 2,3-trans-dihydrobenzofuranoids (Formulas 4.1 and 4.2), the 3-$^{13}CH_3$ resonates at δ16-17. Hence, not only the 2-Ar, but also the 3a-OMe of 4.3, do not contribute a significant γ-effect on 3-Me; in opposition to the 3a-substituents of 4.4 and 4.5 (3-$^{13}CH_3$ δ7-8). In view of the reciprocity of the γ-effect, the α-methylene of the allyl group of 4.5 is shielded by 7 ppm, in contrast with the same group of 4.6. In compounds of this 2,3-cis-dihydrobenzofuranoid series, however, the 2-Ar induces a γ-effect of the 3-Me (3-$^{13}CH_3$ δ12) (57). The relative configuration at C-5 of compounds of Formula 4.2, however, is not amenable to analysis by ^{13}C NMR, and was established jointly with the absolute configuration of all chiral centers by the following sequence of arguments.

The absolute configurations of the 2S,3S (Formulas 5.1 - 5.3) and 2R,3R (Formula 5.4) groups of trans-dihydrobenzofuran neolignans were deduced by correlations with representatives of established structure by ORD curves. The cis-dihydrobenzofuran neolignans (Formulas 5.5, 5.6) and the 2R,3R-derivatives (Formula 5.4) show identically

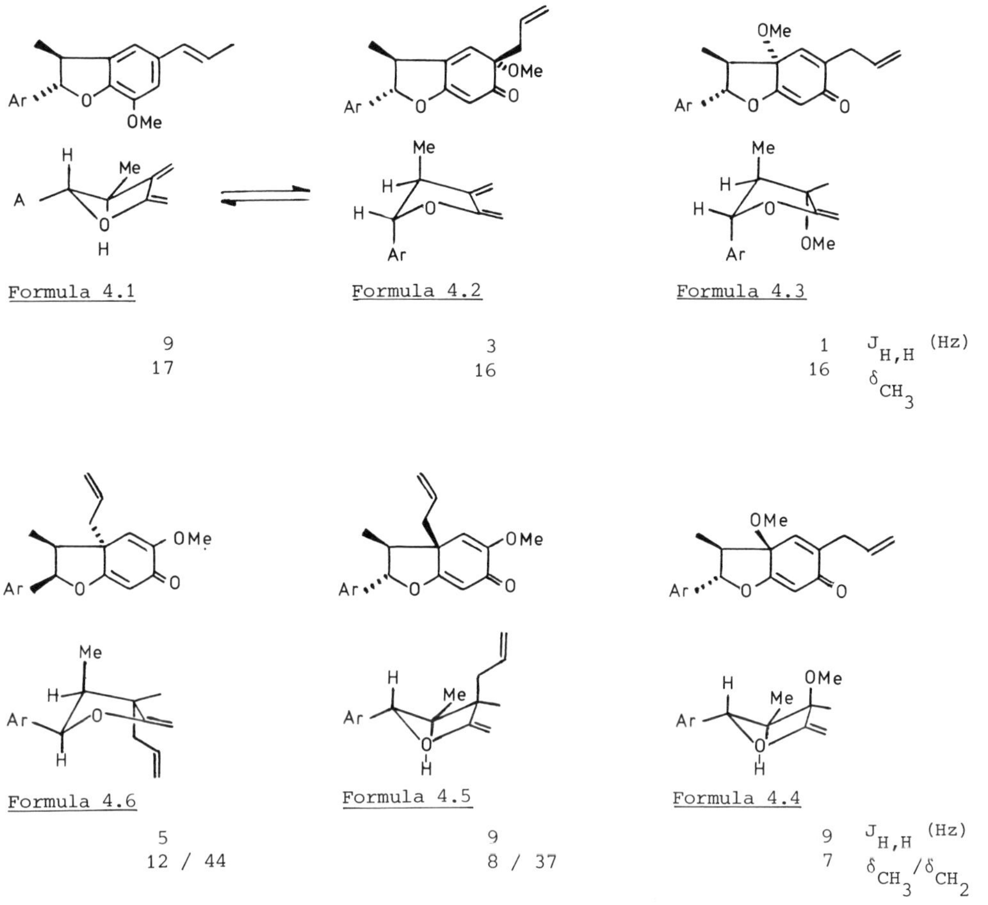

Fig. 4. Conformational and configurational analysis of di- and tetrahydrobenzofuran neolignans by ^{1}H and ^{13}C NMR spectroscopy

directed Cotton effects and thus both support the 2-aryl chromophores in identical configuration. It is consequently to be expected that isomerization by acid of products of Formula 5.5 should lead to products of Formula 5.2 and this was indeed observed (11).

At this stage, thus, the absolute configurations of compound types 6.1 - 6.3 and 6.10 - 6.12 and the relative configurations of compounds with the 3 vicinal chiral centers 2,3,3a (Formulas 6.4 - 6.9) were known. The hydrogenolytic (12), pyrolytic (4,8) and photolytic (8) interconversions featured in Fig. 6 allow, consequently, assignment of absolute stereochemistry to Formulas 6.4, 6.7 - 6.9. The Cotton effects related to the aryl (295 nm) and dienone (260 nm) chromophores of representatives of these types were analyzed and subsequently used in the assignment of absolute stereochemistry to compounds of series Formula 6.5 and 6.6 without recourse to chemical interconversions.

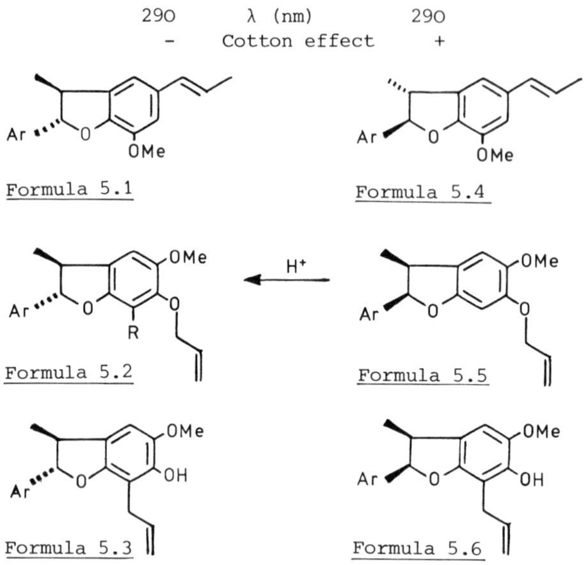

Fig. 5. Configurational analysis of 2,3-dihydro-benzofuran neolignans by ORD

The absolute configuration of the heterocycles of compounds of series 7.5 were again deduced by pyrolytic conversion to 2,3-dihydrobenzofurans (Formulas 7.2, 7.3) of established stereochemistry (4). The Cotton effect related to the aryl chromophore (280 nm) of compounds of Formula 7.5 was analyzed and subsequently used in the assignment of absolute stereochemistry at C-2 of compounds of series 7.4 and 7.6. The stage was thus set for the solution of the problem concerning the chirality at C-5 of compounds belonging to series 7.4 - 7.6. Indeed, the absolute stereochemistry of compounds of Formulas 7.1 and 7.7 being known, their thermal Cope rearrangement products, which must originate by suprafacial allyl migration, can only be represented, respectively, as shown in Formulas 7.4 and 7.6 (6, 11) and again, the Cotton effects related to the dienone chromophore (315 nm) of 7.4 and 7.6 was analyzed and subsequently used in the assignment of the absolute stereochemistry at C-5 of compounds of Formula 7.5.

The NMR shift reagent $Pr(fod)_3$ associates strongly with carbonyls. It was hoped, therefore, that the relative geometry of the substituents around the CO-group of the oxo-tetrahydrobenzofuran neolignans (Formulas 8.1 - 8.6) might be amenable to confirmation by a LIS study. Indeed, relatively strong Δ values were observed for the OCH_3-5 or CH_2-5 signals of compounds of Formulas 8.1 - 8.3 in which OMe or CH_2 and CO are coplaner (Fig. 8). The carbonyl is probably tilted towards the α-face of the molecules, since the Δ values for $CH_2CH{=}CH_2$ and H-2 signals are larger in compounds (Formula 8.3), which have these units on this face, than in compounds (Formula 8.1), which sustain these units on the β-face. This is clearly also the case with respect to H-2 for compounds of Formulas 8.4 and 8.6. In compounds of these series, the relative configuration of methoxyl and allyl at C-5 does not seem to cause differential shifts of other signals which conform to expectation (31).

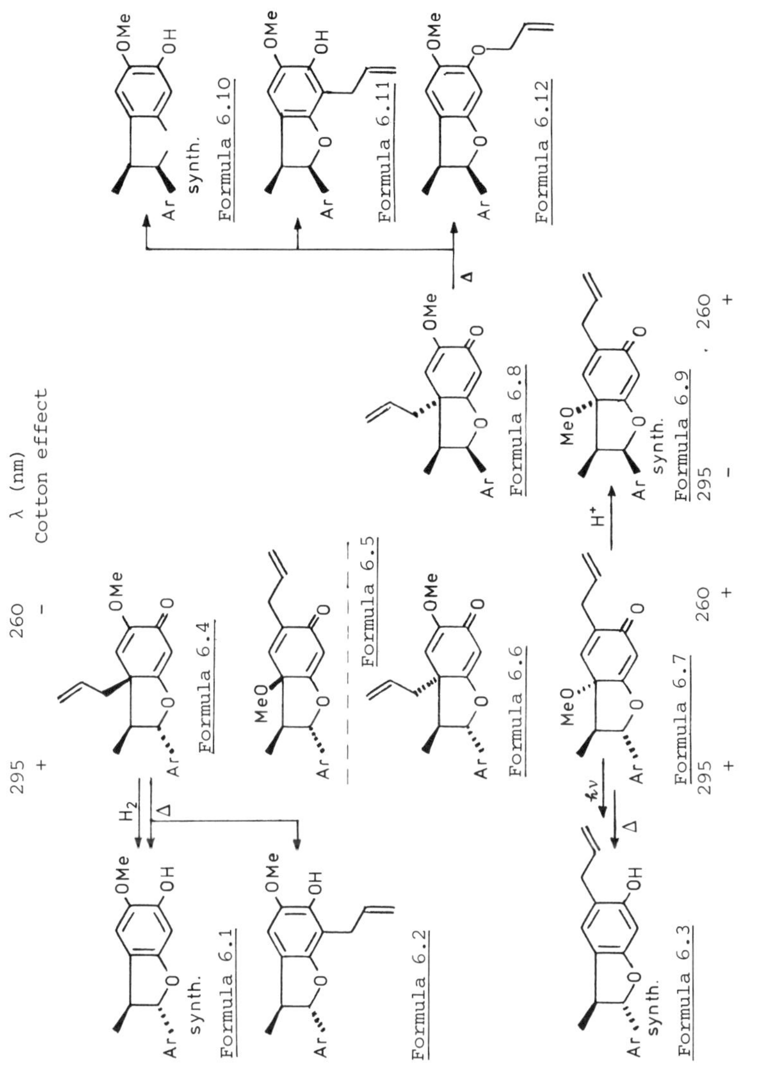

Fig. 6. Configurational analysis of 2,3,3a,6-tetrahydro-6-ozobenzofuran neolignans by ORD

II. Hexahydrobenzofurans

The original structural proposal (Formula 9.1) for porosin was based on ^{1}H NMR and MS evidence, as well as biogenetic reasoning (2). All ^{1}H NMR data are, however, equally interpretable on grounds of structure (Formula 9.2) in which the oxymethine hydrogen, assigned to C-7a in Formula 9.1, occupies C-5. Indeed $Pr(fod)_3$ ^{1}H NMR shifts are relatively feeble in the case of porosin, and, thus, incompatible with the existence of the planar CH=C.OMe.CO.

Further evidence for the validity of structure (Formula 9.2) for porosin was obtained by indirect and direct UV evidence. The indirect method relied on the argument that elimination of a methoxyl from a double bond of an α,β-unsaturated carbonyl system (such as in Formula 9.1) would modify the UV absorption, while removal of the methoxyl from

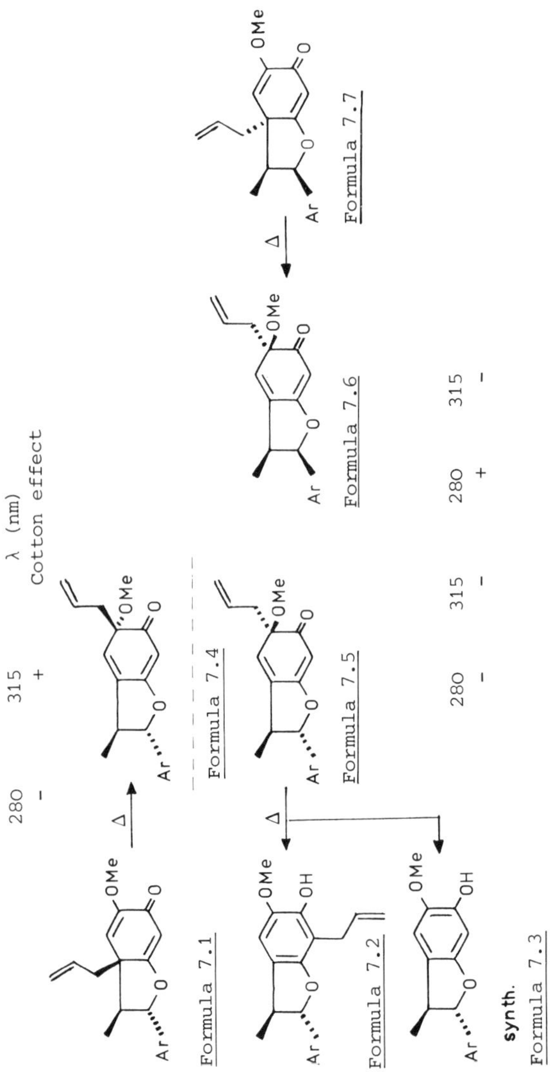

Fig. 7. Configurational analysis of 2,3,5,6-tetrahydro-6-oxobenzofuran neolignans by ORD

a saturated C should not modify the chromophore of Formula 9.2; and, indeed, the UV spectra of porosin (Formula 9.2) and of its photoproduct (Formula 9.4) were found to be superimposable.

The direct method relied on UV spectra of model compounds (Formulas 10.1, 10.2 and 10.3). The addition curve for 10.1 and 10.2, and not for 10.1 and 10.3, proved to be close to the spectrum of porosin, which, thus, must possess the constitution shown in Formula 10.2 and not in Formula 10.1 (10). Porosin is easily oxidized to 9.3 and hence possesses the 2,3-cis geometry.

Having the furanoid substituents in the same configuration as the already discussed compounds of Formula 11.1, porosin is restricted to the conformation of Formula 11.2. The axiality of H-5 (J 5 and 12 Hz) induces a γ-effect on the methylene C, which is absent from compounds of Formula 11.1 (57).

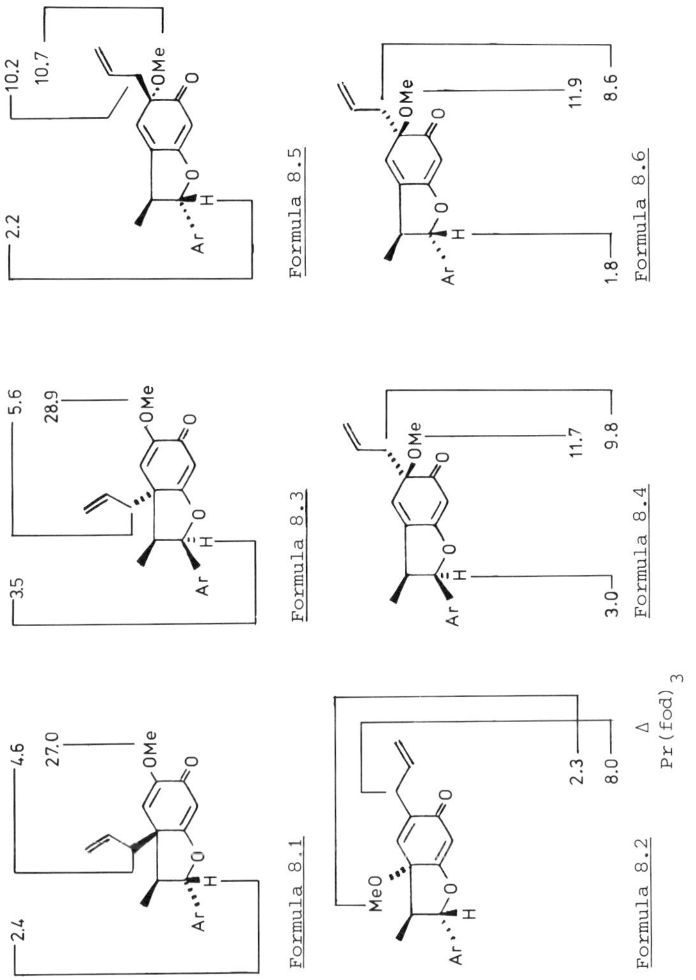

Fig. 8. Ccnfigurational analysis of 2,3,3a,6- and 2,3,5,6-tetrahydro-6-oxobenzofuran neolignans by LIS of ^{1}H NMR signals (Δ values in ppm obtained by graphic extrapolation of experimental shifts to 1:1 $Pr(fod)_3$ - substrate ratio)

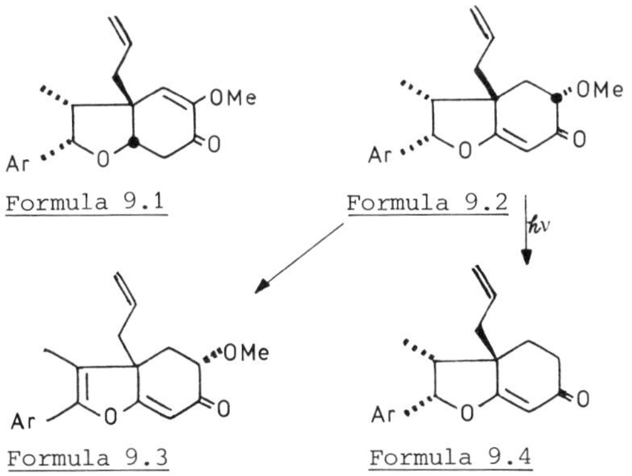

Fig. 9. Structure and reactions of the 2,3,3a,4,5,6-hexahydro-6-oxobenzofuran neolignan porosin (Formula 9.2)

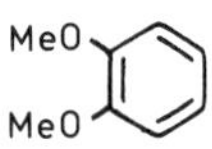

Formula 10.1

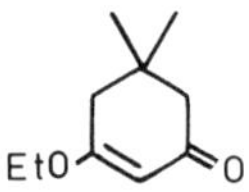

Formula 10.2

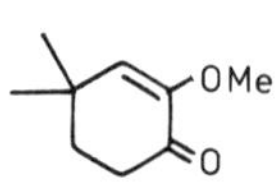

Formula 10.3

Fig. 10. Model compounds (Formulas 10.1, 10.2, 10.3) for the construction of UV absorption spectra of Formulas 9.1 and 9.2 (porosin)

Work on canellin-B (26) and other neolignans of the porosin type (9) is in progress.

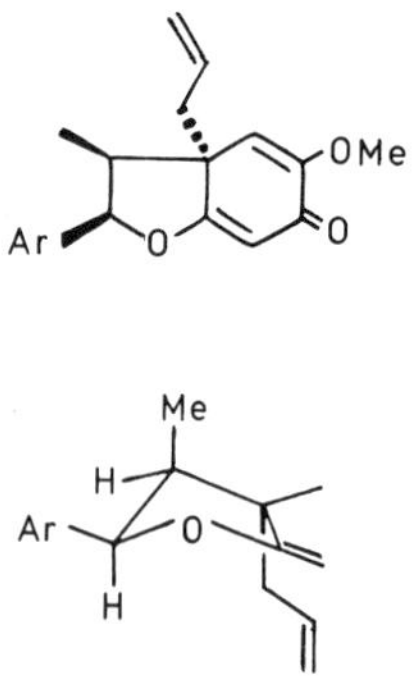

Formula 11.1

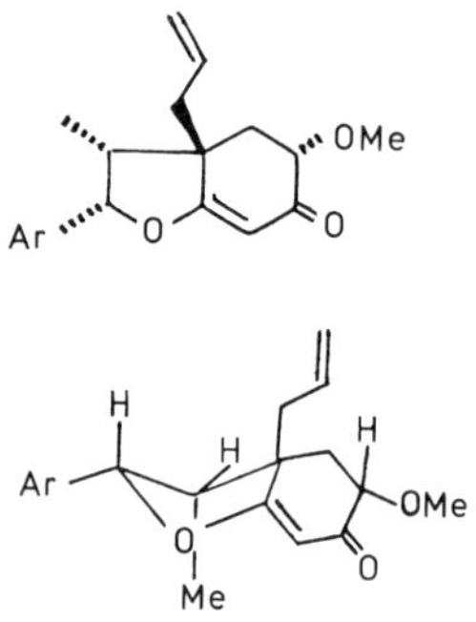

Formula 11.2

Formula 11.1	Formula 11.2	
5	5	$J_{H,H}$ (Hz)
12 / 44	12 / 39	$\delta_{CH_3}/\delta_{CH_2}$

Fig. 11. Conformational and configurational analysis of the 2,3,3a,4,5,6-hexahydro-6-oxobenzofuran neolignan porosin (Formula 11.2)

C. Benzodioxane and Other Neolignans

Structural proposals for eusiderin were based mainly on recognition that no phenolic degradation products were observed other than pyrogallol derivatives. Thus under demethylation conditions the dihydroderivative gave 5-n-propylpyrogallol, indicating that eusiderin arises from the oxidative coupling through oxygen of two C_6-C_3 phenols. Since, however, a series of attempted additional classical reactions were either without effect on eusiderin or yielded impurifiable products, no decision was possible among two benzodioxane alternatives (Formulas 12.2, 12.3) and even the isomeric structure of Formula 12.1 was stated to possess all the observed attributes of eusiderin (35).

Reexamination of this problem by modern spectrometric techniques invalidated any but the benzodioxane formulae (30), Formula 12.3 constituting the favored alternative upon consideration of biosynthetic mechanism (28, 42) and a biogenetically patterned, but not unambiguous, synthesis (Formulas 12.4 and 12.5) of the racemate (42). This postulate was confirmed by a study of the ^1H NMR spectral behavior of eusiderin (Formula 12.3) and eusiderin-B (Formula 12.6) in presence of $Pr(fod)_3$ (17).

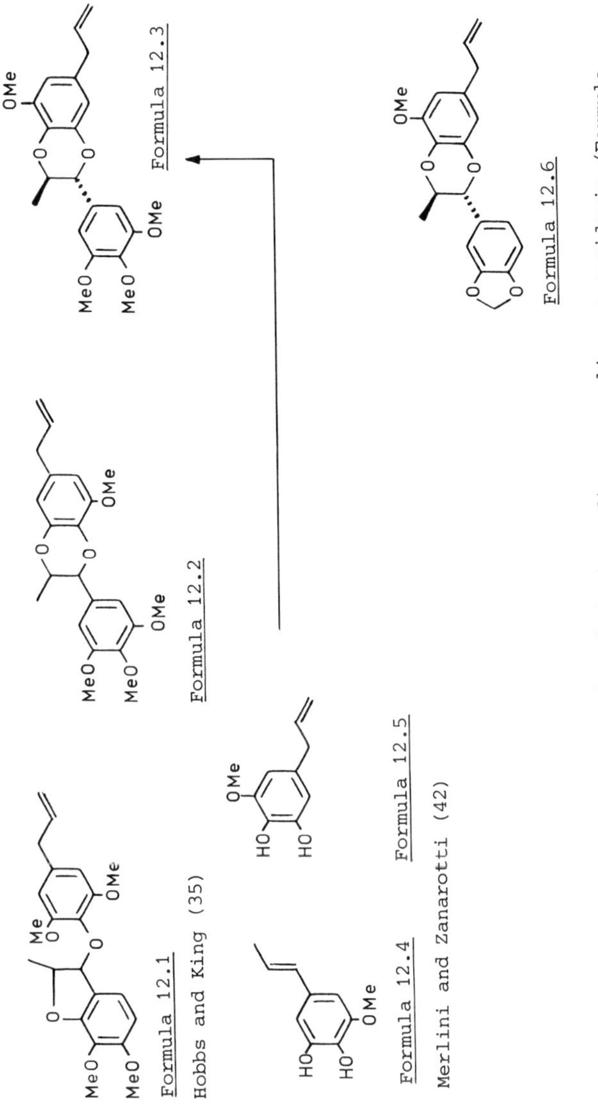

Fig. 12. Constitutions and synthesis of the benzodioxane neolignans eusiderin (Formula 12.3) and eusiderin-B (Formula 12.6)

Isolated aromatic ethers associate only weakly with this NMR shift reagent. The same occurs with ortho diethers in which the oxy-functions are part of an additional ring (e.g. in methylenedioxybenzene and benzodioxane), unless an OR group substitutes at least one of the vicinal positions. Ortho di- and triethers associate strongly with the reagent.

These facts lend significance to LIS data concerning eusiderin-B (Formula 13.2). Coordination with Pr affects H-2 (Δ 9.2 ppm) less strongly than H-3 (Δ 19.2 ppm), and the methoxyl must, thus, be located closer to the latter site and not to the former. Structure 13.2 for eusiderin-B was corroborated examining LIS data for licarin-B (Formula 13.4) (3). Here the Δvalues for H-2 (12.0 ppm) and H-3 (6.2 ppm) show, as expected, that the methoxyl is closer to the former site. While absolute Δvalues are not as useful in such correlations as calculated percentual values (Fig. 13), they indicate that the complexation ratio in 13.2 (Δ_{OMe} 16.2 ppm) is higher than in 13.4 (Δ_{OMe} 10.9 ppm) by a factor of 1.5. Turning to the case of eusiderin (Formula 13.1), the complexation ratio at the oxy-methoxy site (Δ_{OMe} 4.6 ppm) is also higher than in licarin-C (Formula 13.3) (7) (Δ_{OMe} 3.0 ppm), and again by a factor of 1.5. Since this phenomenon is here as clearly linked to differential steric hindrance at the coordination site as it was in the case of 13.2 vs. 13.4, only Formula 13.1 can represent correctly the structure of eusiderin.

4.6	5.6	6.0	4.6	2.4	2.0	OBS.	0.9	4.8	2.8	3.0	1.8	0.8
4.1	4.0	4.8	-	-	1.0	COR.	0.4	3.2	1.4	-	-	-
89	87	104	100	52	22	%	13	107	47	100	60	27

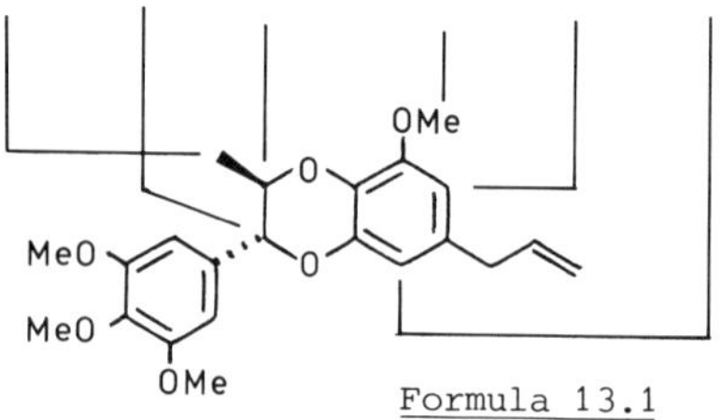

Formula 13.1

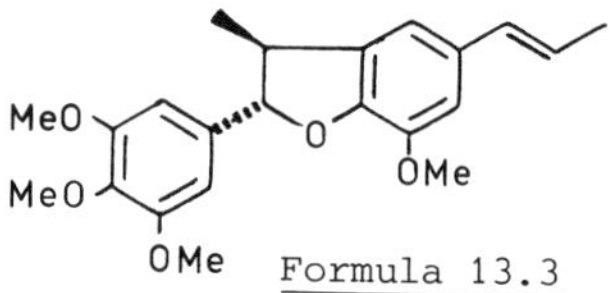

Formula 13.3

16.6	9.2	19.2	16.2	8.8	3.6	OBS.	1.6	12.0	6.2	10.9	6.6	2.5
-	-	-	-	-	-	COR.	-	-	-	-	-	-
102	57	119	100	54	22	%	15	110	57	100	61	23

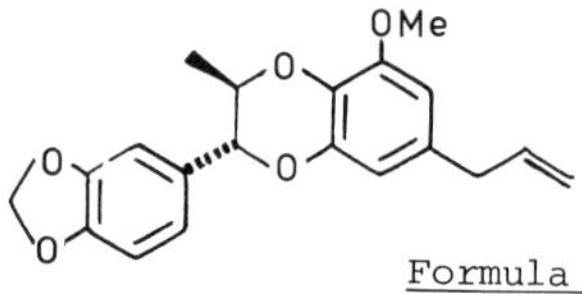

Formula 13.2

Δ
$Pr(fod)_3$

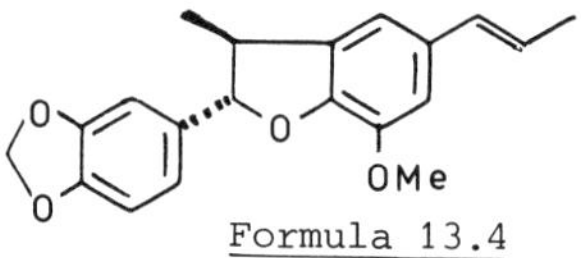

Formula 13.4

Fig. 13. Structural analysis of benzodioxane neolignans eusiderin (Formula 13.1) and eusiderin-B (Formula 13.2) by LIS of ^1H NMR signals (Observed Δ values in ppm obtained by graphic extrapolation of experimental shifts to 1:1 $Pr(fod)_3$ - substrate ratio; Corrected Δ values in ppm (and in % relative to Δ_{OMe}) calculated by subtraction of the increment due to Pr-coordination at the trimethoxy site gauged on model compounds)

The trans-arrangement of the substituents at C-2 and C-3 of the eusiderins was consistent with ^1H NMR data (30) and inferred through the ^{13}C NMR spectrum. This showed, in comparison with model neolignan spectra, that Me-3 must be beyond the nonbonded interaction range of the Ar-2 substituent (57).

The structural determination of surinamensin (Formula 14.4) relied on ^1H and ^{13}C NMR evidence. The reaction of α-bromo-3,4,5-trimethoxypropiophenone (Formula 14.1) with sodium isoeugenolate (Formula 14.2) and $NaBH_4$ reduction of the resulting product (Formula 14.3) led to a mixture of threo- and erythro- compounds, the former predominating in surinamensin (13).

The structure of aurein (Formula 14.5) was deduced from MS, ^{1}H NMR (30) and ^{13}C NMR (57) data. It shows an O-allyl which is easily cleaved by pyrolysis (to 14.6) and acid treatment (to 14.7). The former reaction is relevant, since loss of the allyl group demonstrates that the ortho and para positions relative to the O-allyl group are substituted (30).

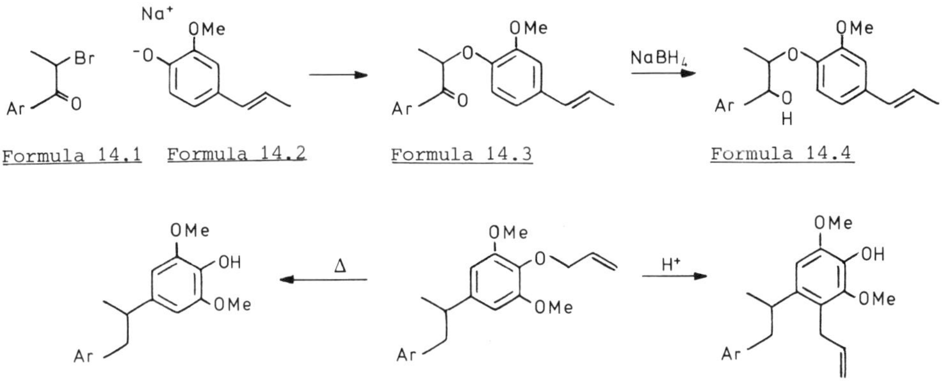

Formula 14.1 Formula 14.2 Formula 14.3 Formula 14.4

Formula 14.6 Formula 14.5 Formula 14.7

Fig. 14. Synthesis of surinamensin (Formula 14.4); reactions of aurein (Formula 14.5)

D. Bicyclo [3,2,1]octanoid Neolignans

The existence of bicyclo [3,2,1]octanoid neolignans was recognized through the isolation of guianin (Formula 15.5) (18), whose gross structural features were ascertained by MS. Guianin is cleaved cleanly into two C_{10}-fragments. The structural moieties responsible for the generation of these ions were formulated on grounds of IR and ^{1}H NMR spectra.

The orientation of the hydroxyl towards the pentacycle became evident upon consideration of ^{1}H NMR coupling and dihedral angle involving the CHOH-CH system. Since this hydroxyl is easily acetylated at room temperature (Formulas 16.1 $\longrightarrow$ 16.2) and addition of hydrogen on the β-side of the molecule is favored, the voluminous aryl group should be located on the endo-face.

The structural proposals for 15.1 and 15.2 were based on spectral data and conversion of 15.1 to 15.2 by Bi_2O_3. It was anticipated that 15.3, the methyl ether of 15.2, should be of the guianin (Formula 15.5) type. Comparison of IR and ^{1}H NMR spectra (in $CDCl_3$), as well as of ORD curves, showed that this was not the case. The conspicuous spectral differences (e.g. H-2: Formulas 15.3 τ 4.33, 15.5 τ 3.90) were interpreted in terms of configurational disparity. Indeed, C_5D_5N-induced solvent shifts, though identical for the common cyclohexenone parts of the molecules, are stronger for H-6 and Me-7 when they are exo situated, as is known for 15.5, than when they are endo situated, as in 15.3.

The ORD curves of 15.3 and 15.4 (negative Cotton effects) and of 15.5 and 15.6 (positive Cotton effects) were antipodal in the region of absorption of the α,β-unsaturated carbonyl chromophore (325 nm) and thus indicate opposite stereochemistries at the bridgeheads. The absolute configurations of compounds are as written, since the major product of acid isomerization of the known tetrahydrobenzofuranoid neolignan of Formula 15.7 is identical, inclusively by m.m.p.and ORD, with 15.4, the oxidation product of 15.3 (11).

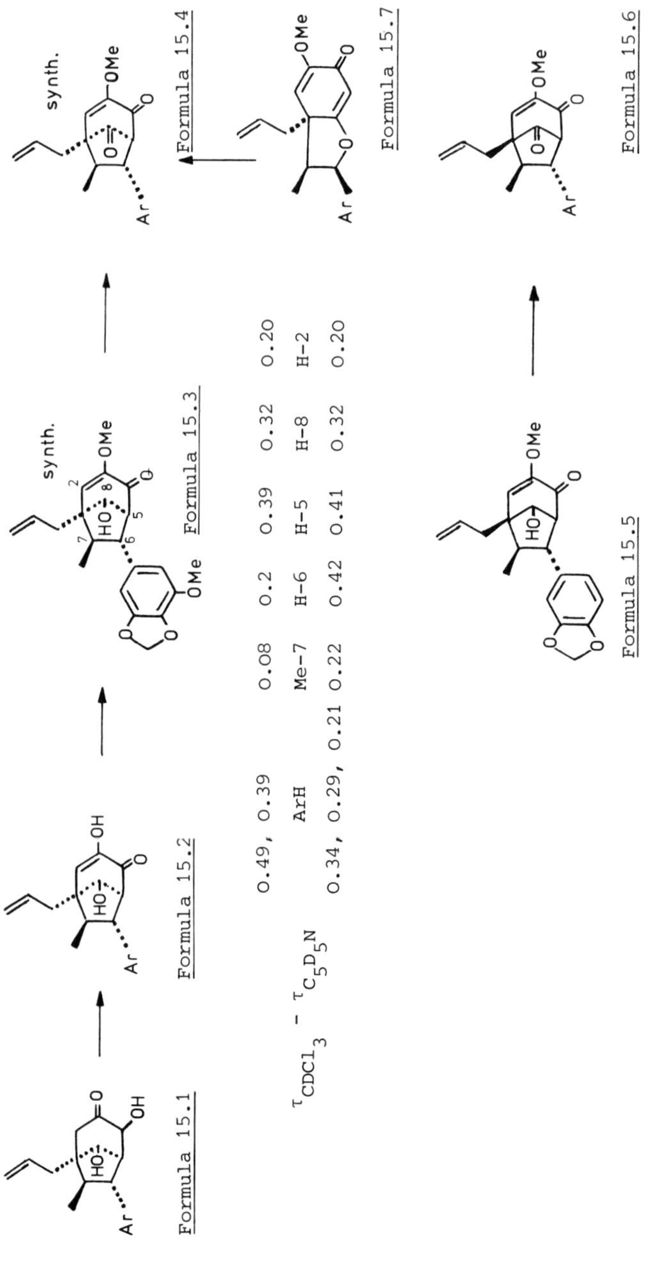

$\tau_{CDCl_3} - \tau_{C_5D_5N}$	ArH	Me-7	H-6	H-5	H-8	H-2
	0.49, 0.39	0.08	0.2	0.39	0.32	0.20
	0.34, 0.29, 0.21	0.22	0.42	0.41	0.32	0.20

Fig. 15. Reactions and ^{1}H NMR data of the bicycle [3,2,1]octanoid neolignans Formulas 15.1, 15.2 and 15.5 (guianin); conversion of benzofuranoid (Formula 15.7) into bicyclo [3,2,1]octanoid (Formula 15.4) neolignans

Formulation of a structural proposal for macrophyllin (Formula 16.7) met with difficulties. There was no doubt that the aliphatic methoxyls are situated on tetrasubstituted carbons. Since, however, no differential shielding of these groups occurred, due to the endo-arrangement of the aryl group, it was impossible to know in which way the C_3-bridge is connected, and Formula 16.7 is only one of two alternative representations of macrophyllin. Evidence for the endo-arrangement, which requires an exo-methyl ($J_{H-7,H-8}$ 8.7 Hz), was seen in the fact that the hydroxyl is as completely acetylated (Formula 16.8) at room temperature as that of guianin (Formula 16.1) (25). Guianin acetate (Formula 16.2) and the oxidation product (Formula 16.3) are also naturally occurring compounds.

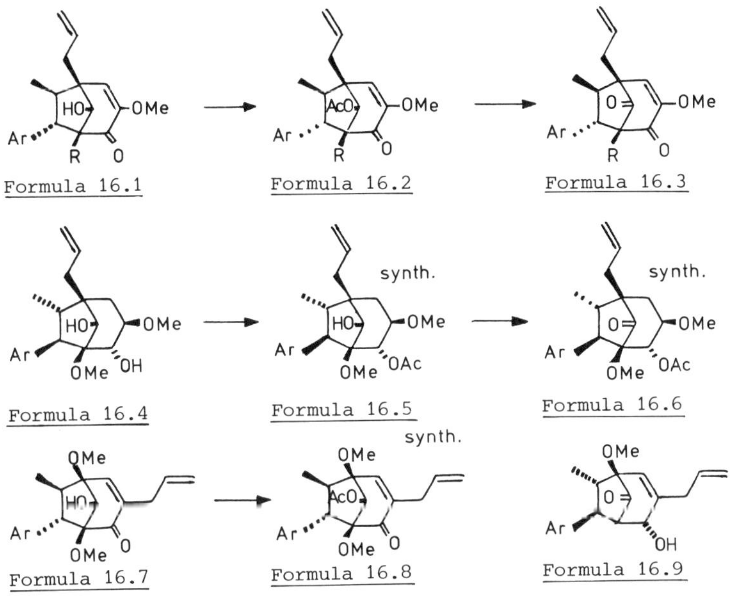

Fig. 16. Reactions of bicyclo [3,2,1] octanoid neolignans Formulas 16.1 (guianin etc.), 16.2, 16.3, 16.4 (canellin-A etc.), 16.7 (macrophyllin) and 16.9 .

Compound 16.9 diverges from macrophyllin not only in aromatic substitution and the lack of an aliphatic methyl, but also by the presence of the carbonyl and carbinol functions at interchanged positions, facts which were deduced by the comparison of IR and ^1H NMR spectra. Doubts about its constitution and configuration were dispelled by allylic oxidation with MnO_2. While this left the CH_3-7, H-7, ArH and OCH_3-1 resonances practically unaffected, the signal due to the benzylic proton suffered a 0.28 ppm diamagnetic shift. The newly introduced carbonyl and H-6 must, thus, be situated at a short distance and on the same side of the molecule (16).

Room temperature acetylation of compounds of the canellin-A type (Formula 16.4) (21, 26) affected only one of the hydroxyls, evidence for the cis relation between the other OH and the aryl groups. Here (Formula 16.4), as in macrophyllin (Formula 16.7), both bridgeheads are tetrasubstituted. Gratifyingly, however, analogous analytical difficulties were not encountered. The monoacetate of canellin-A (Formula 16.5) (26) was oxidized to a five-membered ring ketone (Formula 16.6 , ν_{max} 1760 cm^{-1}). This transformation, featured for dihydro-derivatives (Formulas 17.1 ⟶ 17.2), was accompanied by a stronger ^{1}H NMR paramagnetic shift of one methoxy signal, indicating its correlation to the bridgehead methoxyl. Since in 17.1 it is this same signal which suffers a $CDCl_3/CCl_4$ solvent shift, the bridgehead methoxyl (and not the allyl) is located in the vicinity of the aryl which can be differentially solvated.

Acetylation of the hydroxyl at C-4 of dihydrocanellin-A leaves the ArH and H-7 signals unaffected, but causes significant shifts of the H-6 (Δ -0.40 ppm) and H-3 (Δ - 1.00 ppm) signals. The modified group must thus occupy the endo face of the molecule (Formula 17.1) and, since the proton at C-4 is axial, as shown by its axial-axial interaction (J 6.5 Hz) with the neighboring H-3, the 6-membered ring occurs in the chair conformation. The equatorial conformation of the acetoxyl is consistent with the relative resistance of 17.2 to hydrolysis which requires hot 5 % aq NaOH. The ^{1}H NMR spectrum of the resulting alcohol (Formula 17.3) showed, besides the expected changes, the carbinolic proton signal with an unexpectedly small J (ca. 2 Hz) and the OMe-5 signal at an unexpectedly high field (τ 7.20). These facts probably reflect displacement of OAc through OH. The consequent inversion at C-4 pushes the H-4 into the equatorial position (hence diminishing $J_{H-3,H-4}$) and the methyl over the aryl group (hence increasing τ_{OMe}). Finally, acetylation of the hydroxyl at C-8 of 17.1 shifts the H-7 signal (Δ - 0.29 ppm), but leaves the signals due to the protons of the six-membered ring unaltered. Its orientation towards the five-membered ring is, consequently, indicated. Only in this configuration would it be able to contribute towards the molecular asymmetry sensed by the α and β faces of the aryl group and portrayed by the slight nonequivalence of the methylenedioxy protons (Formula 17.1, AB system, τ4.11 and 4.12). This nonequivalence would be expected to be enhanced through substitution of the C-8 carbinol by a carbonyl and this is indeed the case (Formula 17.2, AB system, τ4.19 and 4.21) (26).

E. Biogenesis of Neolignans

The biogenesis of 124 out of 130 known neolignans can be explained by oxidative coupling of a propenylphenol (Formula 18.1)-derived starter (Formula 18.4 with either propenylphenol (Formula 18.1)-derived or allylphenol (Formula 18.5)-derived termination units (respectively Formulas 18.2, 18.3, 18.4, and 18.6, 18.7, 18.8). Of the remaining six cases, four should involve the coupling of two identical propenylphenol derived (Formula 18.3) or allylphenol derived (Formula 18.7) units, while the biogenesis of asatone (skeletal type Formula 2.5) and isoasatone (skeletal type Formula 2.6) may follow a rather different route, involving an oxidized 4-allyl-2,6-dimethoxyphenol as precursor (49, 59). The relative proneness to oxidation of propenylphenols is to be expected in view of the higher stabilization of the derived radical. Indeed, stability of reactive species and number of neolignans it generates, as well as their natural distribution, seem to correlate quite well (Fig. 18).

As originally postulated by Erdtman (23, 28), the coupling step should produce quinone methide intermediates (Formulas 19.11, 19.15) which may add water, hydroxyl, hydride or carbanion. The coupling step appears to be fairly selective for a family (Fig. 18). The follow-

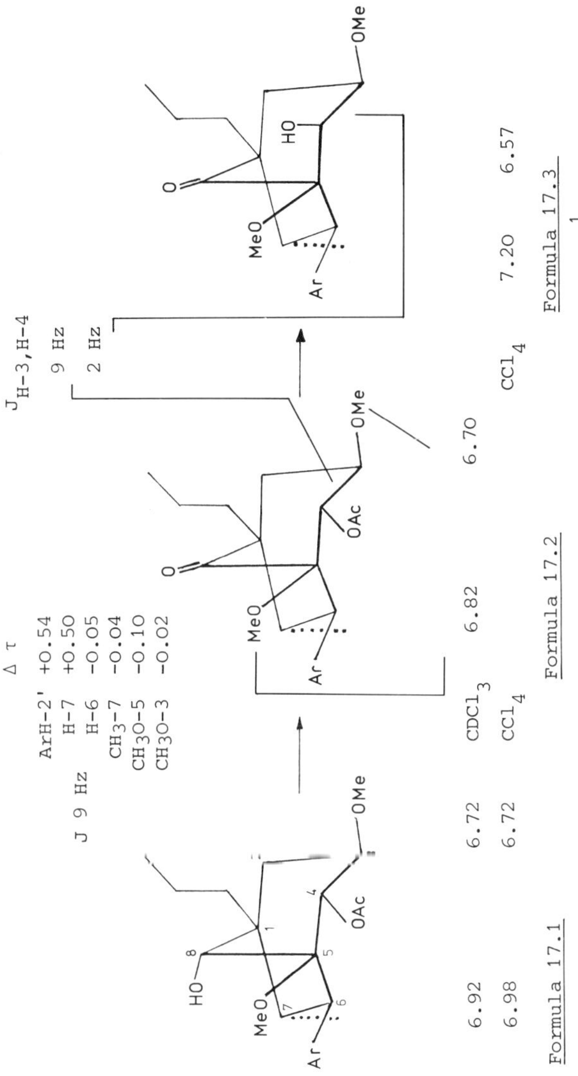

Fig. 17. Configurational analysis of dihydrocanellin-A derivatives by ^{1}H NMR spectroscopy

ing-up steps are of general occurrence, e.g. attack of hydroxyl leads to hydrocoumarans in *Aniba* (Formula 19.12 etc.) and *Nectandra* (Formula 19.16) and to bicycloöctanoids in *Aniba* (Formula 19.10 etc.) and *Nectandra* (Formula 19.14 etc.). The pathway 19.15 → 19.16 → 19.4 seems, thus, to be a more plausible route than 19.11 → 19.12 → 19.8 → 19.4 to this constituent (Formula 19.4) of *Nectandra miranda* (8). The allylic rearrangement of the methoxyl involved in the step 19.16 → 19.4, however, was not achieved in vitro by pyrolysis, in contradistinction to the transposition of the allyl group required in 19.8 → 19.4 which proceeds with ease (6, 11).

In vitro analogies and cooccurrences thus led to the postulate that compounds belonging to type 19.8 are responsible for the biosynthesis of the representatives of types 19.4, 19.3, 19,2 and 19.1 by successive

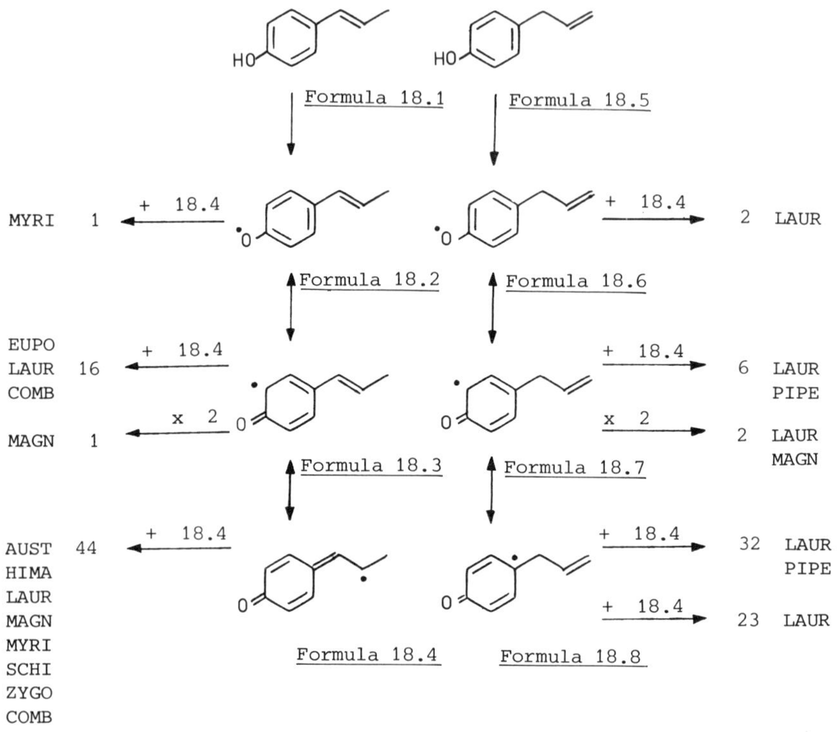

Fig. 18. Biogenetic routes to the indicated number of neolignans isolated from families of the Magnoliidae (Austrobaileyaceae, Eupomatiaceae, Himantandraceae, Lauraceae, Magnoliaceae, Myristicaceae, Piperaceae, Schizandraceae) and Rosidae (Combretaceae, Zygophyllaceae)

Cope, retro-Claisen and Claisen rearrangements and dehydrogenation (4). Such rearrangements, which rationalize also the biogenesis of aurein (Formulas 20.1 → 20.2) (30), recall the dienone-phenol rearrangement (Formulas 20.3 → 20.4) to thyroxin (20) during which, however, the C_3-substituent is lost.

F. Conclusion

Structural variation and chemical reactivity make the neolignans a most interesting group of natural products from the standpoint of potential biological activity. Is the list of skeletal variants, which includes additionally Formulas 2.4 (22), 2.5 (59), 2.6 (49) and 2.14 (45) not illustrated in this lecture and their derivatives, nearing completion?

Many neolignans are difficult to crystallize and their isolation from plant extracts is very tedious. It is possible, consequently, that they have been frequently overlooked in fractionation work. This kind of difficulty will presumably accrue with increasing molecular weight of the products. Clearly, however, oligomeric lignoids, lignans and neolignans, will eventually be isolated from the viscous masses which

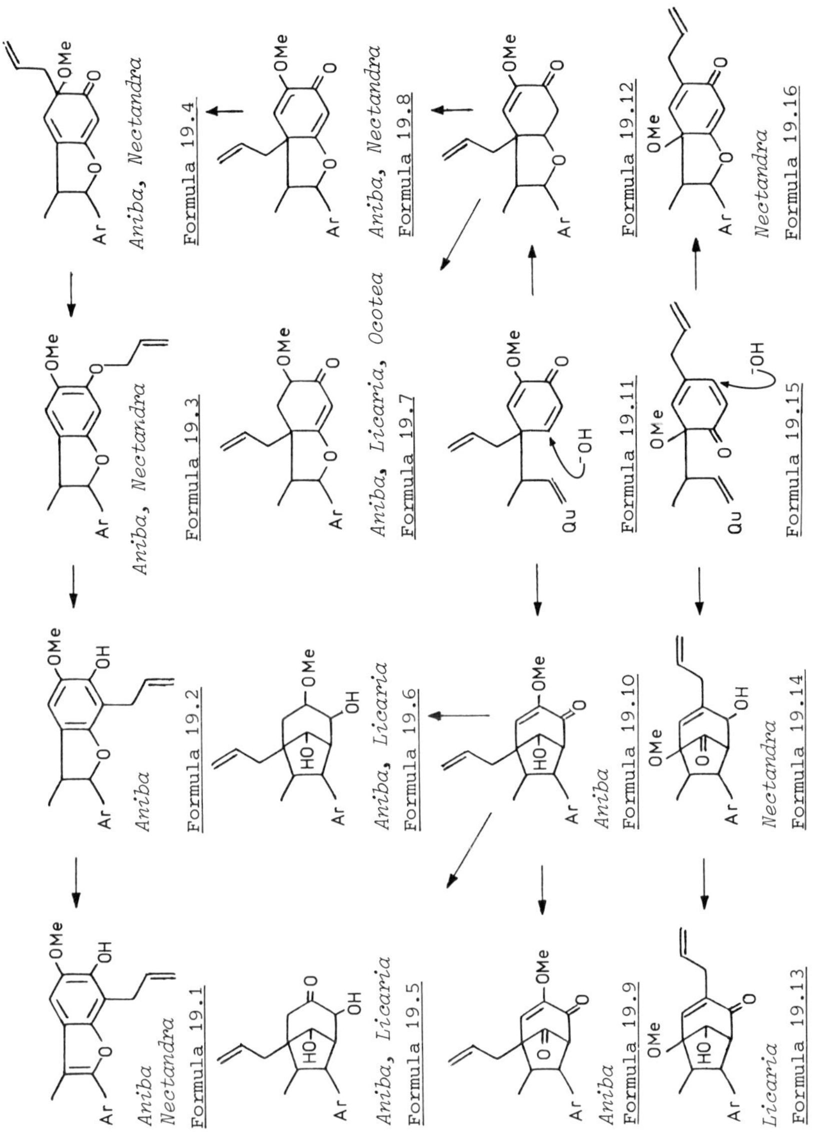

Fig. 19. Biogenetic routes to the benzofuranoid and bicyclo [3,2,1]octanoid neolignans of Lauraceae genera

form large parts of the extractives of tropical woods. Indeed, trimeric and tetrameric lignans have recently been encountered (54). The presently known compounds are thus considered to be merely representative of a domain of natural products chemistry whose delimitations are not yet in sight.

Acknowledgment. This work was sponsored by Fundação de Amparo à Pesquisa do Estado de São Paulo.

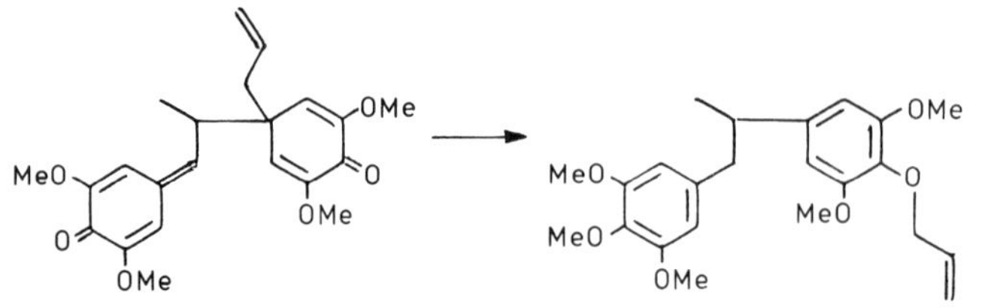

Formula 20.1 Formula 20.2

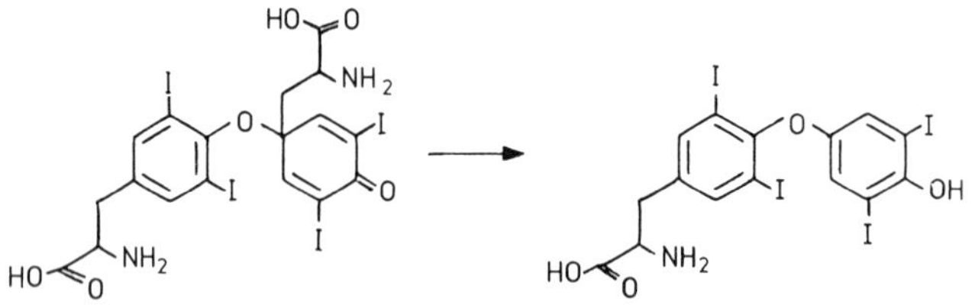

Formula 20.3 Formula 20.4

Fig. 20. Biogenetic routes to aurein (Formula 20.2) and thyroxin (Formula 20.4)

References

1. Adjangba, M.S.: Progrès récents dans la chimie des lignanes. Bull. Soc. Chim. France 1963, 2344
2. Aiba, C.J., Braz, Fo., R., Gottlieb, O.R.: The chemistry of Brazilian Lauraceae. XX. Porosin: a neolignan from *Ocotea porosa*. Phytochemistry 12, 413 (1973)
3. Aiba, C.J., Corrêa, R.G.C., Gottlieb, O.R.: The chemistry of Brazilian Lauraceae. XXII. Natural occurrence of Erdtman's dehydrodiisoeugenol. Phytochemistry 12, 1163 (1973)
4. Aiba, C.J., Fernandes, J.B., Gottlieb, O.R., Maia, J.G.S.: The chemistry of Brazilian Lauraceae. XXX. Neolignans from an *Aniba* species. Phytochemistry 14, 1597 (1975)
5. Aiba, C.J., Gottlieb, O.R.: The chemistry of Brazilian Lauraceae. XXVIII. Synthesis of (±)-licarin-B. Phytochemistry 14, 253 (1975)
6. Aiba, C.J., Gottlieb, O.R., Kamphausen, U., Magalhães, M.T., Yoshida, M.: Unpublished work (1976)
7. Aiba, C.J., Gottlieb, O.R., Pagliosa, F.M., Magalhães, M.T., Yoshida, M.: The chemistry of Brazilian Lauraceae. XXXVII. Neolignans from *Nectandra miranda*. Phytochemistry, in press
8. Aiba, C.J., Gottlieb, O.R., Pagliosa, F.M., Yoshida, M., Rosenstein, R.D., Tomita, K.: Unpublished work (1976)
9. Aiba, C.J., Gottlieb, O.R., Trevisan, L.M.V.: Unpublished work (1976)
10. Aiba, C.J., Gottlieb, O.R., Yoshida, M., Mourão, J.C., Gottlieb, H.E.: The chemistry of Brazilian Lauraceae. XXXV. The structure of porosin. Phytochemistry 15, 1031 (1976)
11. Alvarenga, M.A.de, Castro, C.O., Gottlieb, O.R., Maia, J.G.S.: Unpublished work (1976)
12. Araújo Lima, O., Gottlieb, O.R., Magalhães, M.T.: The chemistry of Brazilian Lauraceae. XX. Burchellin, a neolignan from *Aniba burchellii*. Phytochemistry 11, 2031 (1972)
13. Barata, L.E.S., Baker, P.M., Gottlieb, O.R., Ruveda, E.: Unpublished work (1976)

14. Bowden, B.F., Ritchie, E., Taylor, W.C.: Constituents of *Eupomatia* species. II. Isolation and structure determination of further eupomatenoid lignans from the bark of *Eupomatia laurina*. Australian J. Chem. 25, 2659 (1972)
15. Braz, Fo., R., Andrade, C.H.S., Gottlieb, O.R., Maia, J.G.S.: Unpublished work (1976)
16. Braz, Fo., R., Figliuolo, R., Gottlieb, O.R., Maia, J.G.S.: Unpublished work (1976)
17. Braz Fo., R., Mourão, J.C., Gottlieb, O.R., Maia, J.G.S.: Lanthanide induced shifts as aid in the structural determination of eusiderins. Tetrahedron Lett. 1976, 1157
18. Bülow, M.V. von, Franca, N.C., Gottlieb, O.R., Puentes Suarez, A.M.: The chemistry of Brazilian Lauraceae. XXIV. Guianin: a neolignan from *Aniba guianensis*. Phytochemistry 12, 1805 (1973)
19. Burk, D., Woods, M.: Hydrogen peroxide, catalase, glutathione peroxidase, quinones, nordihydroguaiaretic acid, and phosphopyridine nucleotides in relation to X-ray action on cancer cells. Radiation Res. Suppl. 3, 212 (1963); apud. Chem. Abstr. 59, 1934 (1963)
20. Cahnmann, H.J.: Nonenzymic Model Reactions for the Biosynthesis of the Thyroid Hormones. Annual Report. Osaka: Tanabe Amino Acid Research Foundation, 1971, p. 5
21. Dias, S.M.C., Fernandes, J.B., Gottlieb, O.R., Maia, J.G.S.: Unpublished work (1975)
22. Doskotch, R.W., Flom, M.S.: Acuminatin, a new bis-phenylpropide from *Magnolia acuminata* L. Tetrahedron 28, 4711 (1972)
23. Erdtman, H.: Dehydrierungen in der coniferylreihe. II. Dehydro-di-isoeugenol. Liebigs Ann. Chem. 503, 283 (1933)
24. Fernandes, J.B., Gottlieb, O.R., Maia, J.G.S.: The chemistry of Brazilian Lauraceae. XXXIV. Neolignans from an *Aniba* species. Phytochemistry 15, 1033 (1976)
25. Franca, N.C., Gottlieb, O.R., Maia, J.G.S.: The chemistry of Brazilian Lauraceae. XXVII. Macrophyllin, a neolignan from *Licaria macrophylla*. Phytochemistry 13, 2839 (1974)
26. Giesbrecht, A.M., Franca, N.C., Gottlieb, O.R., Rocha, A.I.: The chemistry of Brazilian Lauraceae. XXVI. The neolignans of *Licaria canella*. Phytochemistry 13, 2285 (1974)
27. Gilchrist, T., Hodges, R., Porte, A.L.: The structure of otobain. J. Chem. Soc. (London) 1962, 1780
28. Gottlieb, O.R.: Chemosystematics of the Lauraceae. Phytochemistry 11, 1537 (1972)
29. Gottlieb, O.R.: Lignans and neolignans. Revista Latinoamericana de Quimica 5, 1 (1974)
30. Gottlieb, O.R., Maia, J.G.S., Mourão, J.C.: The chemistry of Brazilian Lauraceae. XXXVI. Neolignans from a *Licaria* species. Phytochemistry 15, 1289 (1976)
31. Gottlieb, O.R., Mourão, J.C., Yoshida, M.: Unpublished work (1976)
32. Gottlieb, O.R., Silva, M.L. da, Ferreira, Z.S.: The chemistry of Brazilian Lauraceae. XXXI. Neolignans from *Aniba terminalis*. Phytochemistry 14, 1825 (1975)
33. Hartwell, J.L., Schrecker, A.W.: The chemistry of podophyllum. In: Fortschr. Chem. Organ. Naturstoffe. Zechmeister, L. (ed.). Berlin-Heidelberg-New York: Springer, 1958, Vol. XV, p. 83
34. Haworth, R.D.: The chemistry of the lignan group of natural products. J. Chem. Soc. (London) 1942, 448
35. Hobbs, J.J., King, F.E.: The chemistry of extractives from hardwoods. XXIX. Eusiderin, a possible by-product of lignin sythesis in *Eusideroxylon zwageri*. J. Chem. Soc. (London) 1960, 4732
36. Jewers, K., Manchands, A.H., Rose, H.M.: Naturally occurring antitumor agents. In: Progress in Medicinal Chemistry. Ellis, G.P., West, G.B. (eds.). London: Butterworths, 1971, Vol. IX, p. 33
37. Kotchetkov, N.K., Khorlin, A.Ya., Chizhov, O.S.: Chemical study of *Schizandra chinensis*. I. Schizandrin and related compounds. Zhurn. Obshchei Khimii (USSR) 31, 3454 (1961); apud. Chem. Abstr. 57, 3334 (1962)

38. Kotchetkov, N.K., Khorlin, A.Ya., Chizhov, O.S., Sheichenko, V.I.: Schizandrin - lignan of unusual structure. Tetrahedron Lett. 1961, 730
39. Kupchan, M.S., Britton, R.W., Ziegler, M.F., Gilmore, C.J., Restivo, R.J., Bryan, R.F.: Steganacin and steganagin, novel antileukemic lignan lactones from *Steganotaenia araliacea*. J. Am. Chem. Soc. 95, 1335 (1973)
40. Lebedev, A.A., Kamilov, I.K.: Schizandrin pharmacology. Med. Zh. Uzb. 1966 (9), 60; apud Chem. Abstr. 66, 74744 (1967)
41. Matsui, K., Munakata, K.: The structure of piperenone, a new antifeeding substance from *Piper futokadzura*. Tetrahedron Lett. 1975, 1905
42. Merlini, L., Zanarotti, A.: A biogenetically patterned synthesis of (±)-eusiderin. Tetrehedron Lett. 1975, 3621
43. Meyer, W.: *Podophyllum peltatum* - May apple. A potential new cash-crop plant of Eastern North America. Economic Botany 28, 68 (1974)
44. Nasirov, S.Kh., Lebedev, A.A., Ishmukhamedov, N.A., Kamilov, I.K.: Electrophysiological analysis of the schizandrin effect on the central nervous system. Med. Zh. Uzb. 1967 (5), 34; apud Chem. Abstr. 68, 20792 (1968)
45. Ogiso, A., Kurabayashi, M., Mishima, H., Woods, M.C.: The structure of futoenone, a novel spiro-cyclohexadienone derivative. Tetrahedron Lett. 1968, 2003
46. Oliveto, E.P.: Nordihydroguaiaretic acid. A naturally occurring antioxidant. Chem. Ind. 1972, 677
47. Pardini, R.S., Heidker, J.C., Fletcher, D.C.: Inhibition of mitochondrial electron transport by nor-dihydroguaiaretic acid (NDGA). Biochem. Pharmac. 19, 2695 (1970)
48. Picker, K., Ritchie, E., Taylor, W.C.: Constituents of *Eupomatia* species. III. New eupomatenoid lignans from the leaves and wood of *Eupomatia laurina*. Australian J. Chem. 26, 1111 (1973)
49. Sasaki, K., Hirata, Y., Yamamura, S., Chen, Y.-P., Hong, M., Hsu, H.-Y.: The isolation and structure of isoasatone. Tetrahedron Lett. 1973, 4881
50. Shipochliev, T., Ilieva, St.: Pharmacologic study of Bulgarian *Schizandra chinensis*. Farmatsiya (Sofia) 17, 56 (1967); apud Chem. Abstr. 68, 1870 (1968)
51. Stoessel, A.: The antifungal factors in barley - The constitutions of hordatines A and B. Tetrahedron Lett. 1966, 2287
52. Titlyanov, A.A.: Biologically Active Substances of Chinese Magnolia Vine Fruit. Tr. Vses. Semin. Biol. Aktiv. (Lech.) Veshchestvam Plodov Yagod (Edited by L.I. Vigorov, Ural. Lesotekh. Inst., Sverdlovsk, USSR), 3rd ed., p. 363 (1966, publ. 1968); apud Chem. Abstr. 73, 91186 (1970)
53. Volicer, L., Sramka, M., Janku, I., Capek, R., Smetana, R., Ditteova, V.: Some pharmacological effects of *Schizandra chinensis*. Arch. Intern. Pharmacodyn. Ther. 163, 249 (1966); apud Chem. Abstr. 66, 1413 (1967)
54. Wagner, H., Wittmann, D., Schäfer, W.: Zur chemischen Struktur der Lithospermsäure aus *Lithospermum officinale* L. Tetrahedron Lett. 1975, 547
55. Waller, C.W., Gisvold, O.: A phytochemical investigation of *Larrea divaricata* Cav. J. Am. Pharm. Assoc. 34, 78 (1945)
56. Weinges, K.: Über einige neue Lignane und stereochemische Zusammenhänge in der Lignangruppe. Ber. Deut. Chem. Ges. 94, 2522 (1961)
57. Wenkert, E., Gottlieb, H.E., Gottlieb, O.R., Pereira, M.O. da, S., Formiga, M.D.: Carbon-13 nuclear magnetic spectroscopy of naturally occurring substances. XIV. ^{13}C NMR spectroscopy of neolignans. Phytochemistry 15, 1547 (1976)
58. Yamaguchi, K.: Spectral Data of Natural Products. Amsterdam-London-New York: Elsevier, 1970, Vol. I, p. 439
59. Yamamura, S., Terada, Y., Chen, Y.-P., Hsu, H.-Y., Hirata, Y.: Photochemical conversion of asatone to isoasatone. The revised structure of asatone. Tetrahedron Lett. 1975, 1903

Natural Substances with Effects on the Liver

G. VOGEL

Until recently it has been accepted almost as dogma that there was not and could not be any pharmacological treatment for liver diseases. The only drugs used at all were corticosteroids or immunosuppressive agents, sometimes in very high dosage. Now, however, as a result of the discovery of a new group of substances (1, 15, 16, 18, 21, 22, 58 - 62), the flavanolignans - isolated from the milk thistle, *Silybum marianum* - the situation has altered and there is now a substantial body of evidence indicating that the flavanolignans can exert an almost specific influence on the liver parenchyma.

If you refer to the list of pharmaceutical products marketed in Germany and look up the natural substances which are most frequently employed for the treatment of liver disease, in the widest sense of that term, you will find a number of plants, which I will list in alphabetical order: *Aloe, Absinthium officinale, Calamus (Acorus calamus* L.*), Curcuma xanthorrhiza, Cynara scolymus, Foeniculum officinale, Fumaria officinalis, Juniperus communis, Mentha piperita, Silybum marianum* (L.) Gaertn., *Taraxacum officinalis*. In some cases the active principles of these plants are known, but not in others. In my experience the only plant product which has an antihepatotoxic action in the true sense of the word - that is 'A Protective Effect On The Liver' - is the seed of the milk thistle. The seeds contain the flavanolignans silybin, silydianin and silychristin, which are isomers and are lumped together under the collective designation silymarin. The structural formulae of these compounds are shown in Figures 1, 2 and 3.

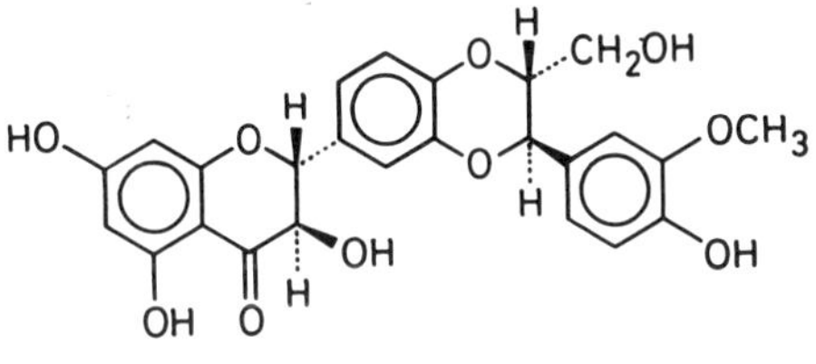

Fig. 1. Structural formula of silybin

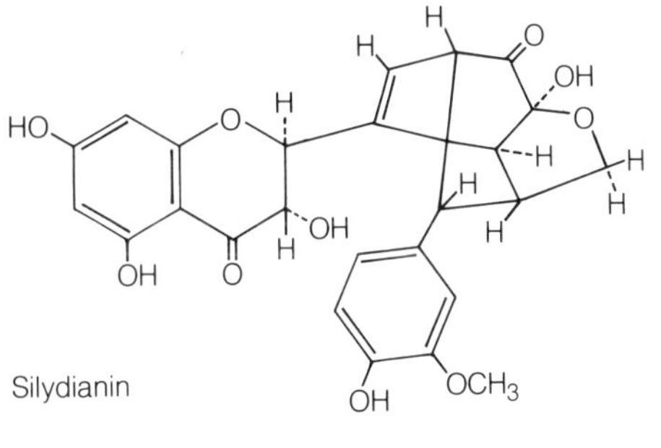

Fig. 2. Structural formula of silydianin

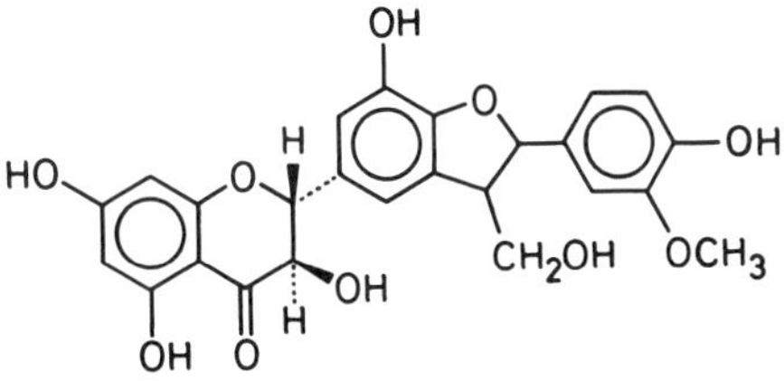

Fig. 3. Structural formula of silychristin

Eighteen years ago, a more or less harmless product for liver diseases under the name "Hepata"® was on the market (Dr. Madaus and Co.). It contained a mixture of imprecisely defined preparations from various plants, among them the milk thistle. Now, throughout its history the company has specialized in pharmaceutical preparations of plant origin and we therefore wanted to know: What is or are the active principles in the milk thistle? Once we know the nature of the active substance our next aim was to produce it in pure form and to market the pure substance as a pharmaceutical product. At first we tackled the problem in a routine way and perhaps rather half heartedly, handicapped as we were by not having any suitable experimental screening tests. We attempted in fact to neutralize the necrosis-inducing effect of allyl alcohol, for which purpose we had to use histological techniques. The main disadvantages of this approach are first the difficulty of quantitatively assessing of the effect, and secondly the fact that one can never be sure that the sample of liver tissue taken for examination is truly representative of the organ as a whole - a difficulty which also arises in connection with needle biopsy of the liver. As already said, we did not make much progress in this work nor indeed in the chemical researches. In 1967 we received a substance isolated by H. Wagner and his co-workers in Munich and we were asked to test it.

At this point I must say something about the screening test which we had adopted in the meantime. What are the requirements of such a screening test if it is to give usable results? First of all, the test must be reasonably quick, so that within the shortest possible time one can apply the test to a large enough number of animals to give statistically valid results. Secondly, the test must be reasonably simple; a test which demands highly qualified staff is no use for our purposes. Thirdly, the test must not be too expensive, because sometimes it will be necessary to test large numbers of substances. Our test - measurement of the hexobarbital sleeping time in rats - met all these requirements. Now, what about its theoretical background? As hexobarbital is metabolized exclusively in the liver, the sleeping time after a given dose is a measure of hepatic metabolism. If there is any preexisting liver damage, associated for example with a reduction in the number of functioning liver cells, or affecting mainly the rough endoplasmic reticulum - the site of the enzyme system which breaks down foreign substances - the sleeping time after a given dose of hexobarbital will be prolonged, because the amount of the hypnotic broken down in unit time will be less. This is the case, for example, after poisoning with carbon tetrachloride. Now, if the rats, besides being poisoned with carbon tetrachloride, are also treated with an antihepatotoxic substance, the sleeping-time-prolonging effect of the carbon tetrachloride will be neutralized, in other words, the sleeping-time will shorten again, and will be restored wholly or partially to normal (see Fig. 4).

The substance from Wagner's laboratory proved effective when tested in this way, and gave consistent results when the test was repeated several times. We then went on to make a further experiment. Paraoxyphenyl pyruvic acid (pOPh) is metabolized exclusively in the liver. In animals with liver damage - induced for example with CCl_4 - an increased percentage of a given dose of pOPh is excreted unchanged in the urine. Treatment of the rats with the milk thistle preparation induced a state in which it was as if they had received no carbon tetrachloride at all. In this test also, therefore, the new substance had a 100 % neutralizing effect on carbon tetrachloride intoxications (14).

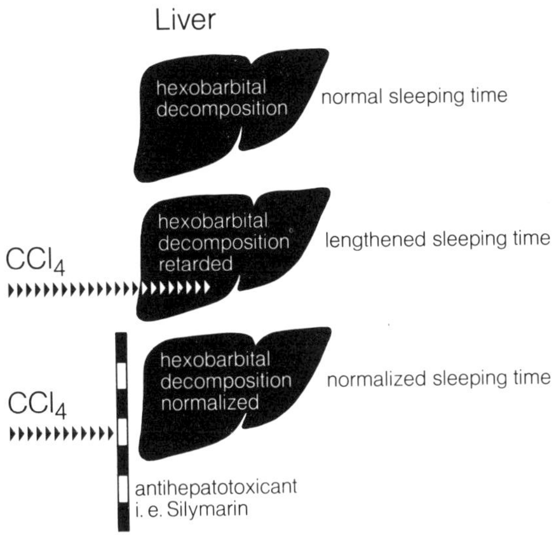

Fig. 4. Hexobarbital sleeping time as a parameter for the determination of the effectiveness of antihepatotoxic substances. The administration of hepatotoxic substances e.g. CCl_4 prolongs hexobarbital sleeping time due to a reduction in the ability of the liver to metabolize barbiturates. Antihepatotoxic substances e.g. silymarin prevent this prolongation of sleeping time

Yet another experiment: long-term administration of thioacetamide (TAA) to rats in their food produces a liver lesion which histologically resembles hepatic cirrhosis. Over the course of three to four months the rats lose weight drastically and, if untreated, 90 to 100 % of them die. Concurrent long-term treatment with the test substance prevented weight loss, the effect being dose-dependent, and greatly reduced mortality (14).

When we had obtained these results, we decided to test this substance we have named silymarin, against the most potent known liver poisons. These are the amatoxins, phalloidine (Fig. 5) and α-amanitine (Fig. 6) from the death-cap toadstool *Amanita phalloides*. The

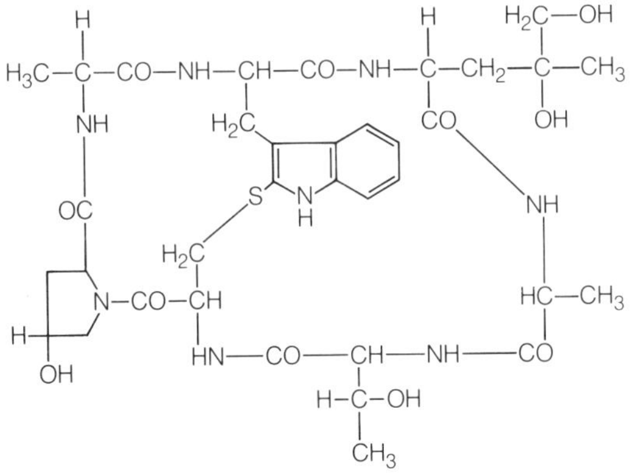

Fig. 5. Structural formula of phalloidine

only one who could provide these toxins was at that time Professor Th. Wieland, organic chemist on the University of Frankfurt am Main (now Heidelberg). He gave me a few milligrams of phalloidine and α-amanitine. In the ensuing experiments we showed that silymarin probably antagonized α-amanitine poisoning, but because so little of the toxin was available we were unable to settle this point beyond doubt. Phalloidine poisoning in mice, on the other hand, was undoubtedly counteracted by silymarin, either when given prophylactically or

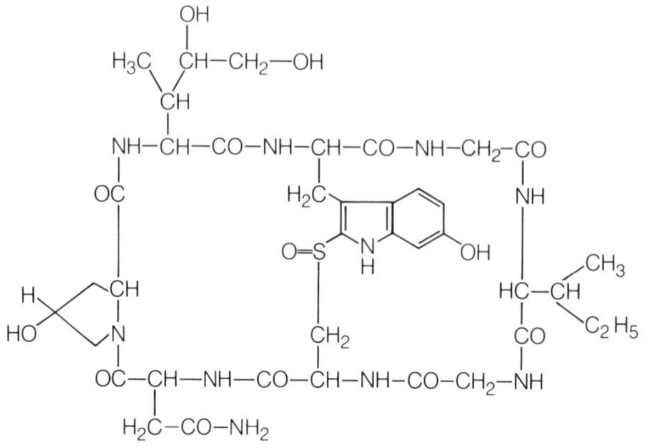

Fig. 6. Structural formula of α-amanitine

therapeutically. In the latter case, however, the effect depended on the interval which elapsed between administration of the toxin and treatment with silymarin (14, 52).

On the basis of the chemical data worked out by Prof. Wagner and his colleagues (61), together with the pharmacological findings outlined above and the results of clinical trials, silymarin was registered with the appropriate office of the German Federal Health Bureau in 1969. This, then, is the historical background behind the use of flavanolignans as antihepatotoxic agents. I now propose to give you an account of our present knowledge of the pharmacology of this group of substances. For this purpose I shall use results from our own laboratories and from research groups outside Dr. Madaus and Co. Most of the latter were motivated to work on silymarin by their spontaneous interest in the subject and subsequently made their results available to us.

After we had demonstrated that silymarin can counteract lethal or sublethal poisoning with the amanita toxins phalloidine and α-amanitine we developed the phalloidine test into our favorite screening test. For the phalloidine test we use mice, first because this species is particularly sensitive and secondly because so little of the toxin is available that we have to work with small animals if we are to have statistically adequate numbers. One reason why it is such a good screening test is that the decision between death or survival is reached within two hours, or at most three hours. On the other hand, after administering α-amanitine the mice do not usually begin to die until the third day. The test may drag on for up to seven days before it is possible to decide which mice will survive and which will not. Before I go on to the mechanism of amatoxin poisoning and the mechanism by which silymarin counteracts it, I should like to show you a few phenomena.

Figure 7 shows the dose-effect relationship for silymarin when given prophylactically one hour before the dose of phalloidine. Whereas 90 % of the untreated mice die, a dose of 50 mg/kg silymarin intravenously gives almost 100 % protection. The duration of the silymarin effect is surprisingly long, bearing in mind the rapidity of metabolic processes in mice. Silymarin exerts its full protective effect when given six hours before administration of the toxin. Thereafter, the protective effect gradually declines. When used therapeutically, i.e. first the toxin and then treatment with silymarin, the protective

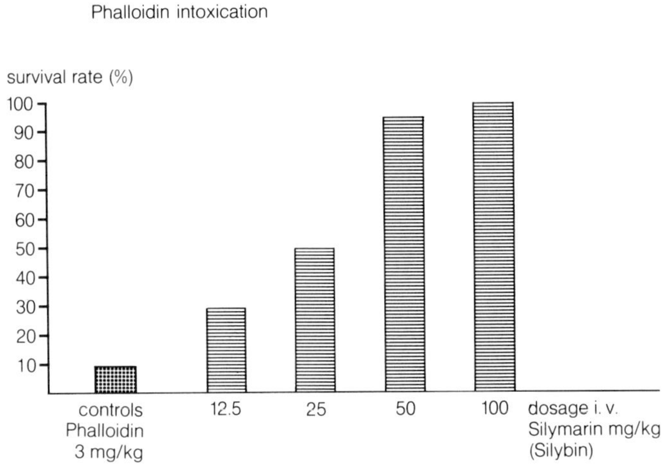

Fig. 7. The dose-dependent, antiphalloidine action of silymarin: the administration of silymarin 50 mg/kg i.v. 1 h before phalloidine 3 mg/kg i.p. results in 100 % of the mice being protected against the lethal toxic effect of phalloidine

effect depends on the interval between poisoning and treatment: 10 min after poisoning protection is complete, 20 min after poisoning 70 % of the mice are protected, while 30 min after poisoning with phalloidine is too late - no protective effect is achieved (Fig. 8).

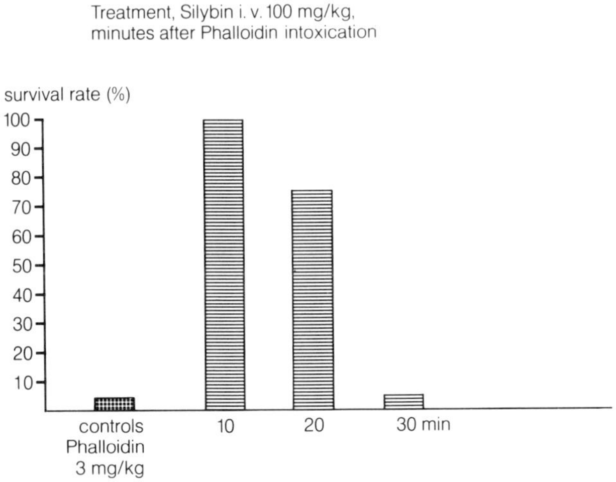

Fig. 8. The therapeutic action of silybin: the administration of silybin 100 mg/kg i.v. 10 min after phalloidine intoxication results in 100 % of the mice being protected against the lethal toxic effect of phalloidine. The administration of silybin 20 min after phalloidine intoxication still protects a proportion of the animals. However, after 30 min silybin offers no protection

Silymarin also confers total protection against α-amanitine, when given a dose of 75 - 100 mg/kg one hour before administration of the toxin (Fig. 9). As in the case of phalloidine poisoning, the protective effect of silymarin given therapeutically falls off with the lapse of time and becomes less and less as the interval between poisoning and treatment lengthens (Fig. 10).

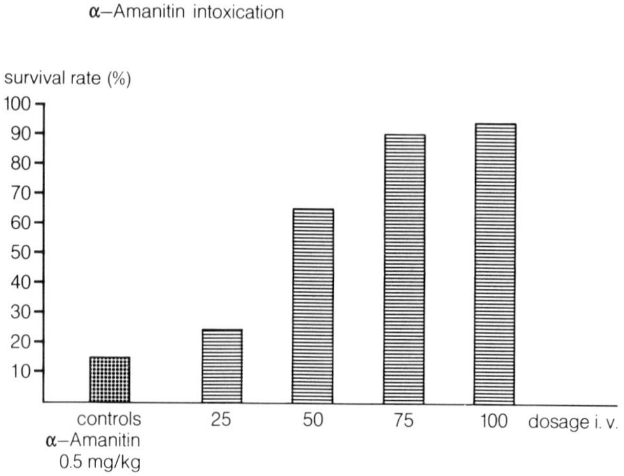

Fig. 9. The dose-dependent anti-α-amanitine action of silymarin: the administration of silymarin 75 mg/kg i.v. 1 h before α-amanitine 0.5 mg/kg i.p. results in nearly 100 % of the mice being protected against the lethal toxic effect of α-amanitine

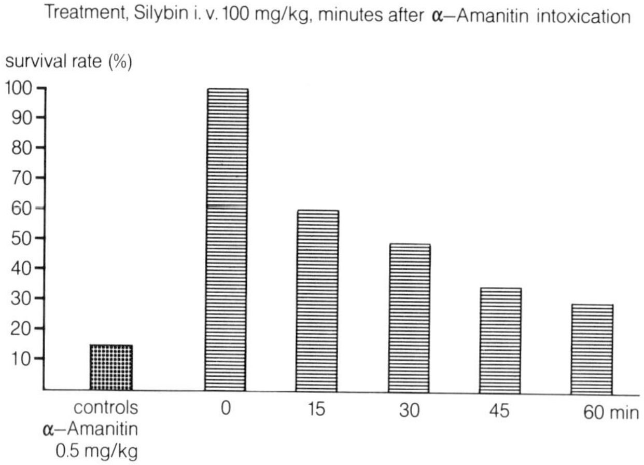

Fig. 10. Therapeutic action of silybin: the administration of silybin 100 mg/kg i.v. 15 min after α-amanitine intoxication results in 60 % of the mice being protected against the lethal toxic effect of α-amanitine. Silybin administered 60 min after α-amanitine intoxication offers no protection

From the time relationship of the silymarin effect against the two amatoxins we can draw the following conclusion: silymarin prevents the toxins from penetrating through the cell membrane or into the interior of the cell by competing with the toxins for the same receptor. If silymarin gets to the receptor before the toxins, phalloidine cannot exert its destructive action on the external cell membrane, while α-amanitine cannot penetrate the cell membrane and hence cannot reach the nucleus, the site where its effect becomes manifest. That this interpretation is in principle correct is shown by the fact that when silymarin is administered *therapeutically* the mortality from a given dose of phalloidine becomes less and less as the therapeutic dose of silymarin is raised (see Fig. 11). This means that silymarin must be capable of displacing phalloidine from the receptor (4 - 9, 44, 45, 49 - 57).

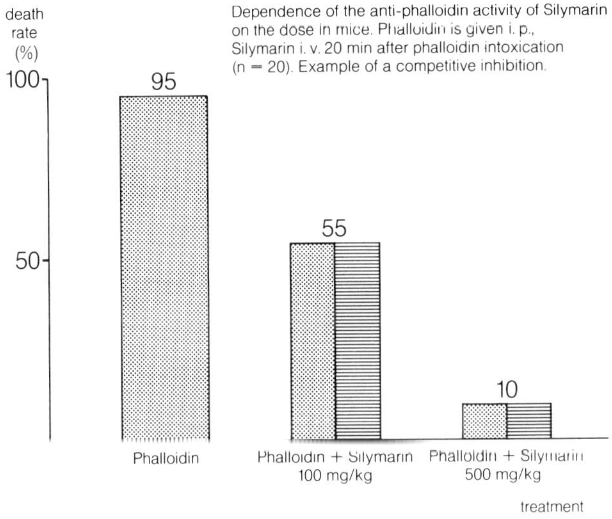

Fig. 11. Evidence that the anti-phalloidine action of silymarin is competitive: when silymarin 100 mg/kg is administered 20 min after phalloidine the mortality rate is reduced from 95 % (controls) to 55 %. By increasing the dose of silymarin to 500 mg/kg 20 min after phalloidine the mortality rate is further reduced to 10 %

Prof. Frimmer from the University of Giessen has made a detailed study of the mechanism of action of phalloidine and has also worked with silymarin. The toxic action of phalloidine is based on its power to nibble holes, so to speak, in the outer cell membrane of hepatocytes, possibly by forming a compound with actin. From his work it is evident that specific phalloidine receptors are present on the outer cell membrane but in very young animals they are not fully developed, their maturation being completed in the later stages of growth. These receptors can be destroyed by tryptic digestion. One of the effects of phalloidine on isolated hepatocytes is the escape of cytoplasm into protuberances on the cell surface - an abnormality which signifies cell death. However, if we treat the hepatocytes with silymarin before exposing them to phalloidine nothing happens.

The next figure (Fig. 12) is taken from a paper by Prof. Frimmer. It shows the changes in potassium concentration in the perfusion fluid pumped through the isolated liver of a rat, a closed system being used. If phalloidine is added to the perfusion fluid, the first manifestation of its toxic action is the breakdown of selective cation permeability with escape of potassium from the cell. The result is a rise of potassium concentration in the perfusion fluid. When silymarin is added in increasing concentration to the perfusion fluid it cuts down the rise in potassium concentration. This effect is dose-dependent, and if enough silymarin is added we reach a state in which the change in potassium concentration is not greater than it is with a healthy liver (10, 11, 63).

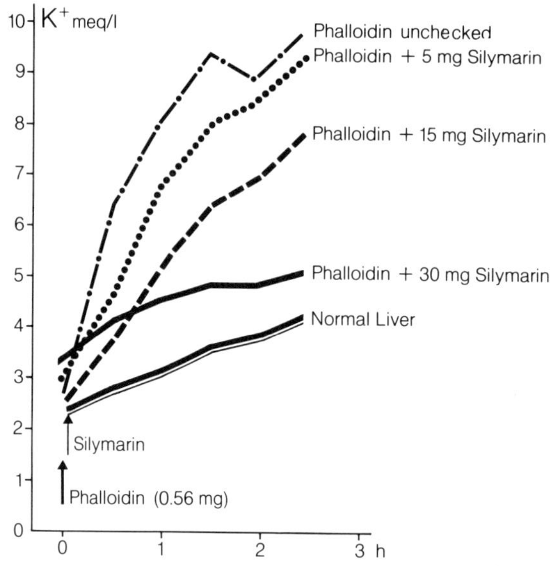

Fig. 12. Increase in potassium content in the perfusate from perfused, isolated rat liver as a method for determining phalloidine damage. The concomitant administration of silymarin dose-dependently antagonizes the toxic effect of phalloidine (graphical representation modified according to Weil and Frimmer (63))

The silymarin as a class of compounds is somewhat disparagingly termed "bioflavonoids". Ever since the US Food and Drug Administration classified bioflavonoids as pharmalogically inert substances silymarin has commonly been tarred with the same brush. For this reason (Fig. 13) we have investigated the question whether compounds chemically related to silymarin such as taxifolin, morin and quercetin have an antiphalloidine effect similar to that of silymarin. 100 % of the control animals died; in those treated with silybin the mortality was from 5 % to zero, while in those treated with coniferyl alcohol, taxifolin, morin or quercetin the mortality was nearly 100 %. These compounds, though resembling silymarin in chemical structure, do not produce anything like the same pharmacological effect. Much the same applies (Fig. 14) to anti-α-amanitine activity: silybin gives 100 % protection, but other flavonoid compounds have no protective effect at all (57).

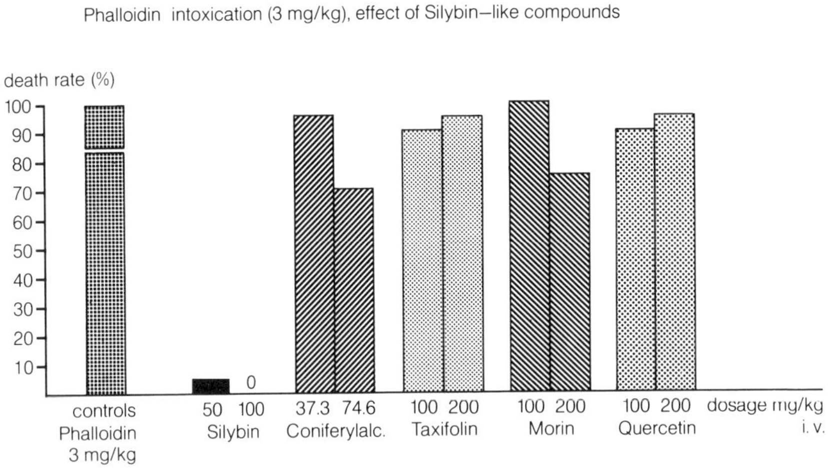

Fig. 13. Evidence that substances whose chemical structures are similar to silymarin do not possess antiphalloidine activity: Morin and quercetin are without activity as are the constituents of silymarin - taxifolin and coniferylalcohol

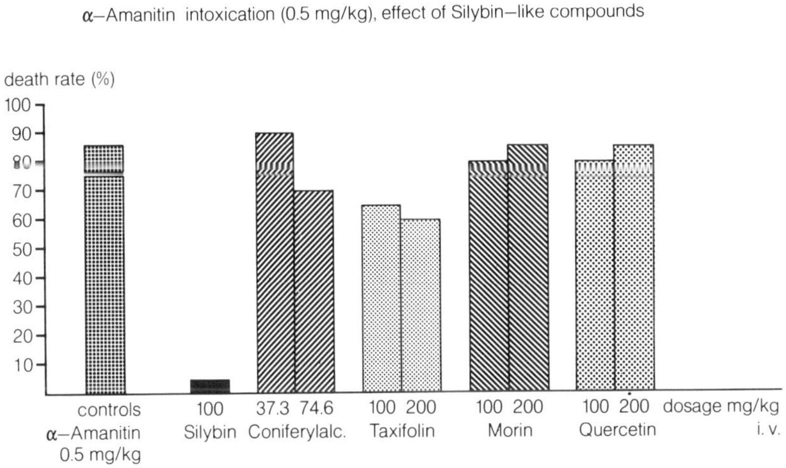

Fig. 14. Like Figure 13 except that α-amanitine is used instead of phalloidine. Also in this case silybin-like compounds are without activity

Many of my critics, in particular those who work in hospitals, have raised the objection that the results obtained in our experimental animals are not necessarily applicable to man. I am of course fully aware of the difficulties of applying the results of animal work to human medicine. Nevertheless, a pharmacologist who works with experimental animals has no option but to set up as many different models of experimental liver damage as possible and to see how the drug under trial behaves in these experimental systems.

Moreover, this approach offers another major advantage, namely that from the spectrum of effects, or in other words, from the different reactions produced by the drug in the various experimental models it may be possible to gain insight into its mechanism of action.

It was with this in mind that we returned yet again to the anticarbon tetrachloride effect. The prolongation of sleeping time produced by carbon tetrachloride is significantly shortened by silymarin and may even be restored to normal (Fig. 15).

Treatment with Silymarin (100 mg/kg iv) 5 min before CCl_4–intoxication (0.15 ml/kg po)

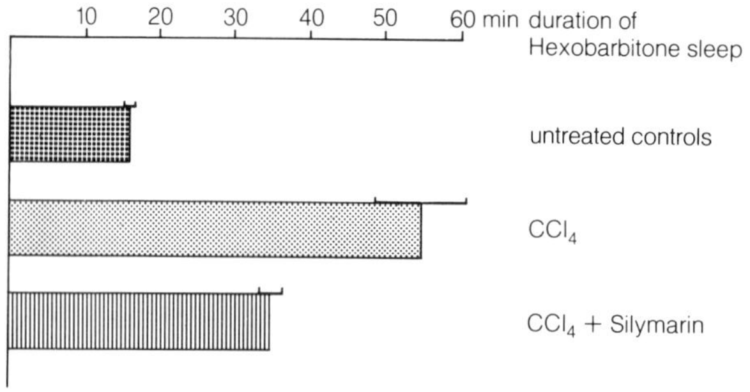

Fig. 15. Antagonism of the prolonged sleeping time produced by hexobarbital following poisoning with CCl_4, by silymarin

Carbon tetrachloride poisoning also raises the serum levels of various enzymes (Fig. 16) but under treatment with silymarin these increases are significantly lessened (3, 20, 25 - 28, 31, 56, 64).

Silymarin likewise neutralizes - though admittedly not completely - the hepatotoxic action of galactosamine (Fig. 17) (23 - 25, 30, 32, 43, 56).

Even more convincing is the power of silymarin to counteract poisoning by the rare earth element praseodymium. This substance produces extensive fatty change in the rat's liver. The rise in serum enzymes induced by praseodymium poisoning is significantly lowered or even completely restored to normal by silymarin (Fig. 18) (46, 47, 56).

Equally impressive is the antiethionine effect of silymarin in preventing hepatic fatty change in rats. These results were kindly made available by my colleague Prof. Antweiler in Düsseldorf (Fig. 19) (2, 12, 48, 56).

Finally, I should mention (Fig. 20) another experiment with thioacetamide. At the end of 120 days all the animals poisoned with TAA had died. However, when silymarin was added to their food in a dose of 35 mg/kg daily, the death rate after 140 days was only 30 % (14, 24, 29, 56).

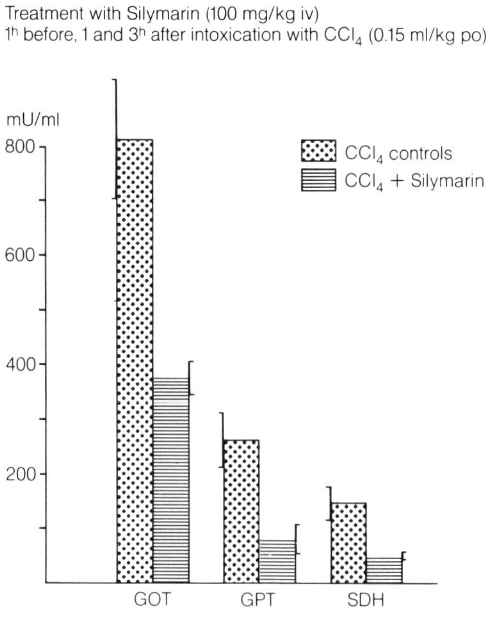

Fig. 16. Following liver damage induced by CCl_4 the serum concentrations of GOT, GPT and SDH rise. Combined prophylactic-therapeutic treatment with silymarin reduces the serum concentrations of these enzymes

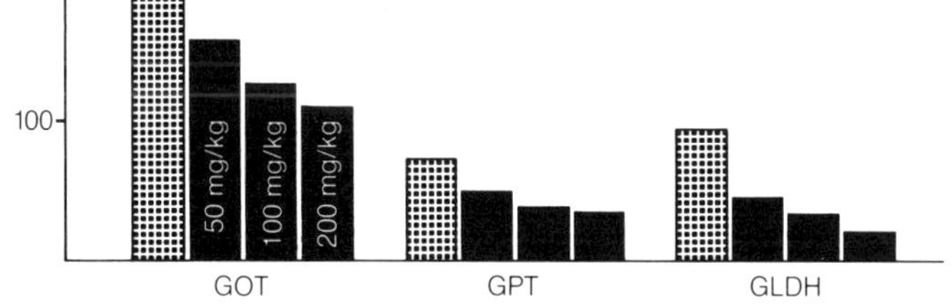

Fig. 17. Following liver damage induced by galactosamine the serum concentrations of GOT, GPT and GLDH rise. Pretreatment of the animals with silymarin partially reduces dose-dependently the serum concentrations of these enzymes

Treatment with Silymarin (100 mg/kg iv) 1h before, 24 and 48h after Praseodymnitrate intoxication (14 mg/kg ip)

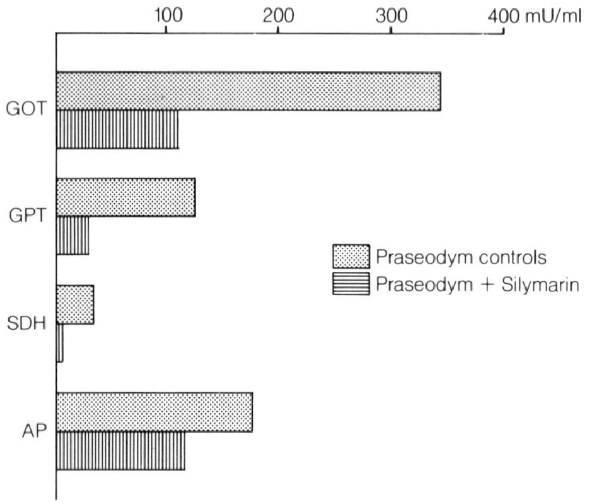

Fig. 18. The pronounced antipraseodymium action of silymarin is measured by the reduction in the serum concentrations of GOT, GPT, SDH and AP

Pretreatment with Silymarin (100 mg/kg iv) 1h before Ethionine intoxication (400 mg/kg ip)

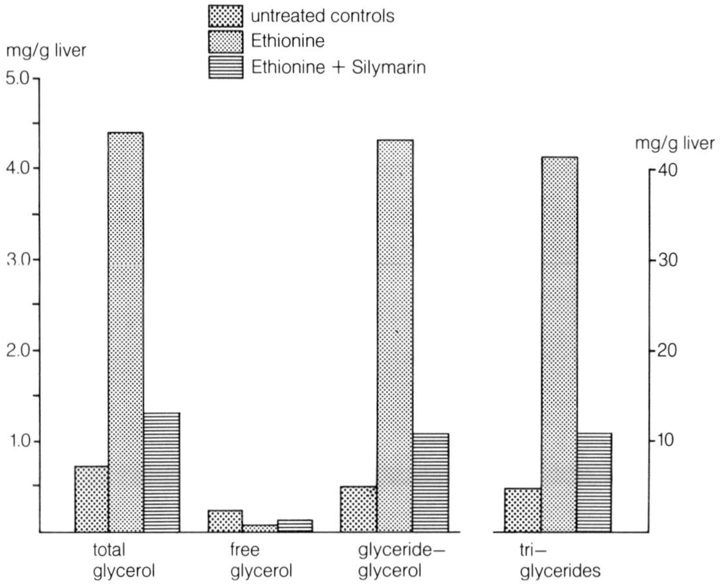

Fig. 19. The marked decrease in ethionine induced fatty liver damage by pretreatment with silymarin [after Antweiler (2)]

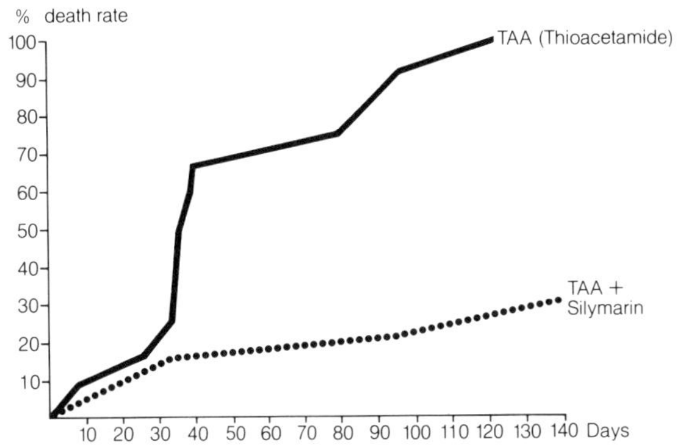

Fig. 20. Mortality rate in rats during chronic administration of TAA. The mortality rate in animals concomitantly treated with silymarin after 120 days is 30 % in comparison with 100 % in the control animals

Now, in order to avoid creating the impression that silymarin is a wonder drug effective against hepatotoxic agents of every kind, I must mention three experiments in which silymarin proved ineffective: hepatic fatty change produced by a single large dose of ethanol, hepatic fatty change induced by yellow phosphorus, and liver damage caused by α-naphthyl isothiocyanate (ANIT) (56).

As silymarin blocks the action of phalloidine on the cell membrane and the penetration of α-amanitine through the cell membrane we have proposed the term "membrane stabilization" to designate its mode of action. The fact that silymarin is capable of modifying the properties of cell membranes has been shown by certain experiments carried out by Prof. Seeger in Würzburg. She found, for instance, that the osmotic resistance of human erythrocytes is increased by silymarin. It also appears to raise the resistance of red cells to thermal haemolysis. Antweiler, who works in Düsseldorf, has shown that it blocks the extrusion of histamine and serotonin containing granules from rat mast cells. He ascribes this to a change in the mechanical properties of the mast cell wall (13, 17, 33 - 37, 56).

Considering all the experiments as a whole one is inescapably left with the impression that silymarin possesses at least *one* site of action on the cell membrane. It seems to modify its properties in such a way that toxic agents can no longer penetrate into cell - or can penetrate only with difficulty. From the standpoint of molecular pharmacology the mode of action of silymarin would hence be interpreted in principle as "prophylactic". Now, there are, however, the findings of Dr. Sonnenbichler, Max Planck Institute of Biochemistry, Munich, which indicate that silymarin has a second site of action, located in the nucleus (38 - 42). Without going into details I should like to present Sonnenbichler's principal finding: Silymarin enhances the activity of polymerase A produced in the nucleolus; this stimulates ribosomal RNA and thus increases protein synthesis within the cell. If we look at a synopsis showing the two effects of silymarin we can see how it is that a *prophylactic* action in the pharmacologists sense is transformed into a *therapeutic* action in the clinical sense. We must of course realize that not every area or every cell in a diseased liver is necessarily in the same state. There are some irreversibly damaged cells, which are degenerating, other cells with reversible damage, and other cells which have not yet been damaged at all. The reversibly damaged cells and those so far undamaged are "stabilized" by silymarin. Stimulation of polymerase A, in other words stimulation of protein synthesis, accelerates the process of regeneration (19). Now, because silymarin has a second site of action on the nucleus, the liver cells protected by silymarin are now able to serve as regeneration centres. They can, therefore, replace the irreversibly damaged cells which have been destroyed. By looking at the two effects of silymarin together - the membrane stabilizing effect and the protein synthesis enhancing effect - we can understand how it is that its action, though primarily prophylactic, can in clinical situations evolve into a therapeutic effect.

This brings me to the end of what I have to represent. I am well aware that our knowledge of the spectrum of effects of the flavanolignans, their mechanism of action and their sites of action is still full of gaps and imperfections. However, it seems to me that our work on flavanolignans has established one point beyond all doubt: the sceptical assertion that there is no effective drug therapy for liver disease is now out of date.

Acknowledgment. The author is indebted to D.P. Winstanley, M.D., Toothill/Essex (England) for the translation of the German text.

References

1. Abraham, D.J., Takagi, S., Rosenstein, R.D., Shiono, R., Wagner, H., Hörhammer, L., Seligmann, O., Farnsworth, N.R.: The structure of silydianin, an isomer of silymarin (silybin), by X-ray analysis. Tetrahedron Lett. 1970, 2675-2678
2. Antweiler, H.: Effects of silymarin on intoxication with ethionine and ethanol. In: Symposium on the Pharmacodynamics of Silymarin, Cologne Nov. 1974. Braatz, R., Schneider, C.C. (eds.). München-Berlin-Wien: Urban and Schwarzenberg, 1976, pp. 80 - 82
3. Aznar Lopez, J., Sanchez de la Cuesta y Alarcon, F., Monfort Albelda, R., Alemany Ontiveros, J.R.: Influencia de la lesion hepatico experimental por tetracloruro de carbono sobre la secrecion acido-peptica estimulada por pentagastrina en la rata y efectos protectores de la silimarina. Med. Esp. 68, 278 - 286 (1972)
4. Braatz, R.: Effects of silybin on phalloidine pretreated mice. In: Symposium on the Pharmacodynamics of Silymarin, Cologne Nov. 1974. Braatz, R., Schneider, C. C. (eds.). München-Berlin-Wien: Urban and Schwarzenberg, 1976, pp. 44-45
5. Desplaces, A.: The effect of silymarin on the histochemical picture in normal liver cells and in phalloidine-intoxicated liver cells. In: Symposium on the Pharmacodynamics of Silymarin, Cologne Nov. 1974. Braatz, R., Schneider, C.C. (eds.). München-Berlin-Wien: Urban and Schwarzenberg, 1976, pp. 103-112
6. Desplaces, A., Choppin, J., Vogel, G., Trost, W.: Histochemical study on the treatment of the liver damage by phalloidine with silymarin, the active principle of the seed of *Silybum marianum* L. Gaertn. Digestion 10, 343-344 (1974)
7. Desplaces, A., Choppin, J., Vogel, G., Trost, W.: The effects of silymarin on experimental phalloidine poisoning. Arzneim.-Forsch. 25, 89-96 (1975)
8. Floersheim, G.L.: Treatment of experimental poisoning by extracts of Amanita phalloides. Toxicol. Appl. Pharmacol. 34, 499-508 (1975)
9. Floersheim, G.L.: Antagonistic effects against single lethal doses of Amanita phalloides. Naunyn-Schmiedebergs Arch. Pharmacol. 293, 171-174 (1976)
10. Frimmer, M.: Comparative studies on effects of silymarin in phalloidine action in perfused livers, isolated hepatocytes and isolated membrane systems. In: Symposium on the Pharmacodynamics of Silymarin, Cologne, Nov. 1974. Braatz, R., Schneider, C.C. (eds.). München-Berlin-Wien: Urban and Schwarzenberg, 1976, pp. 13-19
11. Frimmer, M., Kroker, R.: Phalloidin-Antagonisten. 1. Mitteilung: Wirkung von Silybin-Derivaten an der isoliert perfundierten Rattenleber. Arzneim.-Forsch. 25, 394-396 (1975)

12. Garcia-Pravia, F., Sopena-Dasi, M., Vázquez de Prada, J.R.: Prevención con silimarina de las alteraciones hepáticas inducidas con etionina en ratas. Rev. Esp. Fisiol. 29, 227-232 (1973)
13. Gretzer, K.: Der Einfluß von SMG 11, einem wasserlöslichen Silymarin-Derivat auf die osmotische Resistenz von menschlichen und Rindererythrocyten. Diss. (Med.) Würzburg, 1973
14. Hahn, G., Lehmann, H.D., Kürten, M., Uebel, H., Vogel, G.: Zur Pharmakologie und Toxikologie von Silymarin, des antihepatotoxischen Wirkprinzipes aus *Silybum marianum* (L.) Gaertn. Arzneim.-Forsch. 18, 698-704 (1968)
15. Halbach, G.: Chemistry of silymarin and water-soluble derivatives. In: Symposium on the Pharmacodynamics of Silymarin, Cologne Nov. 1974. Braatz, R., Schneider, C.C. (eds.). München-Berlin-Wien: Urban and Schwarzenberg, 1976, pp. 7-12
16. Hänsel, R., Schulz, J., Pelter, A.: Synthese des Dehydrosilybinpentamethyläthers und verwandter Verbindungen. Chem. Ber. 108, 1482-1501 (1975)
17. Heim, A.: Die Wirkung der wasserlöslichen Silymarinderivate Silymarin-Natrium und SMG 11 auf die thermische Hämolyse, die Digitonin- und die Phallolysin-Hämolyse menschlicher Erythrocyten. Diss. (Zahnmed.) Würzburg, 1972
18. Janiak, B., Hänsel, R.: Phytochemisch-pharmakognostische Untersuchungen über Fructus Cardui Mariae. 1. Mitteilung. Planta Medica (Stuttg.) 8, 71-84 (1960)
19. Magliulo, E., Carosi, P.G., Minoli, L., Gorini, S.: Studies on the regenerative capacity of the liver in rats subjected to partial hepatectomy and treated with silymarin. Arzneim.-Forsch. 23, 161-167 (1973)
20. Monfort Albelda, R., Aznar Lopez, J., Sanchez de la Cuesta y de Alarcon, F.: Influencia de una nueva sustancia hepatoterápica sobre el sueño barbitúrico en ratas lesionadas con tetracloruro de carbono. Rev. Med. Suiza 4, 23-26 (1972)
21. Münster, R.: Strukturaufklärung eines neuen Flavonoidtypes aus den Früchten von *Silybum marianum* G. Diss. Maximilians-Univ. München, 1966
22. Pelter, A., Hänsel, R.: The structure of silybin (Silybum substance E_6), the first flavonolignan. Tetrahedron Lett. 1968, 2911-2916
23. Perings, E.: Workshop Beeinflussung und Verhinderung experimenteller Leberschäden. Freiburg i. Breisgau Okt. 1971, pp. 22-25
24. Rauen, H.M.: The effect of silymarin N-methylglucamine salt on certain disturbances of phospholipid metabolism of rat liver microsomes after intoxication with thioacetamide, and the influence of silybin hemisuccinate on similar alterations after D-galactosamin poisoning. In: Symposium on the Pharmacodynamics of Silymarin, Cologne Nov. 1974. Braatz, R., Schneider, C.C. (eds.). München-Berlin-Wien: Urban and Schwarzenberg, 1976, pp. 65-77
25. Rauen, H.M., Schriewer, H.: Die antihepatotoxische Wirkung von Silymarin bei experimentellen Leberschädigungen der Ratte durch Tetrachlorkohlenstoff, D-Galaktosamin und Allylalkohol. Arzneim.-Forsch. 21, 1194-1201 (1971)
26. Rauen, H.M., Schriewer, H.: Die antihepatotoxische Wirkung von parenteral verabreichtem Silymarin bei der Leberschädigung der Ratte durch CCl_4. Arzneim.-Forsch. 23, 148-149 (1973)
27. Rauen, H.M., Schriewer, H., Tegtbauer, U., Lasana, J.E.: Silymarin verhindert die Lipidperoxydation bei der CCl_4-Leberschädigung. Experientia (Basel) 29, 1372 (1973)
28. Schriewer, H., Badde, R., Roth, G., Rauen, H.M.: Die Pharmakokinetik der antihepatotoxischen Wirkung des Silymarins bei der Leberschädigung der Ratte durch CCl_4 und Desoxycholat. Arzneim.-Forsch. 23, 157-158 (1973)
29. Schriewer, H., Badde, R., Roth, G., Rauen, H.M.: Die antihepatotoxische Wirkung des Silymarins bei der Leberschädigung durch Thioacetamid. Arzneim.-Forsch. 23, 160-161 (1973)
30. Schriewer, H., Lohmann, J., Rauen, H.M.: Die Wirkung von Silybin-dihemisuccinat auf Regulationsstörungen des Phospholipidstoffwechsels bei der akuten Galaktosaminintoxikation der Ratte. Arzneim.-Forsch. 25, 1582-1585 (1975)
31. Schriewer, H., Penin, L., Rahmede, D., Riese, B., Rüther, N., The, L.G., Gebauer, B., Abu Tair, M., Rauen, H.M.: Multivariate Analyse der chronischen Leberschädigung der Ratte durch CCl_4 und die Wirkung des Silymarins. Arzneim.-Forsch. 23, 149-155 (1973)

32. Schriewer, H., Rauen, H.M.: Die antihepatotoxische Wirkung von parenteral verabreichtem Silymarin bei der Galaktosamin-Hepatitis der Ratte. Arzneim.-Forsch. 23, 159 (1973)
33. Seeger, R.: Die Wirkung von Silymarin auf die osmotische Resistenz der Erythrocyten. Arzneim.-Forsch. 21, 1599-1605 (1971)
34. Seeger, R.: Untersuchungen zum Wirkungsmechanismus von Silymarin - Versuche an Erythrozyten. 2. Österr.-Jugoslaw. Symposium über Lebererkrankungen mit dem Thema Hepatitis, Graz/Austria Sept. 1975
35. Seeger, R.: The effect of silymarin on erythrocytes. In: Symposium on the Pharmacodynamics of Silymarin, Cologne Nov. 1974. Braatz, R., Schneider, C.C. (eds.). München-Berlin-Wien: Urban and Schwarzenberg, 1976, pp. 172-174
36. Seeger, R., Beck, G., Gretzer, K., Heim, A.: Der Einfluß von Silymarin-Natriumsalz auf die Hämolyse menschlicher Erythrozyten durch Saponine, Lysolecithin, Natriumdodecylsulfat, Phallolysin und Clostridium welchii-Θ-Toxin. Arzneim.-Forsch. 24, 868-873 (1974)
37. Seeger, R., Rieger, N.: Der Einfluß der Temperatur und des pH-Wertes auf die stabilisierende und lytische Wirkung von Silymarin-Natriumsalz an menschlichen Erythrocyten. Arzneim.-Forsch. 21, 1676-1680 (1971)
38. Sonnenbichler, J.: Stimulierung der RNA-Synthese durch Silybin. Dtsch. Apoth. Ztg. 114, 1813 (1974)
39. Sonnenbichler, J.: Stimulation of RNA synthesis by silybin distribution of radioactive silybin in the rat organism. In: Symposium on the Pharmacodynamics of Silymarin, Cologne Nov. 1974. Braatz, R., Schneider, C.C. (eds.). München-Berlin-Wien: Urban and Schwarzenberg, 1976, pp. 192-200
40. Sonnenbichler, J., Mattersberger, J.: Stimulierung der RNA-Synthese in Rattenleber und in isolierten Hepatocyten durch Silybin, einem antihepatotoxischen Wirkstoff aus *Silybum marianum* L. Gaertn. Hoppe-Seylers Z. Physiol. Chem. 357, 1171-1180 (1976)
41. Sonnenbichler, J., Mattersberger, J., Machicao, F.: Steigerung der RNA-Synthese durch das Flavonolignan Silybin aus *Silybum Marianum*. Dtsch. Apoth. Ztg. 115, 1332 (1975)
42. Sonnenbichler, J., Mattersberger, J., Machicao, F.: Stimulierung der RNA-Polymerase A und der RNA-Synthese in vivo und in vitro durch ein Flavonderivat. Hoppe-Seylers Z. Physiol. Chem. 357, 337 (1976)
43. Stein, U.: Workshop Beeinflussung und Verhinderung experimenteller Leberschäden. Freiburg i. Breisgau Okt. 1971, pp. 15-16
44. Stockinger, L., Trost, W., Uebel, H.: Quantification électronique des lésions hépatiques expérimentales mises en évidence en histologie. Arch. Anat. Cytol. Pathol. 24, 203-209 (1976)
45. Tongiani, R., Malvaldi, G., Chieli, E., Bertelli, A.: Wirkung von Silymarin auf den Gesamtfeststoffgehalt der Leberzellen bei akuter Vergiftung mit Phalloidin und α-Amanitin. Arch. Toxicol. 36, 19-29 (1976)
46. Trost, W.: Effect of silybin on praseodymium nitrate-induced hepatotoxicity in rats. In: Symposium on the Pharmacodynamics of Silymarin, Cologne Nov. 1974. Braatz, R., Schneider, C.C. (eds.). München-Berlin-Wien: Urban and Schwarzenberg, 1976, pp. 58-64
47. Tuchweber, B.: Modification of experimental liver damage by silymarin. In: Symposium on the Pharmacodynamics of Silymarin, Cologne Nov. 1974. Braatz, R., Schneider, C.C. (eds.). München-Berlin-Wien: Urban and Schwarzenberg, 1976, pp. 23-42
48. Vázquez de Prada, J.R.: Estudios experimentales con silimarina. I. Estudio comparado de actividases enzimaticas mitocondriales de higado de ratas tratada con etionina y con etionina mas silimarina. Med. Clin. (Barcelona) 62, 28-30 (1974)
49. Vogel, G.: Silymarin, das antihepatotoxische Wirkprinzip aus *Silybum marianum* (L.) Gaertn., als Antagonist der Phalloidin-Wirkung. Arzneim.-Forsch. 18, 1063-1064 (1968)
50. Vogel, G.: Silymarin as a specific antidote against experimental liver damage induced by the deathcap toxins phalloidine and α-amanitine. International Association for the Study of the Liver, 6th Meeting Acapulco/Mex. Oct. 1974

51. Vogel, G.: Pharmacological properties of silymarin, the antihepatotoxic agent from the seeds of the milk thistle, *Silybum marianum* (L.) Gaertn. In: Symposium on the Pharmacodynamics of Silymarin, Cologne Nov. 1974. Braatz, R., Schneider, C.C. (eds.). München-Berlin-Wien: Urban and Schwarzenberg, 1976, pp. 1-5
52. Vogel, G., Temme, I.: Die curative Antagonisierung des durch Phalloidin hervorgerufenen Leberschadens mit Silymarin als Modell einer antihepatotoxischen Therapie. Arzneim.-Forsch. 19, 613-615 (1969)
53. Vogel, G., Trost, W.: Possibilities to antagonise the experimental poisoning by the toxic components of the toadstool *Amanita phalloides* Fries. Digestion 8, 556 (1973)
54. Vogel, G., Trost, W.: Neutralization of the lethal effects of phalloidine and α-amanitine in animal experiments by substances from the seeds of *Silybum marianum* L. Gaertn. Naunyn-Schmiedebergs Arch. Pharmacol. 282, R 102 (1974)
55. Vogel, G., Trost, W.: Zur Anti-Phalloidin-Aktivität der Silymarine Silybin und Disilybin. Arzneim.-Forsch. 25, 392-393 (1975)
56. Vogel, G., Trost, W., Braatz, R., Odenthal, K.P., Brüsewitz, G., Antweiler, H., Seeger, R.: Untersuchungen zu Pharmakodynamik, Angriffspunkt und Wirkungsmechanismus von Silymarin, dem antihepatotoxischen Prinzip aus *Silybum mar.* (L.) Gaertn. (1. und 2. Mitt.). Arzneim.-Forsch. 25, 82-89, 179-188 (1975)
57. Vogel, G., Trost, W., Halbach, G.: Etude de l'action protectrice de la silymarine vis-à-vis de l'intoxication par la phalloidine chez la souris. Agressologie 15, 263-270 (1974)
58. Wagner, H.: Flavanolignane, ein neuer Verbindungstyp aus *Silybum marianum*. Dtsch. Apoth. Ztg. 114, 93-94 (1973)
59. Wagner, H., Diesel, P., Seitz, M.: Zur Chemie und Analytik von Silymarin aus *Silybum marianum* Gaertn. Arzneim.-Forsch. 24, 466-471 (1974)
60. Wagner, H., Hörhammer, L., Münster, R.: Über die Struktur eines neuen Flavonoids aus den Früchten von *Carduus Marianus* L. (Mariendistel). Naturwissenschaften 52, 305 (1965)
61. Wagner, H., Hörhammer, L., Münster, R.: Zur Chemie des Silymarins (Silybin), des Wirkprinzips der Früchte von *Silybum marianum* (L.) Gaertn. (*Carduus Marianus* L.). Arzneim.-Forsch. 18, 688-696 (1968)
62. Wagner, H., Seligmann, O., Hörhammer, L., Seitz, M., Sonnenbichler, J.: Zur Struktur von Silychristin, einem zweiten Silymarin-Isomeren aus Silybum marianum. Tetrahedron Lett. 1971, 1895-1899
63. Weil, G., Frimmer, M.: Die Wirkung von Silymarin auf die mit Phalloidin vergiftete isolierte perfundierte Rattenleber. Arzneim.-Forsch. 20, 862-863 (1970)
64. Williams, D.E., Priestly, B.G.: Evaluation of prophylactic efficacy of silymarin in CCl_4-induced hepatotoxicity. Res. Commun. Chem. Path. Pharmacol. 6, 185-194 (1973)

The Modification of Natural Substances in the Modern Drug Synthesis

P. W. THIES

A. Introduction

Drugs are remedies which are thought to intervene in disturbed biochemical processes and to repair them.

According to this definition drugs always have something to do with *biochemistry*. Health means that biochemical systems present themselves to the observer by discrete proceedings; this means we can call them "normal." Disease is the unexpected event in a biochemical system, the other, the abnormal, the disturbed, all that has to be regulated and repaired. But is disease also reparable? I do not think disease is reparable in a scientific sense; otherwise, there could never occur the event named death!

Early detection - early analysis and correct diagnosis - may support the disturbed biochemical system in its attempt at self-regulation by the application of a pharmacon. The successful drug can only delay but never block the process towards death. Whenever this retardation is judged not only as a clinical proof of the effect, but experienced by the entire biochemical system - the patient - then we have not only a drug in general, but a true remedy.

The theory of modern drug therapy often presumes that no reasonable medical treatment existed before the year 1875 - the year of the introduction of salicylic acid. Should we really be so presumptuous as to believe that 100 years of pharmaceutical research are enough to the charge natural selection of millions of years, to throw overboard the curative experiences of so-called popular medicine, or to improve in the long run the harmony of symbiosis and immunity?

I am thoroughly convinced that the result of intensive research in biochemistry and natural substances will be drugs which deserve this name, because they help to improve the quality of human life.

How and where does one begin? In publications worthy of being taken seriously the opinion is advocated that nowadays one has to synthesize a minimum of 7000 chemical compounds to have at least a chance to get one new drug. This should be extremely depressing for a pharmaceutical chemist. In fact nobody achieves 7000 new substances during his life as a scientist, and there is really no need to study sciences for ten years to play a game of chance! The fact that responsible agents and representatives of pharmaceutical research make such statistical statements without questioning is really contradictory to the existence of directed planning in pharmaceutics.

Is there actually a lack of reasonable planning in the field of pharmaceutical research? Is there no possibility to reduce the ominous number of 7000 substances by powers of ten? Should the pharmacon of today be only a stroke of luck, or rather the result of multidisciplinary cooperation between creative men and other biochemical systems experienced in evolutions, i.e. microorganisms, plants and animals? I think the latter. Since the isolation of morphine or of the digitalis glycosides, the discovery of penicillin and the production of vaccines against smallpox, polio, diphtheria, whooping cough, measles, and tuberculosis are no lucky hits in a game of chance, but the results of hard work; and according to our present knowledge have contributed more to the relief from human sufferings than some of the so-called synthetics that were discovered as interesting active drug substances by the pharmacological method of screening.

Thus, I am breaking a lance for the use of natural substances in pharmaceutical research. It will be a typical wrong decision, if research managers still decide to cut down on the research of natural substances. Sir Ernest Chain once said to colleagues of Hoechst pharmaceutical research that biochemical research has always led to practical application in clinical medicine, whenever the basic principle was: "Biology first, chemistry second" (1).

B. Main Part

To confirm this working hypothesis I would like to present the examples mentioned earlier. I hope to show you at the same time that the pharmaceutical research of natural substances is a reality.

I. Steroids and Prostanoids

If you leaf through the Index Nominum 1975/76 (2) and then try to estimate which chemically derived or modified natural substances are at present most frequent on the market as therapeutics (3) steroid derivatives, including cardiac glycosides, will be first. However, if you make an analysis in the market of the Federal Republic of Germany to find the leading chemicals according to units and not to sales, you will find a digoxine compound (Novodigal®) among the first five, another - β-methyldigoxine (Lanitop) - among the first ten, and as number ten a combined chemical containing, apart from reserpine and a diuretic, dihydroergocristinmethansulfonate. Surprisingly corticosteroids and steroid hormones range only among the last third of the leading articles on the market.

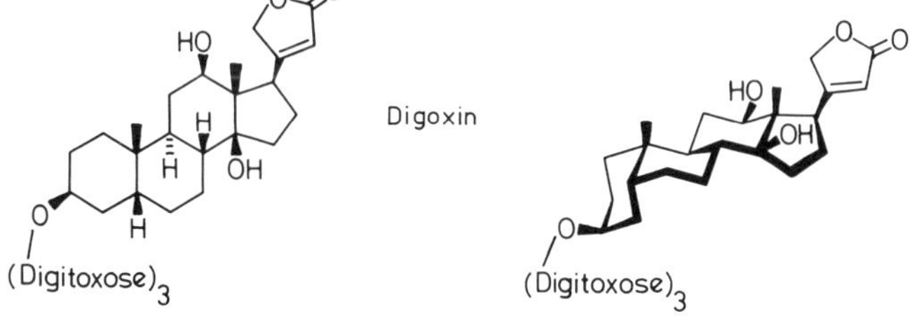

Fig. 1

A concise interpretation of a table on steroid chemistry and therapy by steroid derivatives would go beyond the limits of this lecture. I would only like to point out the synthesis of steroid hormones from steroid sapogenines (4), representing in my opinion still the best example of successful integration of a higher plant into the manufacturing process of highly effective pharmaceutics and, moreover, demonstrating that the substance in the plant must not be a priori the very active one!

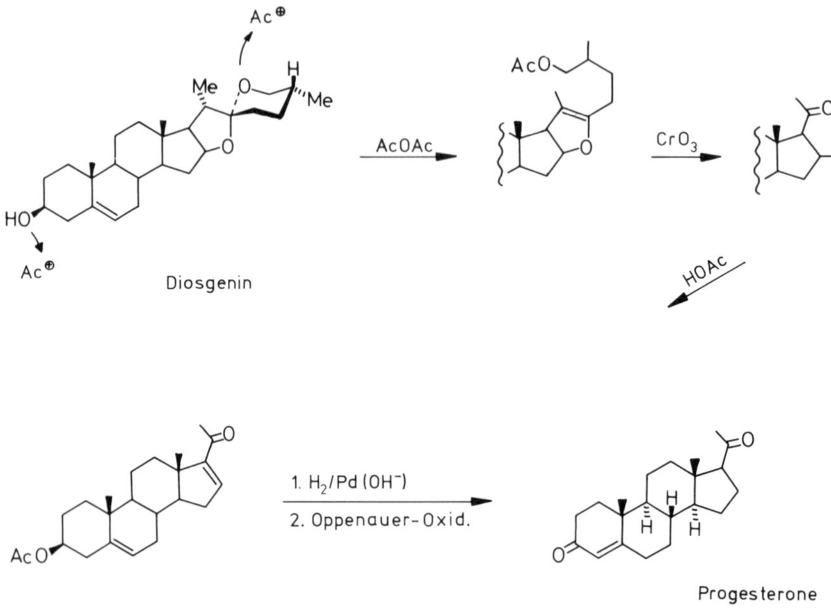

Fig. 2

Another group of natural substances in which almost spectacular chemical syntheses were achieved are the prostanoids (earlier prostaglandines). In comparison with the great chemical success, the results of therapeutical efforts with prostanoids appear rather humble (3, 5 - 7).

$PGF_{2\alpha}$

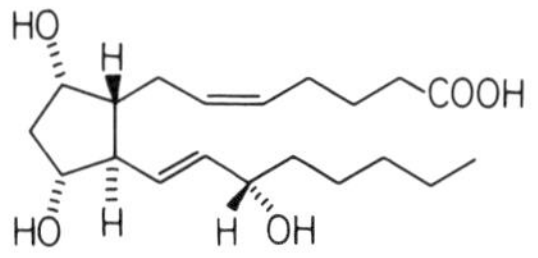

Fig. 3

II. "Chemotherapy"

The domain of natural substances that has brought the greatest therapeutical success of the last thirty years, is, no doubt, the domain of antibiotics. The chemical derivation and modification of penicillins and cephalosporins is an outstanding example of successful cooperation between scientists and microorganisms (cf. Tamm, this vol., 1, 8).

In spite of tremendous successes in this field, there have been some times of resignation whenever the problem of resistance arises. In most cases either so-called pure organic chemistry or immunology and immunotherapy break this resignation. We can recall the investigations by C. Weigert, P. Ehrlich, S. Hata and G. Domagk, F. Mietsch and Mme. Tréfouel, as well as the early works by Robert Koch and Louis Pasteur.

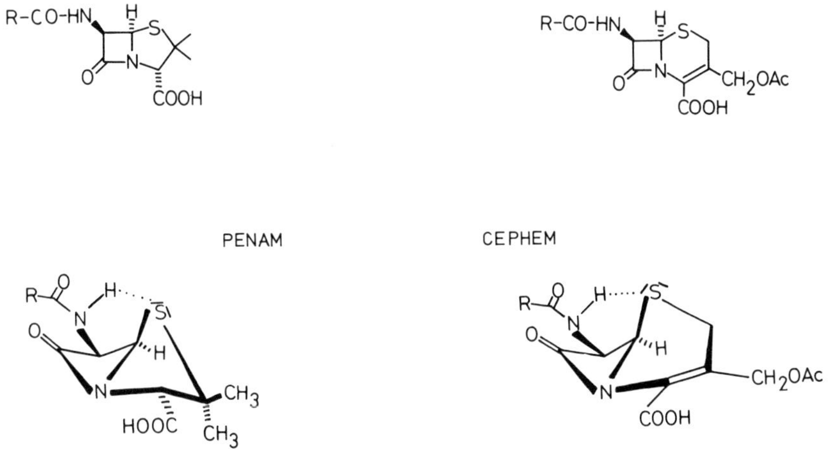

Fig. 4

While the first sulfonamide was discovered by pioneer work with the screening method - because of a false working hypothesis - another example of successful interdisciplinary research with natural substances is the later optimizing of that substance class by means of the so-called long-acting sulfonamides and the sulfonamides with potentiators, and the intensive study of bacterial metabolism and bacterial cell walls, resulting in the surprising development of new chemotherapeutics and finally immunoadjuvants (1, 5).

Of these substances the combination of alanine-derivative MK 641 and cycloserine-derivative MK 642 is still under clinical examination (9). Fluor-deutero-alanine allegedly affects the blocking of the alanine-racemase, which is responsible for the synthesis of alanine, a component of most bacterial walls. 3-Fluor-alanine may function as the antagonist in the biosynthesis of cell walls. Cycloserine is an antibiotic with limited therapeutical qualities because of its high toxicity on the central nervous system. It was discovered, described and synthesized more than 20 years ago by different working groups (10). The new pentandione-derivative (MK 642) is supposed to possess better pharmacokinetic qualities than cycloserine and greater chemical stability.

In spite of this new chemotherapeutical idea and the possibility of another great success in this era (9 - 11), in my opinion, the age of established antibiotics is over (1). The efforts again lean towards the prophylaxis, instead of the treatment of acute infection. The problems of immunotherapy are being more and more intensively discussed all over the world; more and more new immunological research establishments have been developed, leading to the isolation and synthesis of immunostimulants (12) - the components of cell walls such as mycobacteria and *Escherichia coli*, corynebacteria, lactobacilli, etc. These adjuvants were made synthetically accessible! Modifications of the amino acid sequence and the substitution of genuine amino acids by "antimetabolites" should thus reveal new perspectives for a novel therapy! In the meantime even smaller units were found, as fully active as adjuvants, the "smallest synthetic:" N-acetylmuramyl-L-alanyl-D-isoglutamine.

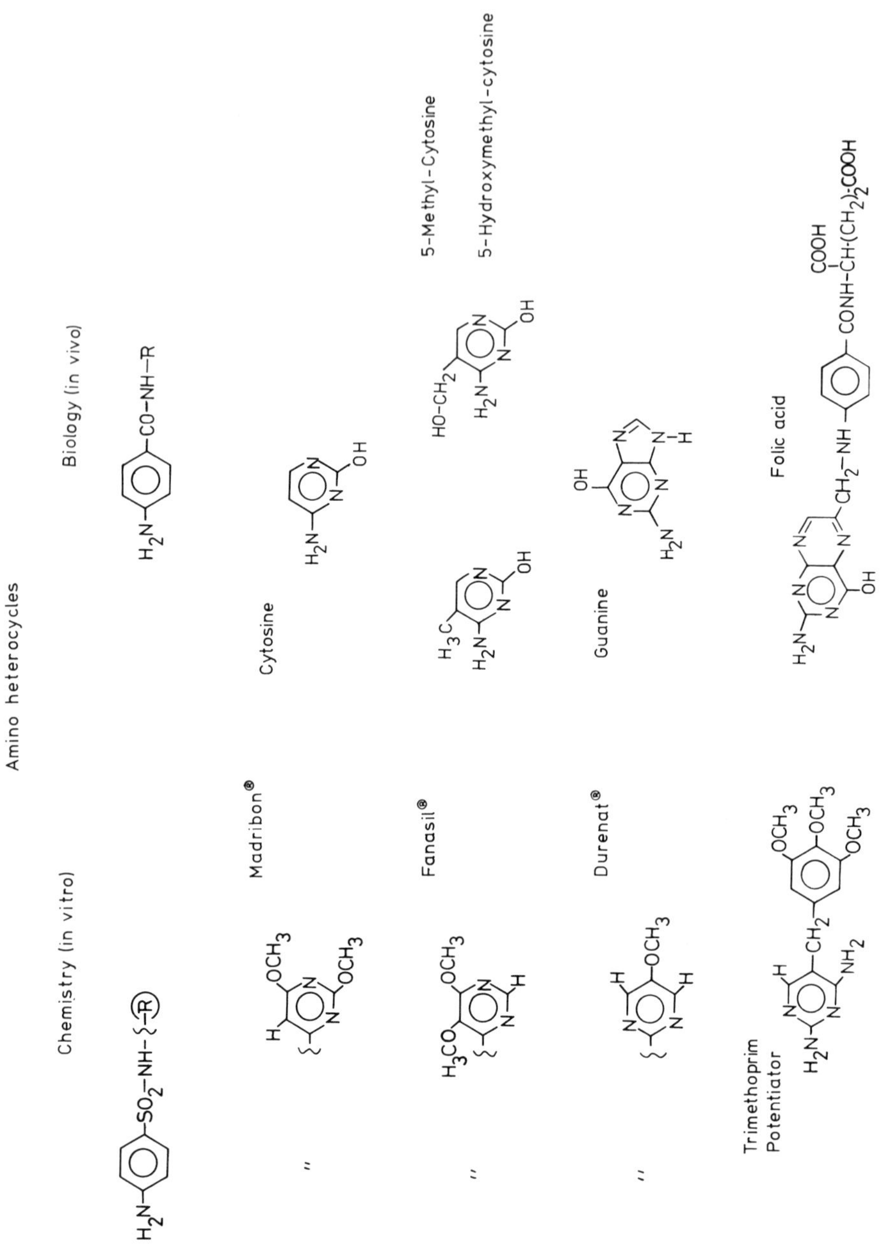

Fig. 5

III. Claviceps Purpurea

Among the first ten best-selling pharmaceutics of this country we can already find three substances from the ergot alkaloid research. Hardly any other modification of natural substances has provided as many pharmacological surprises as the ergot alkaloids. Therefore, I would like to present the most interesting compounds in the ergot research.

Pyrimidines and purines

Nucleosides
(Antitumor/Antivirale)

Chemistry

Biology

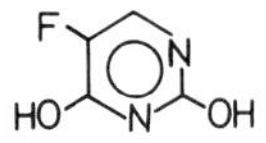

5-Fluoro-uracil

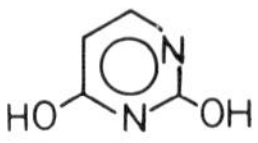

Uracil

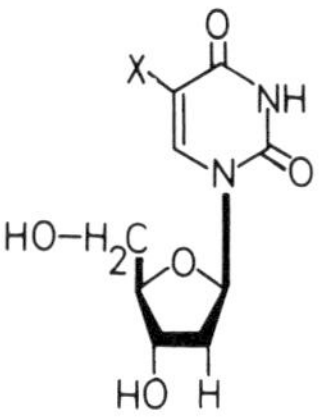

2'-Desoxy-uridine
(X = F/J)

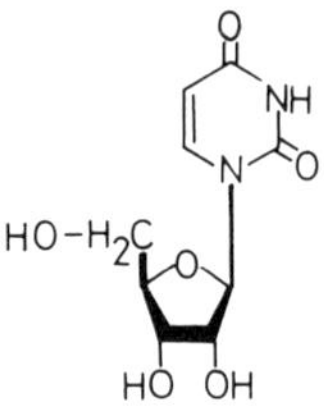

Uridine

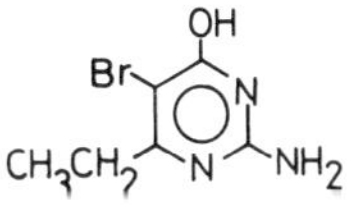

5-Bromo-pyrimidine
Interferoninducer
(virus-synthesis-inhibitor

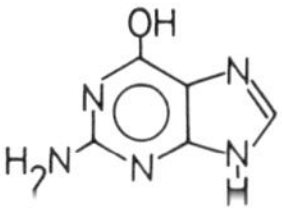

Guanine

Fig. 6

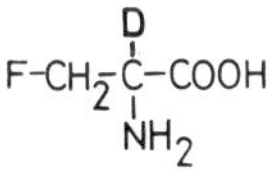

MK 641

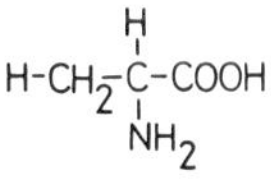

Alanine

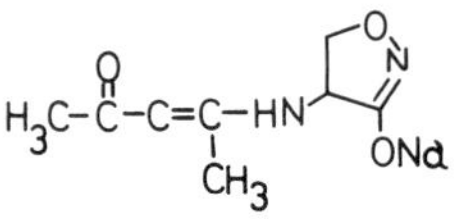

MK 642

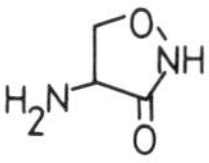

Cycloserine

Fig. 7

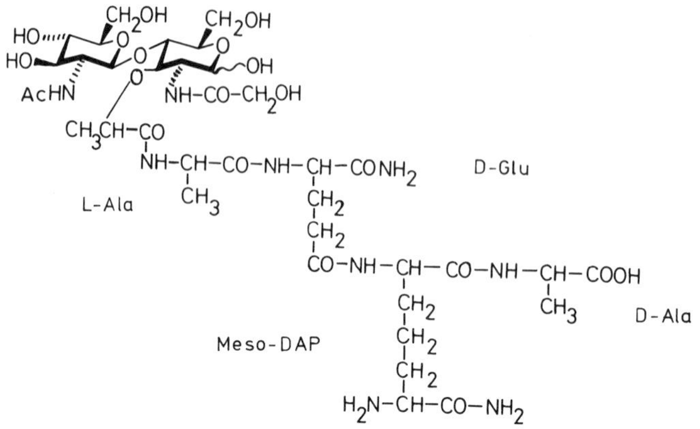

Immunostimulants

Fig. 8 a

Adjuvants

MurNAc – L-Ala – D-Gluc-CONH$_2$ – COOH

from M. tuberculosis

GlcNAc-MurNAc – L-Ala – Glu-NH$_2$ – meso-DAP-NH$_2$ – D-Ala

from E. coli

GlcNAc-MurNAc – L-Ala – D-Glu-CONH$_2$ – L-Lys-L-Thi – D-Ala

from M. roseus

Fig. 8 b

We can define two groups of alkaloids and their derivatives: peptide alkaloids and low molecular lysergic acid derivatives.

1. Peptide Alkaloids (13 - 15)

(a) Ergotamine (2). This genuine alkaloid with primarily uterocontracting effect is still being used in gynecology as Gynergen® (16).

(b) Dihydroergotamine. It was originally the first, non genuine derivative of ergot research. Like ergotamine, but to a higher extent, it has the effect of contracting, constricting veins and is being applied very successfully against migraine and the orthostase-syndrome as Dihydergot®(16).

(c) Dihydroergotoxines. Dihydroergotoxine is not a homogeneous substance, but a defined mixture of hydrated alkaloids, known by the trade name of Hydergen®. In spite of many attacks, this preparation still holds its leading position in the treatment of cerebral vasculous complaints, especially the so-called cerebral insufficiency. These drugs are often controversial because of the complex effects, which can no longer be recorded by the traditional classic methods.

Peptide alkaloids

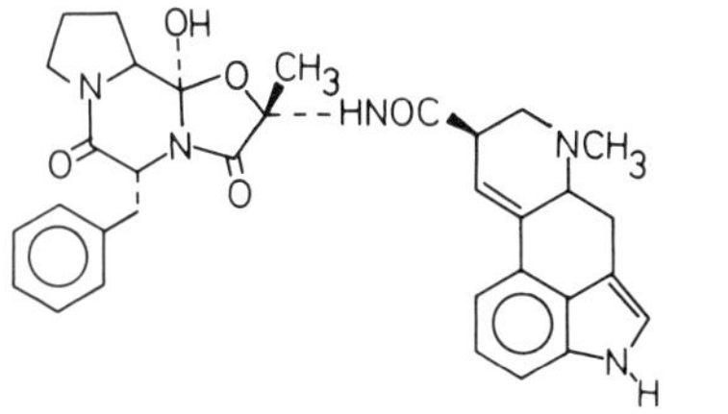

Ergotamine

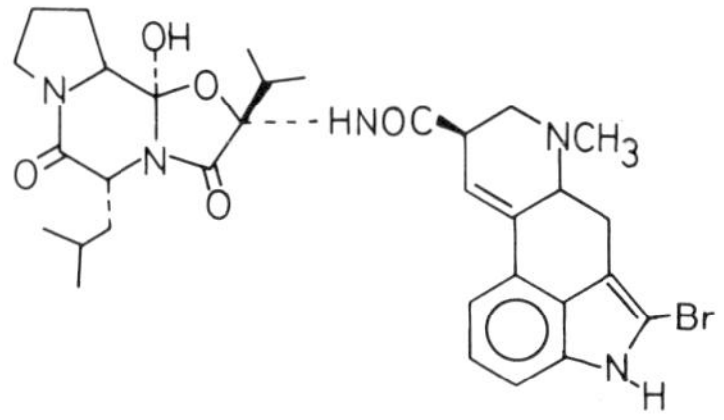

2-Bromo-α-ergocryptine

Fig. 9

(d) 2-Bromo-α-ergocryptine = CB 154 (16). This compound is a new derivative and also an active substance. It is a prolactin inhibitor, which has set new standards for dopaminergic stimulants under the code name of CB 154 and is regarded today as international standard. Since CB 154 also has a considerably high protective effect against mamma tumors in mice with or without the secretion of estrogen, more intensive clinical tests should prove whether CB 154 can effect a regression of human mamma tumors, in the same way as L-Dopa. The substance is in the market as Parlodel® and proved itself extremely successful in the treatment of galactorrhea and morbus Parkinson, i.e. effects connected with dopaminergic stimulation.

2. Low-Molecular Lysergic Acid Derivatives

Lysergic Acid Diethylamide became by far the most famous lysergic acid derivative, known as LSD. Originally the compound was applied in psychiatry to patients with CNS-disorders. It proved itself of considerable value for studying drug-induced disorders (13 - 15). Any further investigation of LSD, however, was more or less swamped by the so-called LSD-wave. Before that however, two other lysergic acid derivatives of this type entered the market, namely:

Methylergobasine which is known as Methergin® (16) and has a strongly selective effect as an uterotonic, and its 1-methylderivative.

Methysergide, known as Deseril® (16), which represents a serotonine antagonist used mainly for the treatment of migraines.

Recently, many research efforts with ergot alkaloid analogs have concentrated on the development of low-molecular prolactine inhibitors and antiparkinsonia (13, 14). From the patent literature, it is obvious that firms such as Sandoz/Basel, Eli-Lilly/USA and Spofa/CSSR have achieved some success in this field. At present a thioether of that group with the appellation CF 25-397 is under clinical

Low-molecular-lysergic acid derivatives

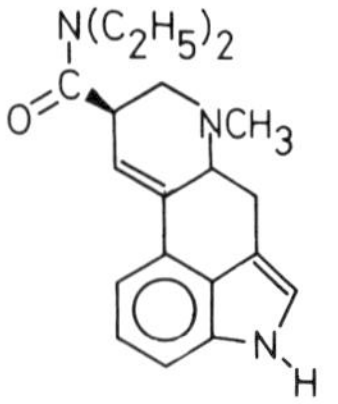

LSD

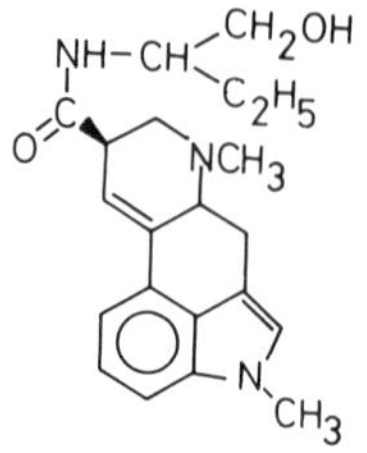

Methysergide

Fig. 10

examination by Sandoz Ltd. as a potential prolactine inhibitor. Spofa developed a urea derivative in this group, which is also under examination (17).

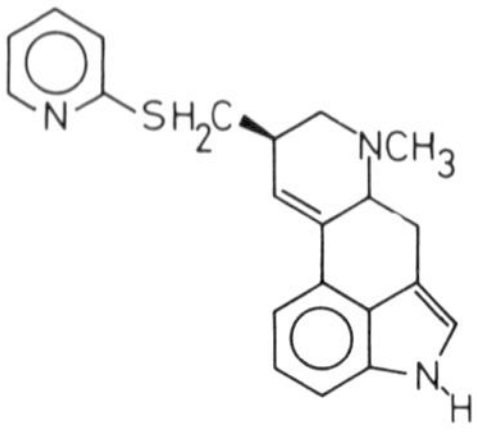

CF 25-397

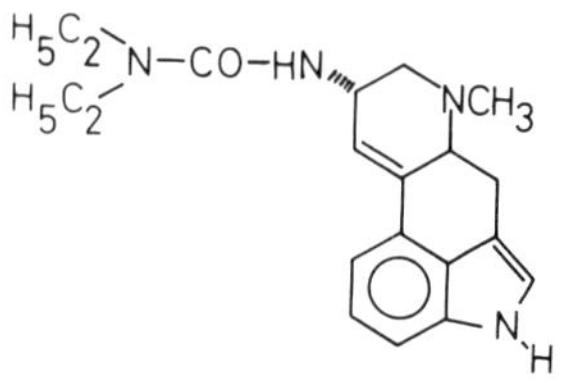

Urea derivative of ergolene

Fig. 11

IV. Opiates

While the results of the modification of ergot alkaloids are good examples of the fact that one can get totally different effects by varying the functions of a basic molecule, the aim of remodeling an already-known active substance, however, can at best be an increase in the effect or a decrease in toxicity or side-effects.

A classical example of this in research is "rocking around" the morphine. Morphine is a challenge for all researchers in the field of the central nervous system. Periodical alternation between hope and resignation is well-known to the expert, who attempts to solve the problem of central analgesia, habituation, addiction, dependence (7). The main questions of the challenge are the following:

1. Is central analgesia possible without addiction?
2. Is it possible to separate the habit-forming effect from the analgesic effectiveness by a modification of morphine?
3. Are structural analogs of morphine always addiction-producing, if they have a strong analgesic effect?

Sertürner isolated morphine in 1804, and since then the "rocking around" the morphine has been an evergreen. After the discovery of the simple derivatives, codeine and heroine, the efforts to functionalize morphine were abandoned unexpectedly. Instead, scientists began developing simple morphine analogs. The success by Eisleb and Schaumann with the piperidine derivative dolantin (18) inaugurated an era of total synthesis of simple morphine analogs. Several hundred piperidine, morphinan and benzomorphan derivatives were synthesized. Then began the era of morphine antagonists - primarily derivatives resulting from the modification of the substituents in ring C and at nitrogen.

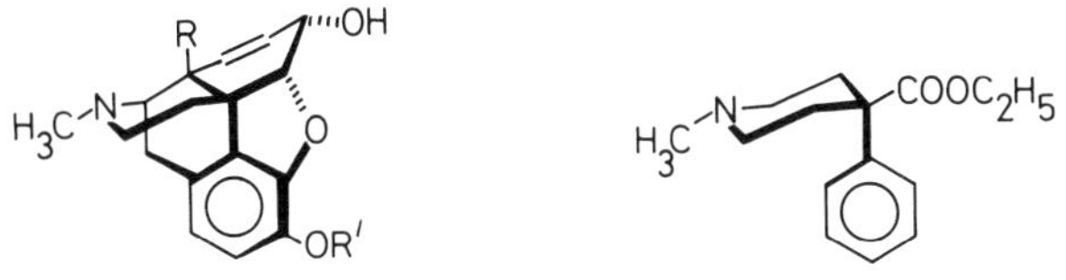

R = R' = H:Morphine
R = H; R' = CH_3:Codeine

Dolantin

Fig. 12. Analgesics

After this work was done, nothing new about morphine-deriving was really expected until the Hungarian working group of Makleit and Bognár undertook a new systematic modification, primarily at ring C (19 - 21).

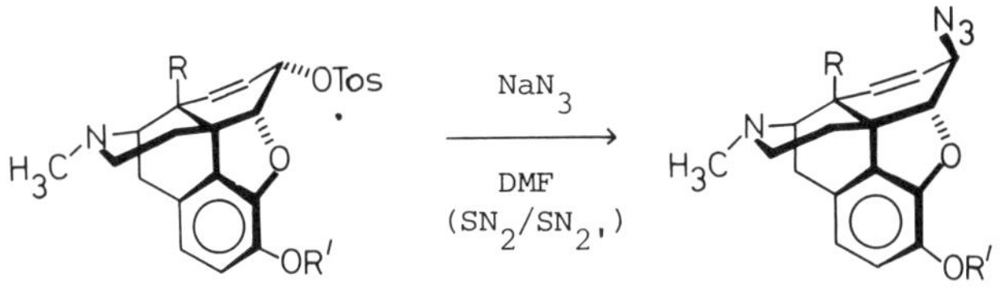

Azidomorphine

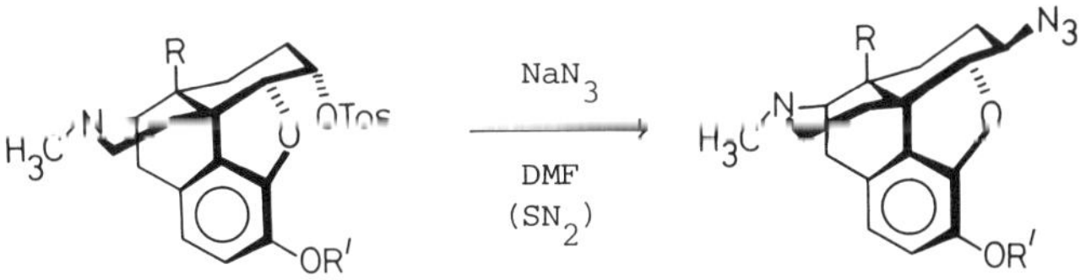

Dihydro-Morphine

Azido-Dihydro-Morphine

Fig. 13. Morphine derivation

By means of 6-O-tosyl- respectively 6-O-mesyl-derivatives of morphine, codeine, dihydromorphine, dihydrocodeine, 14-hydroxy-codeine and 14-hydroxy-dihydrocodeine it was possible to produce new derivatives by nucleophilic substitutions. The substitution of tosylates or mesylates by the azido group led to the so-called azidomorphine derivatives, especially in the dihydro-series.

Pharmacological investigation of these compounds, originally meant to be intermediate products for the synthesis of compounds with an amino group led to totally new perceptions. The analgesic and antitussive effect of these azido derivatives was closely examined by the working group of Professor Knoll at the pharmacological institute of Semmelweis-University (22 - 24). The so-called azidomorphines - azidomorphine itself, azidocodeine, 14-hydroxy-azidomorphine - are not only more effective analgesics than morphine, but also have a wider therapeutical range of action. In animal experiments azidomorphine and 14-hydroxy-azidomorphine are analgesics 300 times stronger than morphine, and the analgesic effect of azidocodeine is about 13 times stronger than that of morphine. In toxicity tests using rats for several weeks, azidomorphine proved to be of significant lower toxicity than morphine or fentanyl, and what is more important, azidomorphine indicated practically no addiction in mice, rats and apes. The clinical data submitted corresponds with the animal experiments.

We should not omit azidodionine (R' = C_2H_5), hitherto the most effective antitussive with oral application, and 60 times more effective than codeine.

In connection with the effect of morphine, I may point out that in the meantime scientists were able to isolate and to characterize the so-called endomorphine, also called enkephaline (7), by studying opiate receptors. It was very surprising that it has the same effect as morphine. Investigations by X-ray structural analysis have proved that the special position of the tyrosine moiety in this pentapeptide apparently is responsible for an effect analogous to morphine. A structural comparison may explain this.

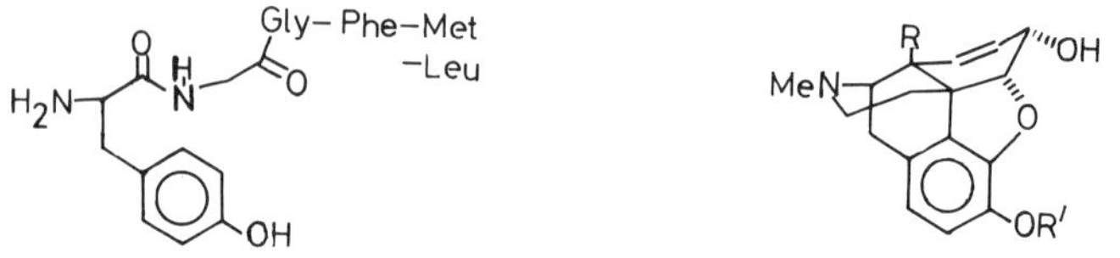

Enkephaline (endomorphine) Morphine Fig. 14

An intensive search for other biological sources of morphine-like substances started because differences appear to exist in the species concerning enkephaline, which differ in the variation of C-terminal amino acid.

Graf and his colleagues (Budapest, Hungary) recently reported that by specific cleavage with trypsin from β-lipotropin of the swine they succeeded in getting a pentapeptide identical with met-enkephaline, corresponding to the sequence of 61 - 65 of LPH and having a 90 % normorphine effect. The intact LPH showed no effect (25).

These works are also good examples for the modification of natural substances and for an efficient synthesis of active molecules.

V. Cannabinoids

It is still impossible with morphine analogs to separate the analgesic effect from the addiction-producing one, and therefore there are more and more experiments with totally different structures. It is quite conceivable that the opiate receptor which is integrated in the analgesic effect is not the same as the bonding and reacting partner, which is responsible for addiction and dependence. Lately great hope has been placed in certain modifications of cannabinol (26 - 28).

The question of whether compound number 7 is addiction-inducing and causes dependence is not yet settled; although the structure has little to do with that of opiates, the morphine antagonist naloxon completely antagonizes their analgesic effect (7). Unlike the narcotic agonist of the morphine series, number 7 has not the ability, however, to com-

Cannabinoids

Δ^9 THC series

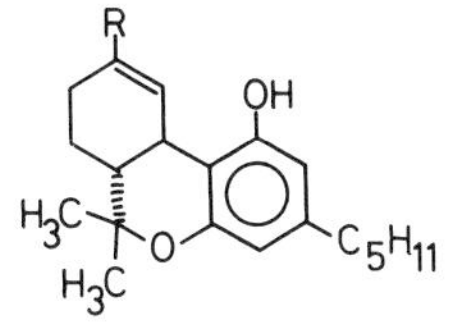

Nr.	R	ED_{50} s.c. hot plate
1	CH_3	9,6 mg/kg
2	CH_2OH	1,9 mg/kg
3	H	> 20 mg/kg

Δ^8 THC series

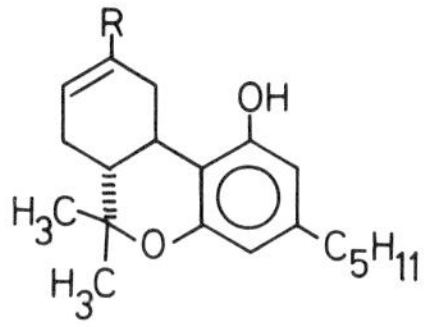

Nr.	R	ED_{50} s.c. hot plate
4	CH_3	8,8 mg/kg
5	CH_2OH	1,9 mg/kg
6	H	> 50 mg/kg

Hexahydro series

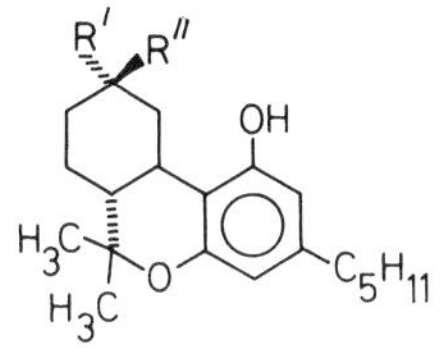

Nr.	R'	R"	ED_{50} s.c. hot plate
7	H	OH	1,6 mg/kg
8	OH	H	> 20 mg/kg
9	= O		> 20 mg/kg

Fig. 15

pensate the symptoms of deprivation on apes addicted to morphine, nor does it react in vitro with the opiate receptor. Heterocyclic modifications of cannabinoids have been known since 1974, with effects said to be analgesic as well as sedatively hypnotic respectively antidepressant (29 - 31).

In animal experiments the compounds do not indicate any dependence analogous to morphine; on the contrary, they even seem to be morphine antagonists. However, clinical examinations have not yet been completed (Eli Lilly & Co.; Smith Kline Corp.; Warner Lambert & Co.; Beecham Inc.; Abbott Laboratories).

VI. Natural Substances in the Role of Raw Material for Drug Synthesis and Biochemical Model Reactions

Up to this point we have assumed that the modification of natural substances is a rational modus operandi for the development of pharmaceutics. The examples cited are orientated, however, according to a priori active substances. But what about trying to modify natural substances without any noticeable pharmacological effects?

The example of steroid saponin - steroid hormone (4) shows one possibility. It is true that the pharmacological effect of saponins was known; the idea to develop a contraceptive by the saponin effect would not have been developed. But the hormone to be synthesized was again already known, and thus the synthesis by diosgenin is on the one hand merely an optimized procedure, and on the other a grand invention; in any case, it is a magnificent creative achievement. The same is true for the most recent example of lipotropin - enkephalin (25). Although

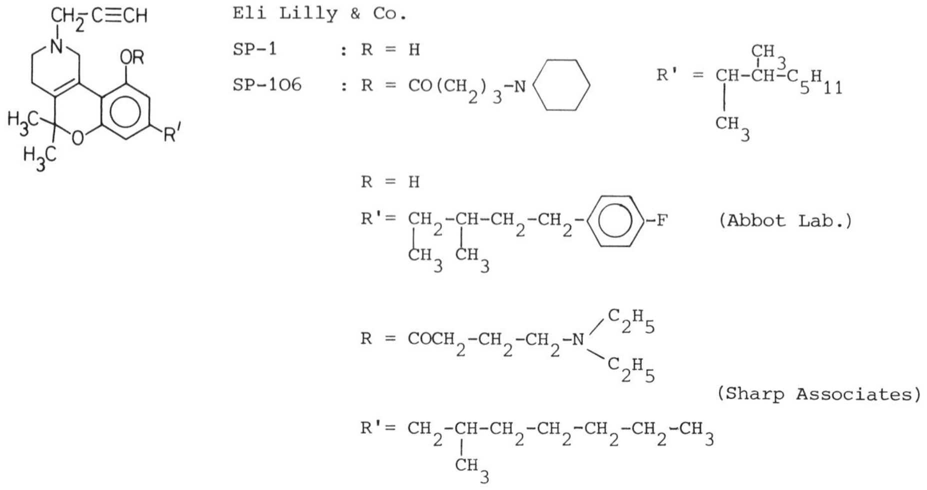

Fig. 16. Heterocyclic modifications of cannabinoids

the biological functions of lipotropin are not exactly known yet, the amino acid sequence is better known. The problem of enkephalin synthesis consisted in a controlled fragmentation of polypeptide to oligopeptide!

What to do now with a natural substance, chemically novel but pharmacologically of no interest? There are really only two possible methods:

1. Modification according to biochemical and physico-chemical conceptions by so-called minor operations to disclose the blocked pharmacodynamic, perhaps by trying to help the potential pharmacon to achieve a better cell permeability perhaps by unveiling the prodrug, to get an active principle.
2. Use the cell origin of the natural substance to reenter the cell, i.e. use the natural substance as a carrier for pharmacophorous groups or molecules.

Both methods have been applied in nature ever since the biosphere existed:

As an example 1. we may mention the enzymatic cleavage of starch by amylase into glucose and the change of L-dopa by decarboxylase into dopamine.
Examples for method 2 include chelating agents, e.g. insulin, hemoglobin, chlorophyll, vitamin B 12 etc., as well as the glucuronization of substances for the purpose of elimination, which means all the possibilities a body or cell may use to take in lose foreign matters or necessary substances. According to both methods highly effective natural substances were also developed, by method (1), for example many highly effective amines and alkaloids, by method (2) the highly effective cardiac glycosides.

You can, of course, also apply both methods for the synthesis of *one* active substance as demonstrated by the alkaloid-bearing plants. The only difficulty is to determine which part of the molecule is pharmacophorous, and which the carrier. This determination is sometimes almost like a world view, as for example in the indole alkaloids. While the amine part nearly always had the priority (actually one speaks of alkaloids only), there is the tendency nowadays to give priority to the nonamine part. According to the above-mentioned ergot alkaloids, it should be quite obvious that the effects of this substance class are mainly due to the tryptamine or arylethyl-amine derivative. Thus, LSD is a competitive serotonine antagonist. Methysergide, however, is used as 5-HT-antagonist against (1) the carcinoid syndrome; (2) the postoperative dumping syndrome and, as mentioned above (3) vascular headache, especially migraine attacks. Other low-molecular ergot-alkaloid derivatives have a dopaminergic effect.

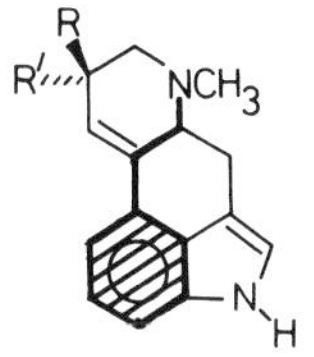

(dopaminergic effect)

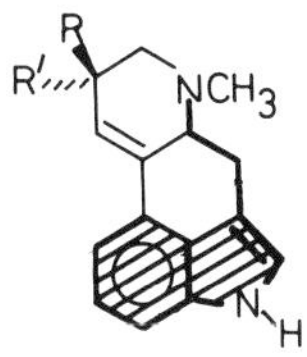

(serotoninergic/tryptaminergic effect)

Fig. 17

This structural comparison makes it evident that ergoline alkaloids do not contain only the tryptamine particle, but also phenylethyl amine, e.g. dopamine, and therefore it is comprehensible that ergoline derivatives can have a serotoninergic (tryptaminergic) effect, as well as a dopaminergic one.

The tryptamine particle of reserpine is quite evident, yet the residual molecule makes such a strong impression that it is difficult to expect the total molecule to have only a tryptaminergic or serotoninergic effect.

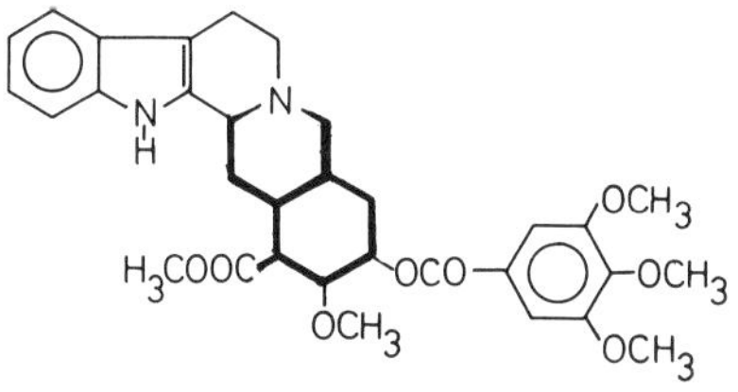

Reserpine

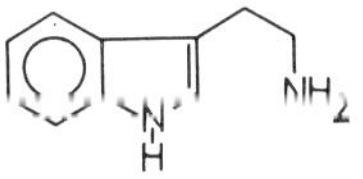

Tryptamine

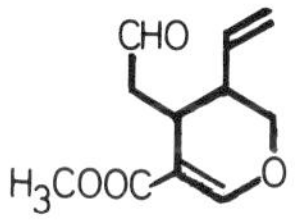

Secologanine

Fig. 18

Today we know that the nonnitrogenous particle of reserpine originates from the iridoid "secologanine."

This iridoid particle is now to be found in very many alkaloids, which are pharmacologically and therapeutically interesting (32 - 34).

Nevertheless, in the field of alkaloid chemistry there have been few modifications besides the amine particle.

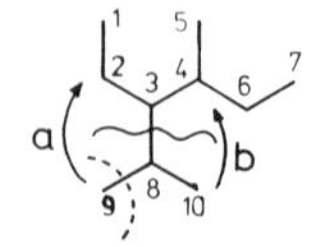

Corynanthe type

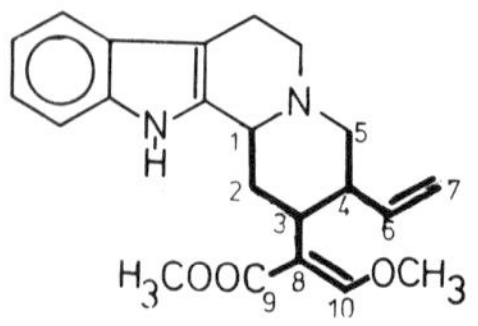

Corynantheine

Geraniol

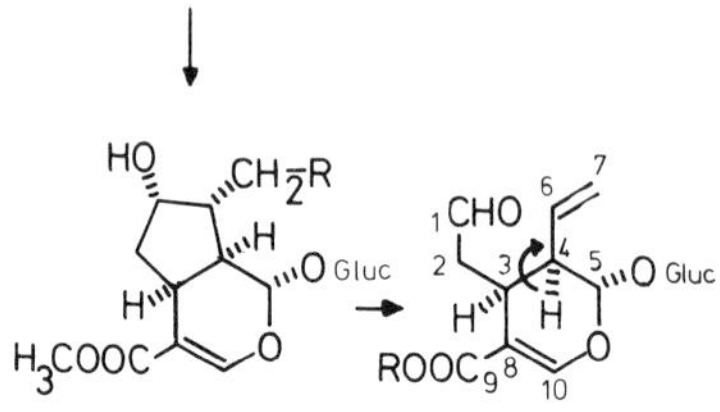

Iridoid compounds

R = H : Loganine
R = OH: Hydroxy-loganine

Secologanine

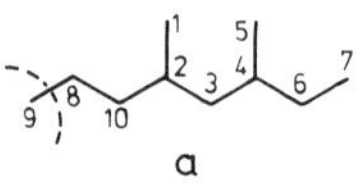

a

Iboga type

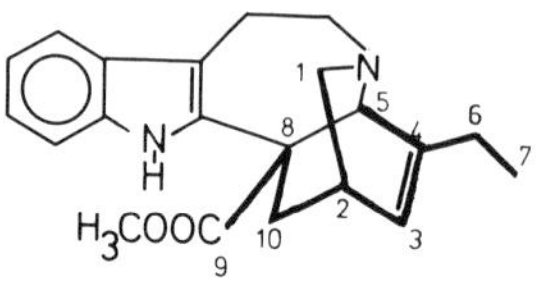

Catharanthine

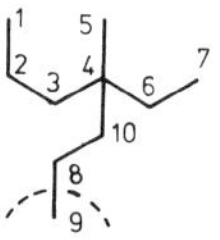

b

Aspidosperma type

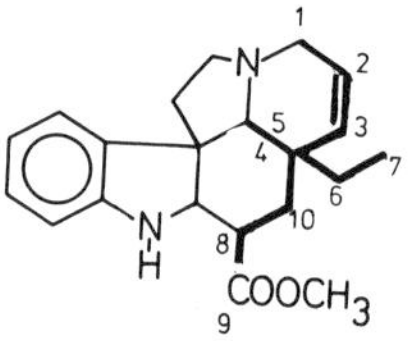

Tabersonine

Fig. 19

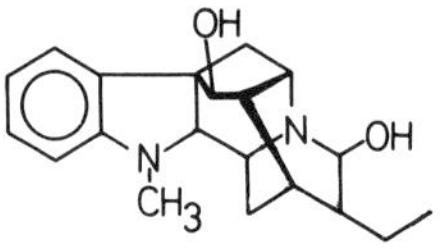

Ajmaline

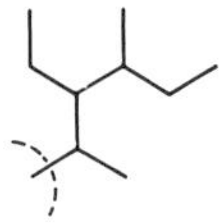

Corynanthe-type

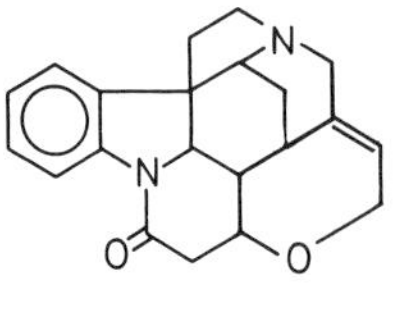

Strychnine

Fig. 20

Although some of the iridoids, for example nepetalactone, matatabi-ether and valepotriates, show pharmacological effects, few have been successful in making nonnitrogenous iridoid modifications with a striking pharmacological effect. The only examples known are the 2,9-dioxatricyclo [4,3,1,0^{3,7}] decanes described by Thies et al. (35), which show interesting effects even without an aminyl-residue.

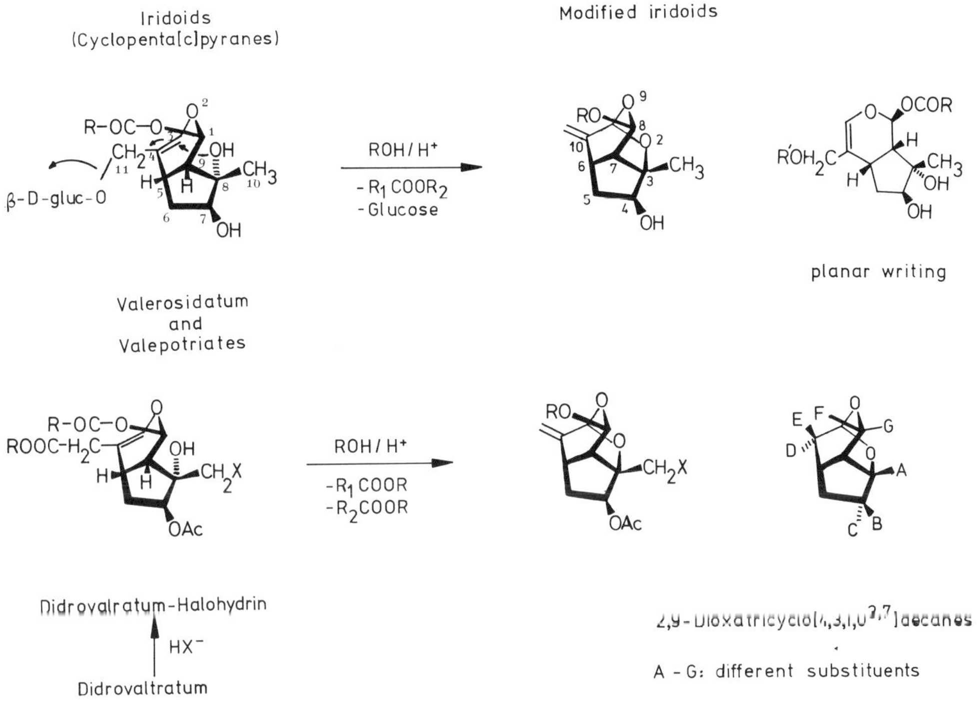

Fig. 21

However, even in this class of compound the functionalization with nitrogenous pharmacophorous groups led to novel alkaloids with profiles of effects unknown till then. We may conclude that the iridoid particle possesses a carrier function rather than a characteristic effect, the nonnitrogenous highly effective compound may not actually reconstruct an alkaloid by synthesis in vivo. This should be of special concern in the study of effects of neuro-hormones, and it should not be forgotten that all transmitter substances as yet known are amines or amino acids (7).

Acknowledgement. I would like to thank my colleague, Dr. Wegener, for drawing up the formulas and for his valuable support in preparing the manuscript for publication.

References

1. Chain, E. Sir: Immunologie und Gesellschaft. Schwick, H.G. (ed.). Stuttgart: Wissenschaftliche Verlagsgesell., 1975
2. Index Nominum 1975/76: Zürich: Wissenschaftliche Zentralstelle des Schweizer Apotheker-Vereins, 1975
3. Wichtl, M.: Wirkstoffsynthese im lebenden Organismus und im Laboratorium, ein Vergleich. Pharmazie in unserer Zeit 2, 33 (1976). IMS-Liste 1. Hj. 1976
4. Goto, T., Ito, S., Nakanishi, K., Natori, S., Nozoe, S.: Natural Products Chemistry. Tokyo: Kodansha Ltd.; London-New York: Academic Press, 1974, Vol. I, pp. 450
5. Horton, E.W.: Prostaglandins. Berlin-Heidelberg-New York: Springer, 1972
6. Goto, T., Ito, S., Nakanishi, K., Natori, S., Nozoe, S.: Natural Products Chemistry. Tokyo: Kodansha Ltd.; London-New York: Academic Press, 1974, Vol. II, pp. 33
7. Hambrecht, B.: Neuronenmodelle. Angew. Chem. 7, 211 (1976)
8. Tamm, Ch.: Recent Advances in the field of antibiotics. Cf. this edition
9. Firmenschrift Merck and Co. Inc., Scrip. 29. Nov. 1975, 10
10. Bretschneider, H., Vetter, W.: Eine Synthese des D,L-4-Amino-3-isoxazolidons (D,L-Cydoserins). Monatsh. Chem. 4-5, 625 (1958)
11. USP 3956-302 (1974), DT-OS 2522-090 (1976)
12. Jolles, P.: Hydrosoluble immunstimulants of bacterial and synthetic origins. Experientia 32, 677 (1976)
13. Auterhoff, H.: Lehrbuch der pharmazeutischen Chemie. Stuttgart: Wissenschaftliche Verlagsgesell., 1976
14. Mutschler, E.: Arzneimittelwirkungen. Stuttgart: Wissenschaftliche Verlagsgesell., 1975
15. Manske, R.H.F.: The Alkaloids. New York-London: Academic Press, 1965
16. Drug by Sandoz Ltd.
17. BE 787026 (DT-OS 2138517)
18. Drug by Hoechst Ltd.
19. Makleit, S.: Acta Universitatis Debreceniensis de Ludovico Kossuth nominatae Series physica et chimica 265 (1972-1973)
20. Bognâr, R., Géza, H., György, G., Peter, K., Zsigmond, D.: Acta Pharm. Hung. 43, 169 (1973)
21. Bognâr, R., Makleit, S.: Acta Chim. Acad. Sci. Hung. 58 (2), 203 (1968)
22. Fürst, Z., Knoll, J.: Acta Physiol. Acad. Sci. Hung. 41, 366 (1972)
23. Fürst, S., Knoll, J., Makleit, S.: The Pharmacologie of 14-hydroxy-azidomorphin. J. Pharm. Pharmac. 27, 99 (1975)
24. Knoll, J.: Azidormorphin and Rymazolium. An approach to the ideal analgesic. Pharmacol. Res. Commun. 5, 175 (1973)
25. Graf, L.: FEBS Lett. 64, (I) 181 (1976)
26. USP 3.944.673
27. Granchelli, F.E., Keller, J.K., Pars, H.G., Razdan, R.K.: Drugs derived from cannabinoids. 1. Nitrogen analogs, benzopyranopyridines and benzopyranopyrroles. J. Med. Chem. 19, 445 (1976)
28. Dalzell, H.C., Handrick, G.R., Howes, J.F., Pars, H.G., Razdan, R.K., Terris, B.Z.: Drugs derived from cannabinoids. 3.[ia]sulfur analogs, [ib]thiopyranobenzopyrans and thienobenzopyrans. J. Med. Chem. 19, 548 (1976)
29. Cannabinoid research may yield new drugs. Chem. and Eng. News 15 (Washington), Sept. 30 (1974)
30. DT-OS 2415698
31. DT-OS 2322960
32. Loew, P., Arigoni, D.: The Biological Conversion of Loganin into Indole Alkaloids. Chem. Commun. 137 (1968)
33. Battersby, A.R., Burnet, A.R., Parsons, P.G.: Alkaloid Biosynthesis. J. Chem. Soc. C 1187 (1969)
34. Scott, A.I., Wright, I.G.: Chem. Commun. 537 (1965)
35. Battersby, A.R., Byrne, J.C., Kapil, R.S., Martin, J.A., Payne, T.G., Arigoni, D., Loew, P.: The Mechanism of Indole Alkaloid Biosynthesis. Chem. Commun. 951 (1968)

36. Luckner, M.: Der Sekundär-Stoffwechsel in Pflanze und Tier. Stuttgart: Fischer, 1969)
37. Thies, P.W.: Pharmacognosy and Phytochemistry. Berlin-Heidelberg-New York: Springer, 1971
38. Thies, P.W., Asai, A.: DT-OS 2129507 (1971, 1972)
39. Thies, P.W., Asai, A.: Notiz über eine vereinfachte Synthese von 2,9-Dioxatricyclo [4,3,1,$0^{3,7}$] decanen aus Didrovaltratum. Chem. Ber. 105, 3491 (1972)
40. Thies, P.W.: DT - OS 2306118 (1973, 1974)
41. Thies, P.W., Finner, E., Rosskopf, R.: Über die Wirkstoffe des Baldrians - X. Tetrahedron 29, 3213 (1973)
42. Inouye, H., Ueda, S., Uesato, S., Shingu, T., Thies, P.W.: Die absolute Konfiguration von Valerosidatum und von Didrovaltratum. Tetrahedron 30, 2317 (1974)

Subject Index

Note: Only the starting pages of the papers are indicated

Plant Tissue Culture and Its Bio-technological Application

Proceedings of the First International Congress on Medicinal Plant Research, Section B, held at the University of Munich, Germany September 6-10, 1976

Editors:
W. BARZ, E. REINHARD, M. H. ZENK

With contributions by numerous experts

199 figures, 60 tables, 419 pages. 1977
(Proceedings in Life Sciences)
ISBN 3-540-08227-1

The Proceedings of Section B of the First International Congress for Research on Medicinal Plants give a comprehensive review of the latest developments of plant tissue culture research.

This work results from the First International Congress for Research on Medicinal Plants, Section B. It presents a broad coverage of present research in all aspects of plant tissue culture. The book also lays emphasis on the importance of interdisciplinary cooperation in investigating, not only research theories, but the various possibilities of practical biotechnical applications, a field whose importance has been observed by the lack of consistent serious scientific research up to the present time.

Contents: Cell Cultures and Secondary Products.-Biochemistry,Physiology and Regulatory Aspects.-Biotransformation.-Catabolism.-General and Analytical Techniques.-Somatic Hybridisation,Fusion and Haploids.-Regeneration and Organogenesis.

Springer-Verlag Berlin · Heidelberg · New York

Lipids and Lipid Polymer in Higher Plants

Editors: M.TEVINI, H.K.LICHTENTHALER

With contributions by B.H.DAVIES, A.H.B.DEAS, W,EICHENBERGER, L.J.GOAD, T.W.GOODWIN, E.HEINZ, F.W.HEMMING, P.J.HOLLOWAY, P.E.KOLATTUKUDY, H.K.LICHTENTHALER, C.LILJENBERG, H.K.MANGOLD, P.MAZLIAK, D.SIEFERMANN-HARMS, P.SITTE, F.SPENER, P.K.STUMPF, M.TEVINI

136 figures, 66 tables, 3o6 pages, 1977.
ISBN 3-54o-o82o1-8

This book contains 16 articles covering the complete field of lipids and lipid polymers in higher plants and is based on the main papers read at the Symposium "Lipids and Lipid Polymers in Higher Plants",held at the botanical Institute of Karlsruhe University in July 1976. The articles of the first part treat the function and organization of biomembranes, which must be considered more and more as the site of biosynthetic and physiologic processes. The second part contains the function and distribution of fatty acids and glycerolipids, including some aspects of physiologic development. Section 3 reports the structure and metabolism of plant sterols, while the fourth part presents five articles on the biochemistry and physiology of prenyl lipids, including chlorophyll formation. The broad spectrum of lipids in higher plants is completed by a highly detailed description of the biosyntheses and breaking down of lipid polymers such as cutin and suberin.

Contents: Functional Organization of Biomembranes.-The Prenyllipids of the Membranes of Higher Plants.-Glyco-and Phospholipids of Biomembranes in Higher Plants.-Lipid Biosynthesis in Developing Seeds.-The Cyclopentenyl Fatty Acids.-Enzymatic Reactions in Galactolipid Biosynthesis.-Light,Function,and Lipids During Plastid Development.-The Biosynthesis of Plant Sterols.-Steryl Glycosides and Acylated Steryl Glycosides.-The Biosynthesis and Biological Significance of Prenols and Their Phosphorylated Derivatives.-Carotenoids in Higher Plants.-The Xanthophyll Cycle in Higher Plants.-Regulation of Prenylquinone Synthesis in Higher Plants.-Chlorophyll Formation: The Phytylation Step.-Biosynthesis and Degradation of Lipid Polymers.-The Intermolecular Structure of Some Plant Cutins.

Springer-Verlag Berlin · Heidelberg · New York